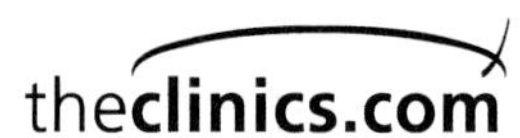

EMERGENCY MEDICINE CLINICS OF NORTH AMERICA

Current Concepts in the Management of the Trauma Patient

GUEST EDITOR
Carrie D. Tibbles, MD

CONSULTING EDITOR
Amal Mattu, MD

August 2007 • Volume 25 • Number 3

SAUNDERS

An Imprint of Elsevier, Inc.
PHILADELPHIA LONDON TORONTO MONTREAL SYDNEY TOKYO

W.B. SAUNDERS COMPANY
A Division of Elsevier Inc.

1600 John F. Kennedy Boulevard, Suite 1800 • Philadelphia, Pennsylvania 19103-2899

http://www.theclinics.com

EMERGENCY MEDICINE CLINICS OF NORTH AMERICA
August 2007
Editor: Patrick Manley

Volume 25, Number 3
ISSN 0733-8627
ISBN-13: 978-1-4160-5065-0
ISBN-10: 1-4160-5065-5

Reprints. For copies of 100 or more, of articles in this publication, please contact the Commercial Reprints Department, Elsevier Inc., 360 Park Avenue South, New York, New York 10010-1710. Tel. (212) 633-3813; Fax: (212) 462-1935; e-mail: reprints@elsevier.com.

Emergency Medicine Clinics of North America (ISSN 0733-8627) is published quarterly by Elsevier Inc., 360 Park Avenue South, New York, NY, 10010-1710. Months of issue are February, May, August, and November. Business and Editorial Offices: 1600 John F. Kennedy Boulevard, Suite 1800, Philadelphia, PA 19103-2899. Customer Service Office: 6277 Sea Harbor Drive, Orlando, FL 32887-4800. Periodicals postage paid at New York, NY, and additional mailing offices. Subscription prices are $193.00 per year (US individuals), $297.00 per year (US institutions), $259.00 per year (international individuals), $351.00 per year (international institutions), $237.00 per year (Canadian individuals), and $351.00 per year (Canadian institutions). International air speed delivery is included in all *Clinics'* subscription prices. All prices are subject to change without notice. POSTMASTER: Send address changes to *Emergency Medicine Clinics of North America*, Elsevier Periodicals Customer Service, 6277 Sea Harbor Drive, Orlando, FL 32887-4800. **Customer Service: 1-800-654-2452 (US). From outside of the US, call 1-407-345-4000. E-mail: hhspcs@harcourt.com.**

Emergency Medicine Clinics of North America is covered in *Index Medicus, Current Contents/Clinical Medicine, EMBASE/Excerpta Medica, BIOSIS, SciSearch, CINAHL, ISI/BIOMED,* and *Research Alert.*

Printed in the United States of America.

CONSULTING EDITOR

AMAL MATTU, MD, Program Director, Emergency Medicine Residency; and Associate Professor, Department of Emergency Medicine, University of Maryland School of Medicine, Baltimore, Maryland

GUEST EDITOR

CARRIE D. TIBBLES, MD, Associate Program Director, Department of Emergency Medicine, Harvard Affiliated Emergency Medicine Residency, Beth Israel Deaconess Medical Center, Boston, Massachusetts

CONTRIBUTORS

JAHN T. AVARELLO, MD, FAAP, Pediatric Emergency Medicine Fellow, Department of Emergency Medicine, SUNY Upstate Medical University, Syracuse, New York

MARIAN BETZ, MD, Harvard Affiliated Emergency Medicine Residency, Department of Emergency Medicine, Beth Israel Deaconess Medical Center, Boston, Massachusetts

MICHELLE BIROS, MD, MS, Research Director; and Professor, Department of Emergency Medicine, Hennepin County Medical Center, University of Minnesota Medical School, Minneapolis, Minnesota

MARK E. BRACKEN, MD, Assistant Professor, Department of Emergency Medicine, Boston Medical Center, Boston University School of Medicine, Boston, Massachusetts

DAVID W. CALLAWAY, MD, Chief Resident, Emergency Medicine, Department of Emergency Medicine, Beth Israel Deaconess Medical Center, Boston, Massachusetts

RICHARD M. CANTOR, MD, FAAP, FACEP, Associate Professor of Emergency Medicine and Pediatrics; and Director, Pediatric Emergency Medicine, Department of Emergency Medicine, SUNY Upstate Medical University; Medical Director, Central New York Poison Center, Syracuse, New York

MICHAEL N. COCCHI, MD, Resident Physician, Department of Emergency Medicine, Harvard-Affiliated Emergency Medicine Residency, Beth Israel Deaconess Medical Center, Boston, Massachusetts

SERIC S. CUSICK, MD, Assistant Professor; and Director of Emergency Ultrasound, Department of Emergency Medicine, UC Davis School of Medicine, Sacramento, California

MICHAEL W. DONNINO, MD, Instructor of Medicine, Harvard School of Medicine; Department of Emergency Medicine; and Department of Medicine, Division of Pulmonary/Critical Care, Beth Israel Deaconess Medical Center, Boston, Massachusetts

WILLIAM HEEGAARD, MD, MPH, Assistant Chief; and Associate Professor, Department of Emergency Medicine, Hennepin County Medical Center, University of Minnesota Medical School, Minneapolis, Minnesota

ROBERT HOCKBERGER, MD, Professor and Chair, Department of Emergency Medicine, Harbor-UCLA Medical Center, Torrance, California

JENNIFER L. ISENHOUR, MD, Associate Program Director, Department of Emergency Medicine, Carolinas Medical Center; Adjunct Assistant Professor, Department of Emergency Medicine, University of North Carolina, Chapel Hill, North Carolina

AMY KAJI, MD, Assistant Clinical Professor, Department of Emergency Medicine, Harbor-UCLA Medical Center, Torrance, California

EDWARD KIMLIN, MD, Resident Physician, Department of Emergency Medicine, Harvard Affiliated Emergency Medicine Residency, Beth Israel Deaconess Medical Center, Boston, Massachusetts

GUOHUA LI, MD, DrPH, Department of Emergency Medicine, Johns Hopkins University School of Medicine, Baltimore, Maryland

JOHN LOVE, MD, Clinical Instructor of Emergency Medicine, Keck School of Medicine and LAC+USC Medical Center, Los Angeles, California; Lieutenant Commander, US Navy

VINCENT J. MARKOVCHICK, MD, FAAEM, Director, Emergency Medical Services, Denver Health; Professor of Surgery, Division of Emergency Medicine, Department of Surgery, University of Colorado Health Sciences Center, Denver, Colorado

JOHN MARX, MD, Chair, Department of Emergency Medicine, Carolinas Medical Center; Adjunct Professor of Emergency Medicine, Department of Emergency Medicine, University of North Carolina, Chapel Hill, North Carolina

JOHN McGILL, MD, Senior Physician, Department of Emergency Medicine, Hennepin County Medical Center; Assistant Professor, Department of Emergency Medicine, University of Minnesota, Minneapolis, Minnesota

DANIEL McGILLICUDDY, MD, Department of Emergency Medicine, Beth Israel Deaconess Medical Center, Boston, Massachusetts

RON MEDZON, MD, Assistant Professor, Department of Emergency Medicine, Boston Medical Center, Boston University School of Medicine, Boston, Massachusetts

ERNEST E. MOORE, MD, FACS, Chief, Surgery and Trauma Service, Denver Health; Vice Chair; and Professor, Department of Surgery, University of Colorado Health Sciences Center, Denver, Colorado

MARIA E. MOREIRA, MD, Associate Program Director, Residency in Emergency Medicine; Staff Physician, Denver Health Medical Center; Instructor of Surgery,

Division of Emergency Medicine, University of Colorado Health Sciences Center, Denver, Colorado

EDWARD J. NEWTON, MD, Professor of Emergency Medicine; and Chairman, Department of Emergency Medicine, Keck School of Medicine, LAC+USC Medical Center, Los Angeles, California

NIELS K. RATHLEV, MD, Associate Professor and Vice Chair, Department of Emergency Medicine, Boston Medical Center, Boston University School of Medicine, Boston, Massachusetts

PHILLIP L. RICE, Jr, MD, Associate Director of Trauma; and Instructor in Medicine, Brigham and Women's Hospital, Boston, Massachusetts

PETER ROSEN, MD, Department of Emergency Medicine, Beth Israel Deaconess Medical Center, Boston, Massachusetts

MELISSA RUDOLPH, MD, Resident Physician, Harvard Affiliated Emergency Medicine Residency, Beth Israel Deaconess Medical Center, Boston, Massachusetts

CARRIE D. TIBBLES, MD, Associate Program Director, Department of Emergency Medicine, Harvard Affiliated Emergency Residency, Beth Israel Deaconess Medical Center, Boston, Massachusetts

MARK WALSH, MD, Clinical Assistant Professor of Medicine, Indiana University School of Medicine—South Bend, South Bend, Indiana

RICHARD WOLFE, MD, Department of Emergency Medicine, Beth Israel Deaconess Medical Center, Boston, Massachusetts

CONTENTS

FORTHCOMING ISSUES

November 2007

Emergencies in the First Year of Life
Ghazala Q. Sharieff, MD and
James E. Colletti, MD, *Guest Editors*

February 2008

Ophthalmologic Emergencies
Joseph H. Kahn, MD
and Brendan Magauran, MD, *Guest Editors*

May 2008

Infectious Disease Emergencies
Daniel R. Martin, MD, *Guest Editor*

RECENT ISSUES

May 2007

Medical Toxicology
Christopher P. Holstege, MD
and Mark A. Kirk, *Guest Editors*

February 2007

Emergency Department Wound Management
LTC John McManus, MD, MCR,
COL Ian Wedmore, MD, and
Richard B. Schwartz, MD, *Guest Editors*

November 2006

Emergency Medicine and the Public's Health
Jon Mark Hirshon, MD, MPH
and David M. Morris, MD, MPH, *Guest Editors*

GOAL STATEMENT

The goal of *Emergency Medicine Clinics of North America* is to keep practicing physicians up to date with current clinical practice in emergency medicine by providing timely articles reviewing the state of the art in patient care.

ACCREDITATION

The *Emergency Medical Clinics of North America* is planned and implemented in accordance with the Essential Areas and Policies of the Accreditation Council for Continuing Medical Education (ACCME) through the joint sponsorship of the University of Virginia School of Medicine and Elsevier. The University of Virginia School of Medicine is accredited by the ACCME to provide continuing medical education for physicians.

The University of Virginia School of Medicine designates this educational activity for a maximum of *15 AMA PRA Category 1 Credits*™. Physicians should only claim credit commensurate with the extent of their participation in the activity.

The Emergency Medicine Clinics of North America CME program is approved by the American College of Emergency Physicians for 60 hours of ACEP Category I Credit per year.

The American Medical Association has determined that physicians not licensed in the US who participate in this CME activity are eligible for *15 AMA PRA Category 1 Credits*™.

Credit can be earned by reading the text material, taking the CME examination online at http://www.theclinics.com/home/cme, and completing the evaluation. After taking the test, you will be required to review any and all incorrect answers. Following completion of the test and evaluation, your credit will be awarded and you may print your certificate.

FACULTY DISCLOSURE/CONFLICT OF INTEREST

The University of Virginia School of Medicine, as an ACCME accredited provider, endorses and strives to comply with the Accreditation Council for Continuing Medical Education (ACCME) Standards of Commercial Support, Commonwealth of Virginia statutes, University of Virginia policies and procedures, and associated federal and private regulations and guidelines on the need for disclosure and monitoring of proprietary and financial interests that may affect the scientific integrity and balance of content delivered in continuing medical education activities under our auspices.

The University of Virginia School of Medicine requires that all CME activities accredited through this institution be developed independently and be scientifically rigorous, balanced and objective in the presentation/discussion of its content, theories and practices.

All authors/editors participating in an accredited CME activity are expected to disclose to the readers relevant financial relationships with commercial entities occurring within the past 12 months (such as grants or research support, employee, consultant, stock holder, member of speakers bureau, etc.). The University of Virginia School of Medicine will employ appropriate mechanisms to resolve potential conflicts of interest to maintain the standards of fair and balanced education to the reader. Questions about specific strategies can be directed to the Office of Continuing Medical Education, University of Virginia School of Medicine, Charlottesville, Virginia.

The authors/editors listed below have identified no professional or financial affiliations for themselves or their spouse/partner:
Jahn T. Avarello, MD, FAAP; Marian Betz, MD; Michelle Biros, MD, MS; Mark E. Bracken, MD; David W. Callaway, MD; Richard M. Cantor, MD, FAAP, FACEP; Michael N. Cocchi, MD; Seric S. Cusick, MD; Michael W. Donnino, MD; William Heegard, MD, MPH; Robert Hockberger, MD; Jennifer L. Isenhour, MD; Amy Kaji, MD; Edward Kimlin, MD; Guohua Li, MD, DrPH; John Love, MD; Patrick Manley (Acquisitions Editor); Vince J. Markovchick, MD, FAAEM; John Marx, MD; Amal Mattu, MD (Consulting Editor); John McGill, MD; Daniel C. McGillicuddy, MD; Ron Medzon, MD; Ernest E. Moore, MD, FACS; Maria E. Moreira, MD; Niels K. Rathlev, MD; Phillip L. Rice, Jr., MD; Peter Rosen, MD; Melissa Rudolph, MD; and, Carrie D. Tibbles, MD (Guest Editor).

The authors/editors listed below have identified the following professional or financial affiliations for themselves of their spouse/partner:
Edward Newton, MD is an independent contractor for Biosite, Inc.
Mark Walsh, MD is on the Advisory Committee/Board of SCOPEMD.
Richard Wolfe, MD is a director of and shareholder in Forerun.

Disclosure of Discussion of non-FDA approved uses for pharmaceutical products and/or medical devices:
The University of Virginia School of Medicine, as an ACCME provider, requires that all faculty presenters identify and disclose any "off label" uses for pharmaceutical and medical device products. The University of Virginia School of Medicine recommends that each physician fully review all the available data on new products or procedures prior to instituting them with patients.

TO ENROLL

To enroll in the Emergency Medicine Clinics of North America Continuing Medical Education program, call customer service at 1-800-654-2452 or visit us online at www.theclinics.com/home/cme. The CME program is available to subscribers for an additional fee of $195.00.

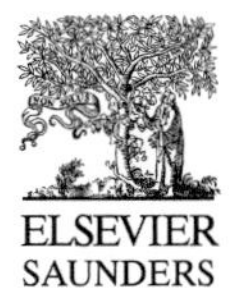

EMERGENCY MEDICINE CLINICS OF NORTH AMERICA

Emerg Med Clin N Am 25 (2007) xv–xvi

Foreword

Trauma in Emergency Medicine

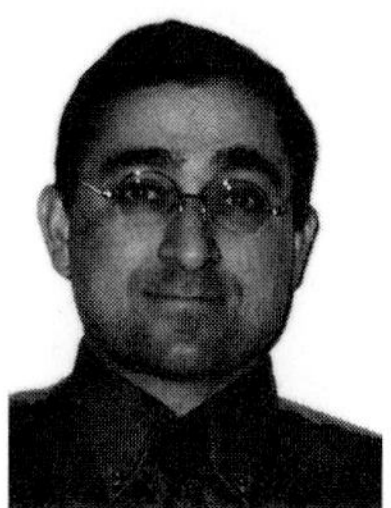

Amal Mattu, MD
Consulting Editor

"A-B-C" is the unofficial mantra of emergency medicine. Students and residents learn to manage every unstable patient from the standpoint of the "A-B-Cs" to focus on the immediate life-threats first. Simulation training and Oral Board Examination testing is also focused on the "A-B-Cs" as a priority. The concept of "A-B-Cs" originated in early Advanced Trauma Life Support (ATLS) courses. Then the "A-B-Cs" of trauma management were extrapolated to management of the adult and pediatric medical patient. An early focus on the "A-B-Cs" is often lifesaving not only for victims of trauma, but also for medically ill emergency patients. Clearly the priorities and practice of trauma management are ingrained in the specialty of emergency medicine.

As the specialty of emergency medicine has progressed, the knowledge base of trauma management in our specialty has advanced far beyond the basic concepts that are taught in ATLS courses. Advanced level resuscitation of victims of trauma is part of the core curriculum in emergency medicine training. Physicians-in-training are routinely taught special airway skills, invasive trauma procedures, and advanced resuscitation of trauma patients. Emergency physicians engage in cutting edge research related to trauma resuscitation both at the clinical and basic science level. Emergency physicians also are actively involved in collaborative efforts designed to advance the quality of trauma care in every practice setting. Although once considered the domain of the surgeon, care of the trauma patients is now clearly recognized as a multidisciplinary responsibility, and emergency physicians are playing a leading role.

0733-8627/07/$ - see front matter
doi:10.1016/j.emc.2007.07.005

In this issue of *Emergency Medicine Clinics of North America*, Guest Editor Dr. Carrie Tibbles has assembled an outstanding group of emergency care providers to bring you the latest in emergency medicine knowledge regarding the care of trauma patients. A comprehensive top down approach is taken, beginning with the airway and progressing through various systems including management of injuries to the brain, neck and spine, chest, abdomen, and extremities. Experts who care for patients in shock discuss this condition as it relates to trauma patients. Management of patients that present special challenges, including pediatric patients, geriatric patients, and pregnant patients, are discussed also. One article is dedicated specifically to wound care, a seemingly basic yet very high-risk aspect of trauma care. Finally, articles regarding trauma system design and injury prevention are provided.

This issue of *Emergency Medicine Clinics of North America* represents an important addition to emergency medicine literature. Dr. Tibbles and her colleagues have provided a cutting edge update of the current knowledge of emergency trauma care. Emergency physicians in every type of practice setting will find this issue immensely useful for the daily care of trauma patients, and this issue will undoubtedly improve the care of those patients. This issue also exemplifies how far our specialty has progressed in trauma care beyond the basics of "A-B-C." Kudos to the contributors for an outstanding issue!

Amal Mattu, MD
Department of Emergency Medicine
University of Maryland School of Medicine
110 S. Paca Street, 6th Floor, Suite 200
Baltimore, Maryland 21201, USA

E-mail address: amattu@smail.umaryland.edu

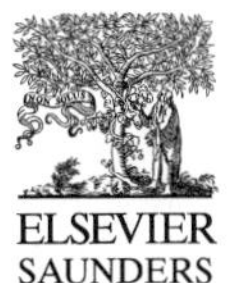

EMERGENCY
MEDICINE
CLINICS OF
NORTH AMERICA

Emerg Med Clin N Am 25 (2007) xvii–xviii

Preface

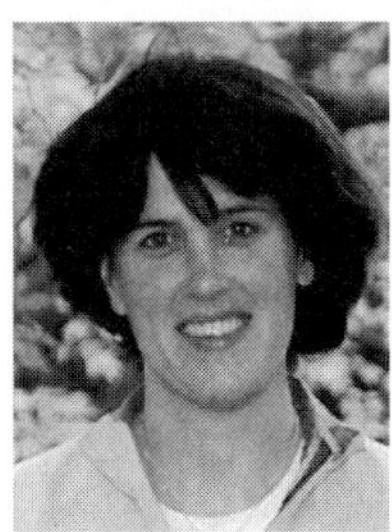

Carrie D. Tibbles, MD
Guest Editor

Trauma remains the fourth leading cause of death in the United States, and it is the number one cause of death in people ages 1 to 44. The fundamental principles of trauma care established by the American College of Surgeons still guide our treatment of trauma patients today. However, with advances in diagnostic imaging and therapies, some of the traditional teachings have become outdated. In this issue of *Emergency Medicine Clinics of North America*, each article focuses on recent developments in the trauma literature and highlights new technologies, novel therapies, or current controversies.

The first article reviews the new airway devices and their role in the management of the difficult trauma airway. The article on the identification and treatment of shock emphasizes the importance of early recognition of shock, including the role of markers of occult perfusion and the importance of aggressive resuscitation. Drs. Moore and Marchovichick provide an interesting article on the development of trauma systems in the United States and the optimal use of trauma management resources from the perspective of both trauma surgery and emergency medicine. The blunt chest trauma article focuses on subtle and challenging diagnoses, such as myocardial contusion and diaphragmatic rupture.

Algorithms for the management of patients who have major abdominal trauma have evolved in recent years with the widespread acceptance of bedside ultrasonography, nonoperative management of solid organ injury, and advances with computed tomography. The article on pelvic trauma describes the new commercially available pelvic binders and discusses the

doi:10.1016/j.emc.2007.07.004

technique of preperitoneal packing: a novel approach for stabilizing a patient following major pelvic trauma. Clinical decision rules to determine which patients require brain and spine imaging have been developed in recent years and these are described in the articles on brain and spine injury. The emergency department management of challenging orthopedic complications, the comprehensive management of neck trauma, and the latest evidence in optimal wound care are also included. The issue concludes with reviews of the unique considerations in managing pediatric, pregnant, and geriatric trauma patients, and an article that focuses on the role of the emergency department in injury prevention and education. Our goal has been to provide the emergency physician with a comprehensive review of the recent trauma literature, highlighting recent developments that impact how we practice. Editing this edition has truly been a rewarding experience, and I thank all the authors for their hard work and commitment to this project and Karen Sorensen and Patrick Manley for their expert editorial guidance.

Carrie D. Tibbles, MD
Associate Program Director
Department of Emergency Medicine
Harvard Affiliated Emergency Medicine Residency
Beth Israel Deaconess Medical Center
One Deaconess Road
West Campus Clinical Center CC2
Boston, MA 02115, USA

E-mail address: ctibbles@bidmc.harvard.edu

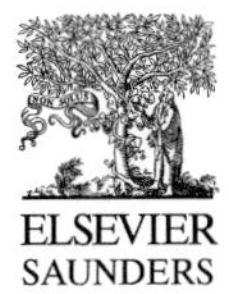

ELSEVIER
SAUNDERS

EMERGENCY MEDICINE CLINICS OF NORTH AMERICA

Emerg Med Clin N Am 25 (2007) 603–622

Airway Management in Trauma: An Update

John McGill, MD[a,b,*]

[a]Department of Emergency Medicine, Hennepin County Medical Center, 701 Park Avenue North, Minneapolis, MN 55415, USA
[b]Department of Emergency Medicine, University of Minnesota, Minneapolis, MN, USA

The past 10 years has seen a proliferation in the number of devices that are designed specifically for the difficult airway. The advantage of most of these devices is that the laryngeal opening can be visualized indirectly; they do not require the head and neck to be positioned so that the oral, pharyngeal, and laryngeal axes line up. This is particularly advantageous in the setting of trauma where movement of the neck can be dangerous. Another major advancement in the management of the airway in trauma has been the development and increasingly widespread use of the laryngeal mask airways, particularly the intubating laryngeal mask airway. These devices have become critical airway adjuncts in the management of patients who are difficult to ventilate or to intubate.

This article reviews the more recent theoretic and practical information that pertains to airway management in trauma. This includes newer airway devices, techniques, or maneuvers that are useful in the trauma setting, though potentially are underused. The algorithmic approach to the difficult airway, which aptly describes the trauma airway, is not discussed because several well-informed algorithms are readily available (www.asahq.org, www.das.uk.com). Each clinician needs to be knowledgeable about the various airway options and then, based on the physician's particular skills and resources, construct an algorithm that works best.

Intubation in the setting of potential cervical spine injury

The safety of inline immobilization of the cervical spine and emergency orotracheal intubation in multiple trauma is well established. Since the

* Department of Emergency Medicine, Hennepin County Medical Center, 701 Park Avenue North, Minneapolis, MN 55415.
E-mail address: john.mcgill@co.hennepin.mn.us

0733-8627/07/$ - see front matter
doi:10.1016/j.emc.2007.06.007

mid-1980s, when this became an accepted practice, there have been only a handful of reports of intubation causing spinal cord injury and, in each case, the head and neck were not immobilized [1–3].

Despite this exceptional safety record, during which time most intubations were performed using direct laryngoscopy, studies continue to be published comparing cervical spine movement during direct laryngoscopy with that observed using other airway interventions. There are two models: the patient with normal airway anatomy undergoing elective intubation in the operating room and cadavers in whom unstable cervical spines were created surgically. Spine movement is documented fluoroscopically or with radiographs. In the normal patients, in whom angulation of the cervical bodies is the sole measurement, most cervical spine movement during intubation occurs in the upper cervical spine, especially the occiput–C1 and atlantoaxial segments, regardless of which device is used [4–9]. Although these studies produce results that are statistically significant, their clinical significance is questionable. Specifically, a clinically significant degree of angulation has not been described (the largest reported angle was 15° at the occiput–C1 junction) [9]; displacement, not angulation, accounts for most spinal cord injuries and; several studies were conducted without immobilization. In the cadaveric model of the unstable cervical spine, there are data to suggest that the lighted stylet and fiber-optically guided nasotracheal intubation cause the least amount of subluxation, but, again, the differences were small and of unknown clinical significance [10–15]. Crosby [16], in a comprehensive review of airway management after cervical spine trauma, concluded that, as of 2006, there was no clearly superior modality for intubation in this setting.

Although the clinical relevance of much of the research on the movement of the C-spine during intubation is unclear, the cadaveric studies served to validate the practice of removing the C-collar and immobilizing the C-spine during intubation. Gerling and colleagues [14], using a C5–6 transection model, reported more subluxation during direct laryngoscopy with the collar than with inline immobilization. Laryngeal visualization also was improved after collar removal. Immediately following intubation, the collar is reapplied. Studies of unstable c-spines also demonstrated that there is as much subluxation with facemask ventilation, the chin lift, and the jaw thrust as with intubation itself [11,12], thus emphasizing the need for immobilization during all airway maneuvers.

Before leaving the topic of inline immobilization, a final comment should be made regarding the concept of "neutral" positioning of the head and neck in adult trauma. Although this term is used commonly, there is no accepted definition. Some studies defined it clinically [9,17], but most major trauma references do not address the subject [18–20]. Schriger and colleagues [17] defined neutral as the position that one assumes when standing and looking straight ahead; they found that a mean of 4 cm of occiput elevation was required to achieve this position. Data from De Lorenzo and colleagues [21], using MRI to determine the optimal elevation of the occiput for maximizing the spinal canal/spinal cord ratio at C5 and C6 (a common level of injury), suggested that at least 2 cm of elevation is desirable in normal individuals. Regardless of how neutral is defined, it is clear that the common practice of leaving the head immobilized on the backboard results in a position that may be far from neutral. This is especially evident in the profile of an obese patient whose thick back puts the cervical spine in hyperextension when the head rests on the backboard. Head elevation needs to be individualized in the morbidly obese and the elderly who may have preexistent lordotic deformities. Optimizing head and neck position, within the constraints of the trauma setting, will improve positioning for intubation while maintaining the integrity of the spinal cord.

Anterior neck maneuvers during intubation

There are two manipulations of the anterior neck that often improve laryngeal visualization during intubation. "BURP" (backward upward right pressure) is applied by an assistant over the lower thyroid cartilage to improve the glottic view when it is found to be suboptimal. The second maneuver, optimal external laryngeal manipulation (OELM), differs primarily in that it is the laryngoscopist who, by reaching around with the right hand, manipulates the anterior neck and identifies the position of the larynx that best exposes the laryngeal inlet. Once identified, the assistant assumes the position of the laryngoscopist's hand so that intubation can be performed.

Although both manipulations improve the laryngeal view [22–24], OELM seems to be superior [25]. Given the frequency of suboptimal laryngeal views during inline immobilization [26], these maneuvers, preferably OELM, should be used whenever visualization is poor. Cricoid pressure, the "Sellick's maneuver," is used to prevent stomach insufflation and regurgitation, yet it may make intubation more difficult [27–29]. Although it is still recommended, cricoid pressure should be relaxed, or even removed, if it is believed to impede intubation significantly.

Tracheal tube introducers

The tracheal tube introducer, originally the gum elastic bougie, was developed decades ago to assist in difficult intubations (Fig. 1). It is a long, thin, semirigid adjunct that, with the aid of a laryngoscope, is passed through the laryngeal inlet and over which an endotracheal (ET) tube is advanced into the trachea. Although ideally used when a portion of the laryngeal inlet is visible, it can be effective when only the epiglottis is seen [30]. This attribute, coupled with the fact that it is not affected by the presence of blood and secretions, makes the bougie well suited in the trauma setting.

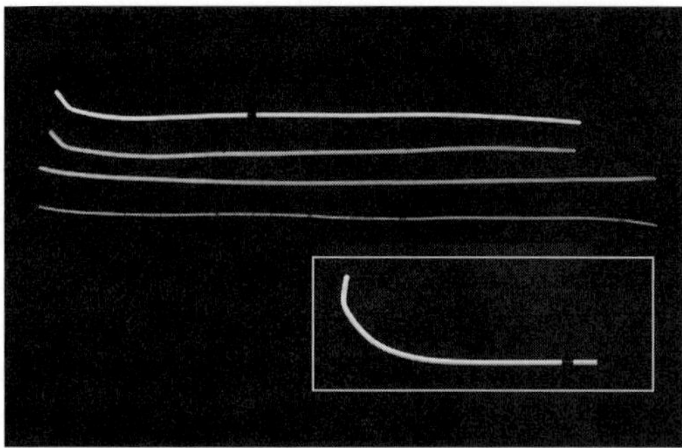

Fig. 1. Several types of tracheal tube introducers. The gum elastic bougie (dark yellow) is reusable and comes in curved- and straight-tip adult forms and a straight pediatric form. The straight bougies are 70 cm, and the curved-tipped bougies are 60 cm. The blue introducer (Flextrach ETTube Guide) is polyethylene, designed for single use, and comes only in a curved-tip adult form (60 cm). The inset demonstrates the 60° optimum curve if none of the laryngeal inlet can be seen on laryngoscopy.

Its efficacy was demonstrated prospectively in difficult intubations in the operating room (OR), as a key component of a difficult airway algorithm in the OR, and it has been compared favorably to conventional laryngoscopy in the emergency department (ED) [31–33]. Despite this track record, the tracheal tube introducer has seen limited use in the United States.

The original adjunct, called the gum elastic bougie or simply "the bougie," is available in reusable form for adults and pediatrics (Eschmann Tracheal Tube Introducer, Portex Sims, Kent, UK). The adult version accommodates a 5.5-mm ET tube, whereas the pediatric version can accommodate a 4.0-mm tube. An adult polyethylene introducer, designed for single use, also is available (Flextrach ETTube Guide, Greenfield Medical Sourcing, Inc., Austin, Texas).

Ideally, tracheal tube introducer-assisted intubation is a two-person procedure, with the assistant handing the introducer to the operator after the best laryngoscopic view has been obtained. If the laryngeal inlet is not visible, a 60° distal bend is placed in the introducer, and it is passed just under the epiglottis and directed anteriorly (see Fig. 1, inset). The assistant slides the ET tube over the introducer, and the operator passes the tube through the larynx. A 90° counterclockwise rotation is recommended just before entering the larynx to avoid the ET tube tip catching on laryngeal structures (Fig. 2) [34]. The laryngoscope is removed only after successful placement of the ET tube.

There are several confirmatory findings after successful introducer placement. Success is indicated, up to 90% of the time, by feeling clicks produced by the angled tip of the introducer as it strikes against the tracheal rings [35]. Also, an assistant usually feels confirmatory movement in the airway if the anterior neck is palpated. If there is any question about whether the introducer is in the airway, it should be advanced at least 40 cm, at which point

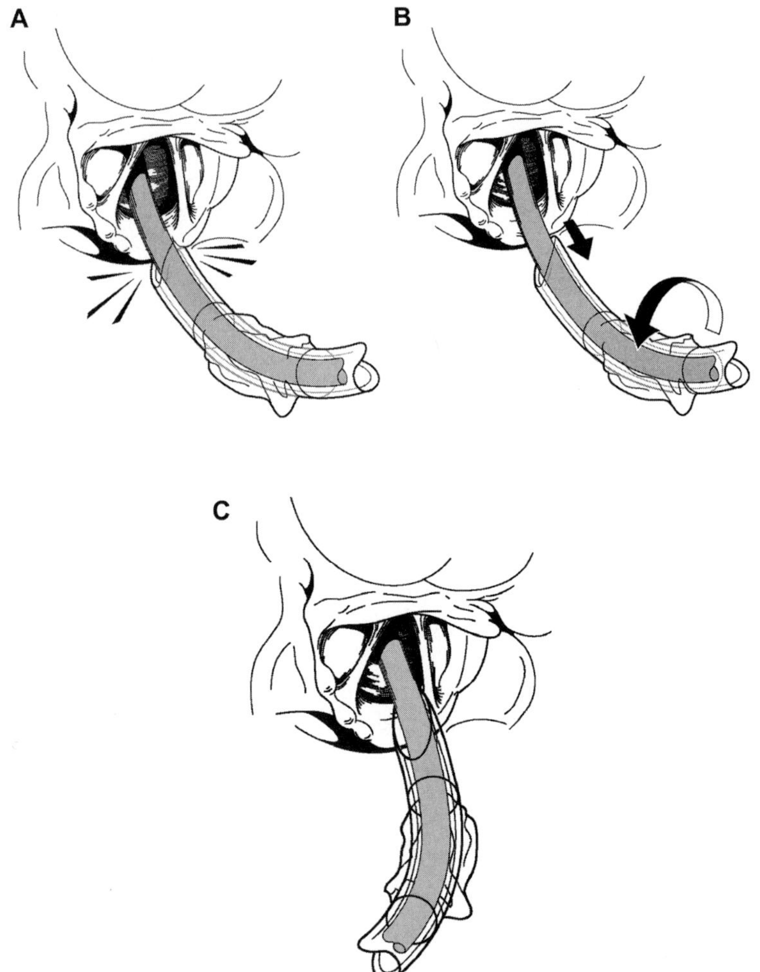

Fig. 2. A common cause of difficulty when railroading an ET tube over a tracheal tube introducer. (*A*) ET tube tip caught on the right arytenoid as it is being railroaded over the introducer. Corrective maneuvers: (*B*) ET tube is withdrawn 2 cm to disengage the arytenoids and counterclockwise rotation of ET tube 90° to orient the bevel posteriorly. (*C*) The bevel of the ET tube is facing posteriorly and allows for smooth passage through the glottis. (*Courtesy of* Department of Emergency Medicine, Hennepin County Medical Center, Minneapolis, MN.)

resistance should be felt as the introducer passes the carina into a main bronchus.

In the prehospital setting, where assistance may not be available, removal of the laryngoscope may be required so the operator can mount the ET tube onto the introducer. Once the tube is on the introducer, the laryngoscope may be reinserted and the tube rotated 90° counterclockwise to ensure successful passage of the tube. Mounting the tube onto the introducer and introducing them as a unit is not advised because it often is difficult to direct the introducer into the laryngeal inlet as it moves within the ET tube.

In addition to its usefulness in multiple trauma, the tracheal tube introducer can be useful when intubating patients who have blunt and penetrating upper airway injury. In this setting, a carefully passed introducer that advances into the trachea without resistance is added assurance that an ET tube will be able to be placed without causing further damage. It also can be used as an introducer for an ET tube being placed through an open neck wound [36] or, as in the author's institution, when performing a cricothyrotomy.

Laryngeal mask airways

The laryngeal mask airway (LMA) and the intubating LMA (ILMA) are excellent rescue devices for the "cannot intubate/cannot ventilate" situation. Both devices are valuable for rescue ventilation, but the ILMA is superior as a conduit for intubation [37]. As ventilatory devices, their reliability has been excellent. The ILMA also is successful when intubating patients with known difficult airways [38,39]. In the OR, blind intubation through the ILMA has an overall success rate of 90%; when aided by fiberoscopy, the success rate approaches 100% [37]. LMAs are contraindicated in patients with less than 2 cm of mouth opening and are unlikely to be successful in patients with grossly distorted supraglottic anatomy from disease processes or postradiation scarring or in patients with an intact gag reflex.

Most intubations through the ILMA are performed blindly, using the designated LMA ET tube or a standard ET tube. If a standard ET tube is used, it should be inserted so that the curve is opposite the normal orientation (Fig. 3A). This results in the ET tube exiting the ILMA at a less acute angle and allows it to pass into the trachea more easily (Fig. 3B) [40]. If difficulty is encountered, a fiber-optic scope can be helpful in guiding intubation.

If an LMA has been placed, blind ET tube placement is not an option. A fiber-optic scope must be used or, better yet, a hollow introducer, such as an Aintree Intubation Catheter (Cook Critical Care, Bloomington, Indiana; www.cookmedical.com) in conjunction with a fiber-optic scope, is placed though the LMA into the trachea (Fig. 4). Once placed, the LMA is removed, and an ET tube is railroaded over the hollow introducer into the trachea. Use of a regular tracheal tube introducer is not recommended because of a high failure rate [41]. If intubation fails, despite the recommended adjustment maneuvers and fiber-optic assistance, definitive airway control—using a retrograde wire or a surgical airway—can be accomplished in a controlled fashion while the patient continues to be ventilated with the laryngeal mask [42]. An excellent resource for troubleshooting LMA difficulties can be found on the company's website (www.lmana.com) under "Insertion Technique and Maneuvers Guide."

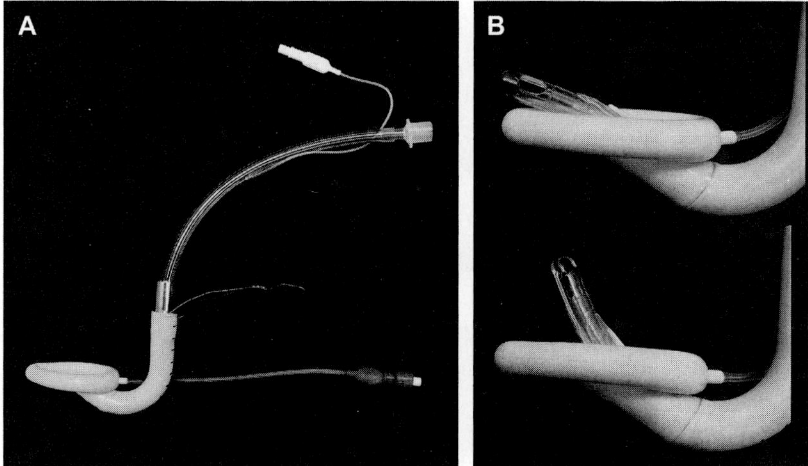

Fig. 3. Intubating through an ILMA using a standard tracheal tube. (*A*) The tracheal tube is inserted so the curve of the tube is opposite the curve of the ILMA. This allows the tube tip to exit the ILMA at an angle more conducive to smooth passage into the trachea. (*B*) Angle of the tracheal tube tip after normal orientation of the ET tube (*lower*) versus the correct "reverse curve" orientation (*upper*).

LMAs provide an excellent means of oxygenating and ventilating when facemask ventilation is difficult or impossible. In addition, the ILMA is particularly useful in managing patients who are difficult to intubate with direct laryngoscopy. Thus, by facilitating the management of difficult/failed ventilation and difficult/failed intubation, the ILMA has become an indispensable component of any difficult airway algorithm.

The Combitube and laryngeal tube

The Esophageal-Tracheal Combitube remains an effective intermediate airway that is used primarily in the prehospital setting. Its popularity has decreased as the use of laryngeal masks has increased. Its biggest drawback is the difficulty establishing a definitive airway after the Combitube has been placed. The laryngeal tube, also known as the King LT, is a new intermediate airway that is replacing the Combitube in some prehospital systems because of its simpler design and availability in a disposable version (Fig. 5). A major difference between the King LT and the Combitube is that it is designed specifically not to go into the trachea.

Lighted stylet intubation

The Trachlight (Laerdal Medical Corp., Wappingers Falls, New York) was introduced in 1995 and is the only lighted stylet, among several

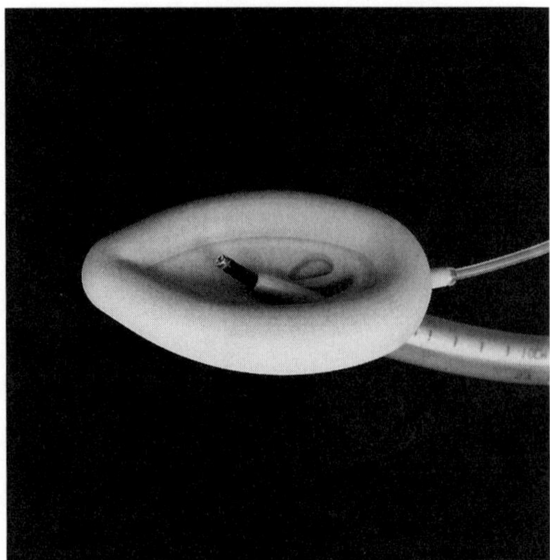

Fig. 4. Facilitating intubation through an LMA: a hollow introducer (Aintree Intubation Catheter, 60 cm) is placed through the LMA and into the trachea and guided by a fiberoptic scope. Then the LMA is railroaded over the introducer into the trachea. (*From* Roberts, Hedges, editors. Tracheal intubation. In: Clinical procedures in emergency medicine. 5th edition. Philadelphia: Elsevier; in press; with permission.)

available today, that has a proven track record. By transilluminating the soft tissues of the neck, the light serves to guide the tube into the larynx (Fig. 6). It compared favorably with direct laryngoscopy in a randomized study of 950 surgical patients [43], and, in another large series, also by

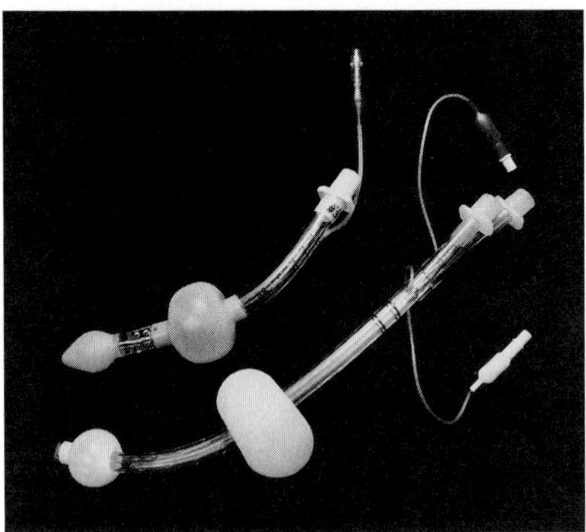

Fig. 5. The Combitube (*bottom*) and the King LT (*top*).

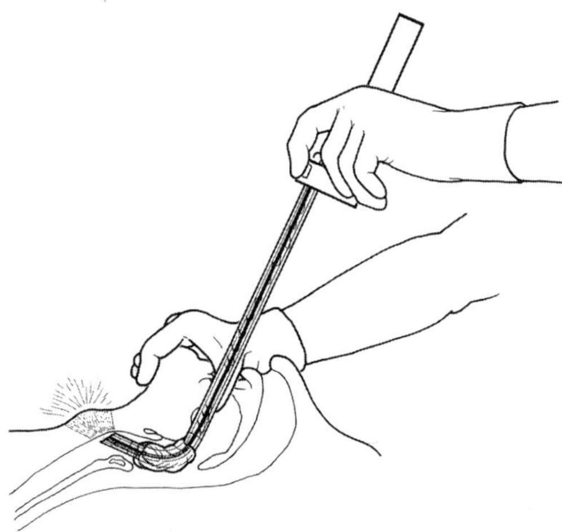

Fig. 6. Lighted stylet intubation. Use of the Trachlight for ET intubation using transillumination of soft tissues as a guide to placement. (*Courtesy of* Department of Emergency Medicine, Hennepin County Medical Center, Minneapolis, MN.)

Hung and colleagues [44], the device was 99% successful in intubating patients who had difficult airways. The stylets come in adult, pediatric, and infant sizes and can accommodate down to a 2.5-mm internal diameter (ID) tube (Fig. 7).

The patient's head and neck are optimally placed in the neutral or, if possible, slightly extended position. This makes the Trachlight well suited for the patient who has experienced trauma, especially given the fact that its success is not impacted by the presence of blood or secretions. Because lighted stylet intubation is a blind approach, it should be avoided in patients with expanding neck masses or laryngopharyngeal trauma. Morbid obesity is the most common cause for failure because of the difficulty transilluminating through generous soft tissue.

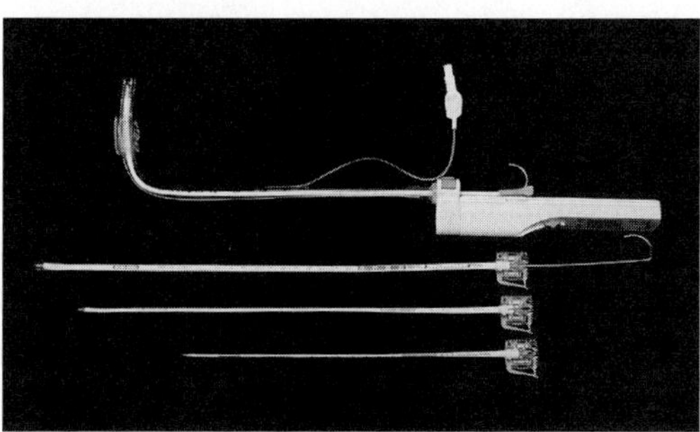

Fig. 7. Trachlight and related stylets. The malleable stylet is bent at a 90° angle, 6.5 to 8.5 cm from the tip (marked on stylet). The smallest stylet accommodates a 2.5-mm ID tube.

The clinician stands at the head of the patient. When this is not possible, the patient can be approached from either side. With the patient's head and neck in the neutral position or slightly extended, the jaw is grasped near the corner of the mouth, between the thumb, index, and middle fingers, and lifted to elevate the tongue and epiglottis (see Fig. 6). A transilluminating glow indicates the location of the tube tip. Application of cricoid pressure may enhance the transillumination [45]. The overhead light often must be dimmed in the obese patient. Positioning is optimal when a light bulb–like glow emanates from the midline, just below the level of the thyroid prominence. In extremely thin patients, it is possible to observe transillumination and still be in the esophagus. The clue is that the glow is diffuse if the tip is in the esophagus, as opposed to the well-circumscribed glow of intralaryngeal placement.

The Trachlight is a safe, effective, rapid, and inexpensive intubating device that is placed with the patient in neutral position and is not affected adversely by blood. These features make it especially amenable to the trauma setting.

Semirigid fiber-optic stylets

A class of devices that incorporate fiber optics into a semirigid metal or metal-reinforced stylet was introduced in the late 1990s. They can be used in conjunction with direct laryngoscopy or alone. They require direct laryngoscopic assistance in 8% to 20% of cases and, in general, are more successful when used in this way [46,47]. In either case, the tip of the fiber-optic stylet, with its overlying ET tube, is passed under the epiglottis and directed through the glottis into the trachea. Visibility can be hampered by blood and secretions, but less so than with flexible fiberoscopy [48]. They also are easier to learn how to use. The Shikani Optical Stylet and Levitan FPS Scope (Clarus Medical, Minneapolis, Minnesota) are examples of these malleable optical stylets (Fig. 8). Most often, the Shikani Stylet is used similarly to the Trachlight, with the added feature of being able to see fiber-optically what is just beyond the tube tip. The Levitan Scope is designed to be used with a laryngoscope, serving as a stylet for the tracheal tube while providing fiber-optic visualization if required. The Levitan stylet can accommodate a minimum tube size of 5.5-mm ID, whereas the Shikani comes in two sizes: the adult, accommodating a 5.5-mm ID tube, and a pediatric version that accommodates a 3.5-mm ID tube.

The semirigid fiber-optic stylets are useful in patients in whom the glottis cannot be seen readily. Blood and secretions may complicate their use, but less so than with flexible fiberoscopy. The Shikani scope was more successful than the gum elastic boogie in simulated Cormack and Lehane Grade 3 views [49]. There are no absolute contraindications and no reported complications with semirigid fiber-optic stylets, other than the failures or prolonged attempts usually related to poor visibility from blood and secretions [46].

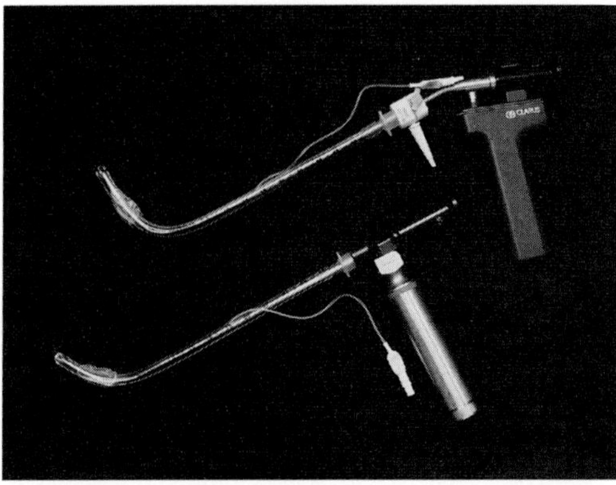

Fig. 8. Examples of semirigid fiber-optic stylets: the Shikani (*top*) and Levitan (*bottom*). The recommended bends when used alone (*top*) and when used with a direct laryngoscope (*bottom*) are demonstrated. The sliding adapter on the Shikani stylet allows for various lengths of tracheal tubes.

Semirigid fiber-optic stylets combine the features of direct and indirect laryngoscopy and provide a valuable tool when one is faced with a difficult airway. They can be used alone or in conjunction with a laryngoscope. They are considerably less expensive than rigid fiber-optic devices and are easier to use than flexible scopes. There are no head-to-head clinical trials with other devices; however, early reports suggest that the semirigid fiber-optic stylets have a role to play in managing the airway in trauma.

Nasal and orotracheal intubation over a flexible fiber-optic bronchoscope

Flexible fiber-optic intubation is cited often in the anesthesia literature as the preferred method for intubating a patient with an unstable C-spine. It also is recommended in patients with suspected or known injury to the upper airway. In a survey at the 1999 annual meeting of the American Society of Anesthesiologists, 75% of respondents said they would use awake fiber-optic intubation in the setting of cervical spine disease, yet only 59% felt competent with this approach [50]. In the ED, the success rate is 50% to 90% [51–53]. Failure is attributed most often to poor visibility from blood, vomitus, and other secretions. Mlinek and coworkers [53] found that successful ED fiber-optic intubations averaged 2 minutes, whereas failures averaged 8 minutes; they recommended considering alternative approaches if intubation attempts take more than 3 minutes.

Fiber-optically guided intubation can be accomplished using the nasal or oral route. The nasal approach is technically easier because the angle of insertion allows for easier visualization of the larynx, with minimal manipulation of the fiberscope, and because patient cooperation is not as critical. Insertion using the oral route can be facilitated by using an oral-intubating airway (Fig. 9). Contraindications to the nasal approach are severe midface trauma and coagulopathy. Active airway bleeding and vomiting are relative contraindications for both approaches because successful intubation is unlikely in these settings. If the clinician is inexperienced in fiber-optic intubation, significant hypoxia is another relative contraindication to its use.

The primary advantages of fiber-optic intubation are the ability to visualize upper airway abnormalities, to negotiate difficult airway anatomy, and to carefully perform tracheal intubation with visual guidance. A major limitation in trauma is the lack of visibility in the presence of blood and secretions. If blood is present, it is best to avoid the fiber-optic scope.

Rigid fiber-optic laryngoscopy

Rigid fiber-optic laryngoscopes are designed to approximate the anatomy of the upper airway and provide indirect fiber-optic visualization of the laryngeal inlet. Examples include the Bullard laryngoscope (Circon Corp., Stamford, Connecticut), the UpsherScope (Mercury Medical, Clearwater, Florida), and the WuScope (Achi Corp., San Jose, California). These devices offer the advantage of a conventional fiber-optic scope but require less training [54]. They are well suited for patients who have potential cervical spine injury because no movement of the neck is necessary. Case reports also suggested their usefulness in patients who had upper airway distortion from mass or hematoma [55,56]. One potential advantage of the WuScope is that its fiber-optic element is relatively protected from blood and secretions by its tubular blade.

The Bullard laryngoscope comes in two sizes: pediatric (newborn to 10 years) and adult. It can be used in awake or unresponsive patients [57]. At least 2 cm of occlusal opening is necessary for the introduction of the scope and an ET tube. The technique for introducing the Bullard

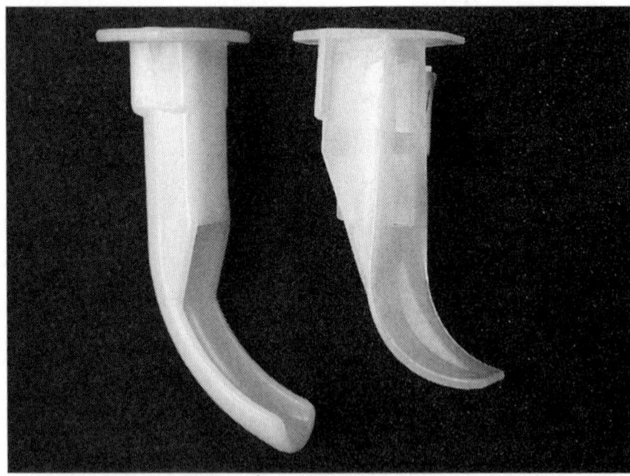

Fig. 9. Examples of oral intubating airways. The Williams Airway Intubator (*left*) cradles the ET tube in an open, curved guide, whereas the Ovassapian Fiberoptic Intubating Airway (*right*) positions the ET tube on the posterior surface of the intubation airway.

laryngoscope blade is similar to that for direct laryngoscopy (Fig. 10). With the glottis in view, the tube is advanced off the attached stylet and into the larynx. Cricoid pressure does not seem to interfere with Bullard scope success [58]. A newer, multifunctional stylet has a hollow lumen that allows an introducer to be passed through it and into the laryngeal inlet and over which the tube can be advanced. Plastic tip extensions are available for the larger patient in whom the epiglottis may be difficult to elevate.

The major difficulty in using rigid fiber-optic laryngoscopes is the inability to visualize the larynx because of blood, emesis, or secretions; a possible exception is the WuScope, with its relatively protected optical element, but it has yet to be studied in this setting. Once visualized, the glottis usually can be intubated, although accessing the inlet and passing the tube occasionally may be difficult.

Video-assisted laryngoscopy

Video-assisted laryngoscopy transmits an image from an optical element located on the laryngoscope blade to a monitor. In addition to providing indirect images that may be unobtainable with direct laryngoscopy, the image is enhanced by magnification and a wide-angle view. The newer devices incorporate miniature video cameras on their blades. The ability to view the images on a monitor provides immediate feedback to an assistant providing

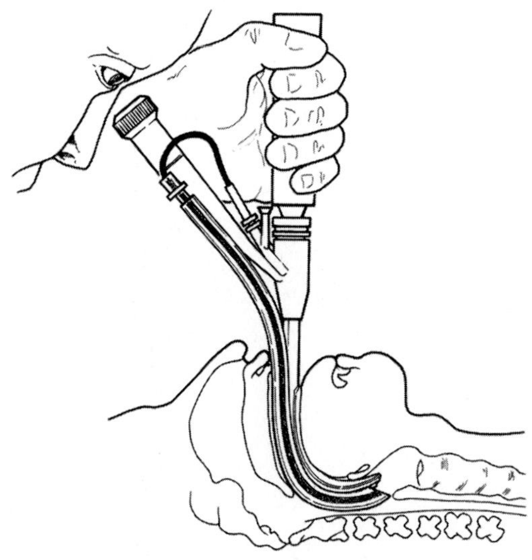

Fig. 10. Bullard laryngoscope. Anatomically shaped laryngoscope visualizing the glottis; tracheal tube is mounted on the attached stylet to facilitate laryngeal placement. (*Courtesy of* Department of Emergency Medicine, Hennepin County Medical Center, Minneapolis, MN.)

external laryngeal manipulation. Video-assisted laryngoscopy also has great potential as a teaching aid.

The GlideScope videolaryngoscope (Verathon, Bothell, Washington), first introduced in 2001, is the first of a new class of video-assisted rigid scopes that provide enhanced video views of the laryngeal inlet while being less likely to be affected by the presence of blood and secretions. There are three sizes: small for neonates and infants, medium for children and small adults, and large for adults. It comes with a small monitor on a stand or a smaller, more portable monitor. The McGrath Portable Video Laryngoscope (Aircraft Medical Ltd., Edinburgh, UK) is a device with similar characteristics, but it is more compact, has an adjustable blade length, and uses disposable blade covers (Fig. 11). It is new, and no studies have been reported on its use.

The GlideScope has a miniature camera embedded midway along the undersurface of the blade that has a 60° midblade angulation (Fig. 12). Blood and secretions are unlikely to compromise laryngeal visualization because of the camera's orientation, its location well away from the blade tip, and its antifogging technology. Visualization of the laryngeal inlet is excellent and is usually less of a problem than placing a tube through it. Difficult laryngoscopic cases are intubated more easily with this scope than with direct laryngoscopy, but easy cases are more time consuming because of difficulties in advancing the tube [59]. A contraindication is a small mouth through which the blade cannot be passed safely (opening less than 2 cm). Learning to use the GlideScope is easy because the overall feel of the device is similar to that of a conventional laryngoscope. The absence of fiber-optic elements increases its durability and decreases inevitable breakage expenses.

The styletted tracheal tube is usually bent to conform to the 60° angle of the GlideScope blade (see Fig. 12). The GlideScope blade is placed into the mouth and, under direct vision, is advanced in the midline. Verifying midline position on the monitor, the uvula is passed as the GlideScope blade

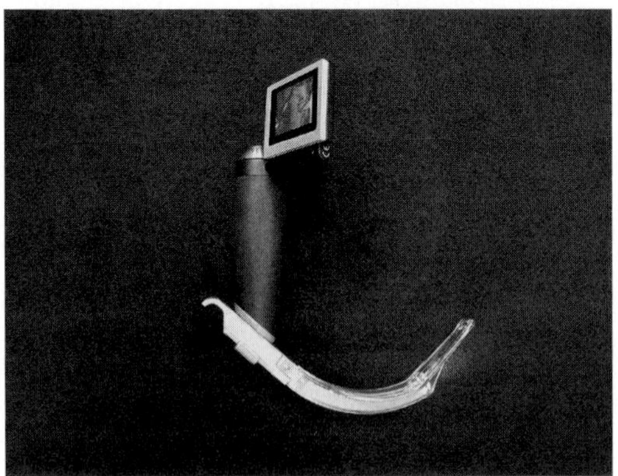

Fig. 11. The McGrath Portable Video Laryngoscope.

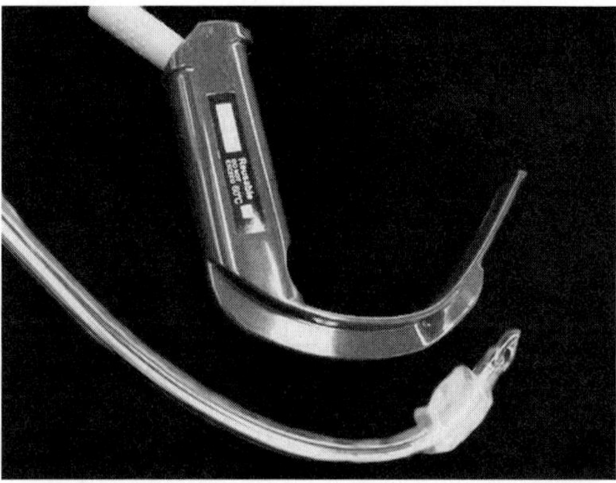

Fig. 12. The GlideScope. The ET tube has the 60° bend recommended by the manufacturer.

is slipped behind the tongue, hugging the tongue base. With a gentle lifting motion, the tip of the blade enters the vallecula, and the epiglottis is seen and elevated out of the way to expose the laryngeal inlet. The ET tube is passed blindly along the side of the blade and into the hypopharynx. When the tip of the ET tube comes into view, it is directed into the glottis and advanced to the appropriate depth. If difficulty is encountered trying to access the laryngeal inlet, success may be achieved by a variety of means, including application of external laryngeal pressure, increasing the bend of the stylet, using a tracheal tube introducer, or using a Parker Flex-It Stylet (Parker Medical, Englewood, Colorado) [60]. This is a new device, but several minor injuries have been reported: two cases of puncture of the right palatopharyngeal arch, with one requiring surgical repair [61].

Video-assisted laryngoscopy is a major advancement in the visualization of the laryngeal inlet. The GlideScope, the first device that incorporates micro video camera technology, provides an improved laryngeal view compared with difficult direct laryngoscopy while avoiding some of the problems associated with fiber-optic bronchoscopy. It has yet to be studied extensively in the setting of difficult intubation, although preliminary reports are promising [62]. Most intubation failures result from the inability to pass the tube through the larynx, despite adequate glottic views [60]. Improvements in the configuration of the tracheal stylet should decrease this problem.

Blind nasotracheal intubation

There are few indications for blind nasotracheal intubation in trauma. One potential circumstance is in the patient with minimal mouth opening, because all of the newer devices that provide an indirect view of the laryngeal inlet require at least 2 cm of mouth opening. In this situation, nasotracheal intubation may be a reasonable option if a surgical airway is not immediately indicated.

Surgical airways

Cricothyrotomy remains the preferred procedure for establishing a definitive emergency surgical airway. The four-step approach, first described in 1996 [63], has gained popularity; in a series of 50 patients [64], the complication rate compared favorably with that found when the more traditional approach was used [65]. This approach begins with a smaller, horizontal stab wound that is carried down through the cricothyroid membrane. The tracheal hook is placed caudally under the cricoid cartilage as opposed to superiorly, under the inferior edge of the thyroid cartilage, as with the traditional approach. Regardless of the approach, a generous vertical incision should be made if there is difficulty identifying the cricothyroid membrane [65,66]. In addition to gaining exposure in the patient with a large neck, this incision permits definitive, digital identification of the membrane and reduces the chances of suprathyroid tube placement. If difficulty is encountered placing a Shiley tracheostomy tube, a tracheal tube introducer can be inserted and a #6 ET tube passed over it into the trachea.

Percutaneous cricothyrotomy is another potential approach for establishing a surgical airway. Schaumann and colleagues [67], in a large, cadaveric study comparing the Seldinger technique (Arndt Emergency Cricothyrotomy Catheter Set, Cook Critical Care, Bloomington, Illinois) to the standard surgical approach, concluded that the Seldinger technique had the advantage of being quicker. They failed to mention, however, that 4 of 100 catheters placed with the Seldinger technique ended up in the subcutaneous tissue. This serious complication results from the insufficient catheter length (6 cm) used in the study; this study, using normal-sized cadavers, undoubtedly underestimates the likelihood of this complication occurring in a patient with a large neck. The Melker Cricothyrotomy Catheter Set (Cook Medical, Inc., Bloomington, Indiana) (9 cm) is long enough for most patients; however, even with a vertical skin incision, sets of this variety can be difficult to place through the tissues of the anterior neck [68]. Thus, although the percutaneous approach is far better than no surgical attempt at all, the approaches that ultimately permit digital identification of the cricothyroid membrane and incorporate a scalpel incision through the membrane remain the preferred surgical approaches for the emergency trauma airway.

Summary

Conceptually, the management of the airway in trauma has not changed significantly in recent years. The safety of inline immobilization and rapid sequence intubation has been reaffirmed clinically. Although the general management has not changed, the choice of airway devices has markedly increased. The most important among these is the ILMA because it can provide effective rescue ventilation and intubation. The newer devices that allow for indirect visualization of the laryngeal inlet also will contribute to effective trauma airway management.

Despite the advances in intubating devices, direct laryngoscopy likely will continue to be the initial approach to intubating the patient after trauma. As with any intubation, preoxygenation is essential and, by extending the apnea time before desaturation, it can make the difference between a successful and a failed intubation. Positioning, another key element in successful intubation, is more complicated in the setting of trauma; however, it can be improved upon, from a neurosurgical and an airway perspective, by elevating the head off the backboard. If the laryngoscopic view is suboptimal, intubation often can be accomplished rapidly using a tracheal tube introducer. External laryngeal manipulation also may be useful at this juncture. These steps should be accomplished rapidly and usually result in successful intubation. If unsuccessful, a device that provides indirect glottic visualization should be used. Alternatively, especially in the setting of oxygen desaturation, an ILMA can be placed to ventilate and intubate the patient. Cricothyrotomy remains the ultimate back-up airway and should be performed using the technique that corresponds best to the patient's body habitus and operator experience.

References

[1] Hastings RH, Kelley SD. Neurologic deterioration associated with airway management in a cervical spine-injured patient. Anesthesiology 1993;78(3):580–3.

[2] Muckart DJ, Bhagwanjee S, van der Merwe R. Spinal cord injury as a result of endotracheal intubation in patients with undiagnosed cervical spine fractures. Anesthesiology 1997;87(2):418–20.

[3] Liang BA, Cheng MA, Tempelhoff R. Efforts at intubation: cervical injury in an emergency circumstance? J Clin Anesth 1999;11:349–52.

[4] Sawin PD, Todd MM, Traynelis VC, et al. Cervical spine motion with direct laryngoscopy and orotracheal intubation. Anesthesiology 1999;85(1):26–36.

[5] Watts ADJ, Gelb AW, Bach DB, et al. Comparison of the Bullard and Macintosh laryngoscopes for endotracheal intubation of patients with a potential cervical spine injury. Anesthesiology 1997;87(6):1335–42.

[6] Shulman GB, Connelly NR. A comparison of the Bullard laryngoscope versus the flexible fiberoptic bronchoscope during intubation in patients afforded inline stabilization. J Clin Anesth 2001;13(3):182–5.

[7] Waltl B, Melischek M, Schuschnig C, et al. Tracheal intubation and cervical spine excursion: direct laryngoscopy vs. intubating laryngeal mask. Anaesthesia 2001;56:221–6.

[8] Sahin A, Salman MA, Erden IA, et al. Upper cervical vertebrae movement during the intubating laryngeal mask, fiberoptic and direct laryngoscopy: a video-fluoroscopic study. Eur J Anaesthesiol 2004;21:819–23.

[9] Turkstra TP, Eng M, Eng P, et al. Cervical spine motion: a fluoroscopic comparison during intubation with lighted stylet, GlideScope, and Macintosh laryngoscope. Anesth Analg 2005;101(3):910–5.

[10] Bilgin H, Bozkurt M. Tracheal intubation using the ILMA, C-Trach or McCoy laryngoscope in patients with simulated cervical spine injury. Anaesthesia 2006;61:685–91.
[11] Brimacombe J, Keller C, Kunzel KH, et al. Cervical spine motion during airway management: a cinefluoroscopic study of the posteriorly destabilized third cervical vertebrae in human cadavers. Anesth Analg 2000;1(5):1274–8.
[12] Donaldson WF III, Heil BV, Donaldson VP, et al. The effect of airway maneuvers on the unstable C1-C2 segment: a cadaver study. Spine 1997;22:1215–8.
[13] Lennarson PJ, Smith DW, Sawin PD, et al. Cervical spine motion during intubation: efficacy of stabilization maneuvers in the setting of complete segmental instability. J Neurosurg 2001; 94:265–70.
[14] Gerling MC, Davis DP, Hamilton RS, et al. Effects of cervical spine immobilization technique and laryngoscope blade selection on an unstable cervical spine in a cadaver model of intubation. Ann Emerg Med 2006;36(4):293–300.
[15] Gerling MC, Davis DP, Hamilton RS, et al. Effect of surgical cricothyrotomy on the unstable cervical spine in a cadaver model of intubation. J Emerg Med 2001;20(1):1–5.
[16] Crosby ET. Airway management in adults after cervical spine trauma. Anesthesiology 2006; 104(6):1293–318.
[17] Schriger DL, Lamon B, LeGassick T, et al. Spinal immobilization on a flat backboard: does it result in neutral position of the cervical spine? Ann Emerg Med 1991;20(8):878–81.
[18] Wilmore DW, Cheung LY, Harken AH, et al, editors. ACS surgery: principles and practice. 3rd edition. New York: WebMD Corp; 2003.
[19] Danne PD, Hunter M, Mackillop AD. Airway control. In: Moore EE, Feliciano DV, Mattox, editors. Trauma. 5th edition. New York: McGraw Hill; 2004. p. 181–2.
[20] Head trauma. In: American College of Surgeons Committee on Trauma. Advanced trauma life support for doctors: student course manual. 7th edition. Chicago: American College of Surgeons; 2004. p. 151–67.
[21] De Lorenzo RA, Olson JE, Boska M, et al. Optimal positioning for cervical immobilization. Ann Emerg Med 1996;28(3):301–8.
[22] Takahata O, Kubota M, Mamiya K, et al. The efficacy of the "BURP" maneuver during a difficult laryngoscopy. Anesth Analg 1997;84:419–21.
[23] Benumof JL, Cooper SD. Quantitative improvement in laryngoscopic view by optimal external laryngeal manipulation. J Clin Anesth 1996;8(2):136–40.
[24] Krill RL. Difficult laryngoscopy made easy with a "BURP". Can J Anaesth 1993;40:798–9.
[25] Levitan RM, Everett WW, Kinkle WC, et al. Pressing on the neck during laryngoscopy: a comparison of cricoid pressure, backward upward rightward pressure, and external laryngeal manipulation. Acad Emerg Med 2005;12(Suppl 1):92.
[26] Nolan JP, Wilson ME. Orotracheal intubation in patients with potential cervical spine injuries. Anaesthesia 1993;48:630–3.
[27] Ho AMH, Wong W, Ling E, et al. Airway difficulties caused by improperly applied cricoid pressure. J Emerg Med 2001;20:29–31.
[28] Brimacombe J, White A, Berry A. Effect of cricoid pressure on the ease of insertion of the laryngeal mask airway. Br J Anaesth 1993;71(6):503–7.
[29] Smith CE, Boyer D. Cricoid pressure decreases ease of tracheal intubation using fiberoptic laryngoscopy (WuScope System). Can J Anaesth 2002;49(6):614–9.
[30] Nolan JP, Wilson ME. An evaluation of the gum elastic bougie. Intubation times and incidence of sore throat. Anaesthesia 1992;47(10):878–81.
[31] Combes X, Le Roux B, Suen P, et al. Unanticipated difficult airway in anesthetized patients: prospective validation of a management algorithm. Anesthesiology 2004;100(5):1146–50.
[32] Latto IP, Stacey M, Mecklenburgh J, et al. Survey of the use of the gum elastic bougie in clinical practice. Anaesthesia 2002;57(4):379–84.
[33] McGill J, Vogel EC, Rodgerson JD. Use of the gum elastic bougie as an adjunct for orotracheal intubation in the emergency department. Acad Emerg Med 2000;7(5):526.

[34] Dogra S, Falconer R, Latto IP. Successful difficult intubation. Tracheal tube placement over a gum-elastic bougie. Anaesthesia 1990;45(9):774–6.
[35] Kidd JF, Dyson A, Latto IP. Successful difficult intubation. Use of the gum elastic bougie. Anaesthesia 1988;43(6):437–8.
[36] Steinfeldt J, Bey TA, Rich JM. Use of a gum elastic bougie (GEB) in a zone II penetrating neck trauma: a case report. J Emerg Med 2003;24(3):267–70.
[37] Brimacombe J. Laryngeal mask anesthesia: principles and practice. 2nd edition. Philadelphia: Saunders; 2005.
[38] Joo H, Rose K. Fastrach–a new intubating laryngeal mask airway: successful use in patients with difficult airways. Can J Anaesth 1998;45(3):253–6.
[39] Langeron O, Semjen F, Bourgain JL, et al. Comparison of the intubating laryngeal mask airway with the fiberoptic intubation in anticipated difficult airway management. Anesthesiology 2001;94(6):968–72.
[40] Joo HS, Rose DK. The intubating laryngeal mask airway with and without fiberoptic guidance. Anesth Analg 1999;88(3):662–6.
[41] Gabbott DA, Sasada MP. Tracheal intubation through the laryngeal mask using a gum elastic bougie in the presence of cricoid pressure and manual in line stabilisation of the neck. Anaesthesia 1996;51(4):389–90.
[42] Harvey SC, Fishman RL, Edwards SM. Retrograde intubation through a laryngeal mask airway. Anesthesiology 1996;85(6):1503–4.
[43] Hung OR, Pytka S, Morris I, et al. Clinical trial of a new lightwand device (Trachlight) to intubate the trachea. Anesthesiology 1995;83(3):509–14.
[44] Hung OR, Pytka S, Morris I, et al. Lightwand intubation: II–clinical trial of a new lightwand for tracheal intubation in patients with difficult airways. Can J Anaesth 1995;42(9):826–30.
[45] Mehta S. Transtracheal illumination for optimal tracheal tube placement. A clinical study. Anaesthesia 1989;44(12):970–2.
[46] Rudolph C, Schlender M. [Clinical experiences with fiberoptic intubation with the Bonfils intubation fiberscope]. Anaesthesiol Reanim 1996;21:127–30 [in German].
[47] Shikani AH. New "seeing" stylet-scope and method for the management of the difficult airway. Otolaryngol Head Neck Surg 1999;120(1):113–6.
[48] Agro F, Cataldo R, Carassiti M, et al. The seeing stylet: a new device for tracheal intubation. Resuscitation 2000;44(3):177–80.
[49] Evans A, Morris S, Petterson J, et al. A comparison of the Seeing Optical Stylet and the gum elastic bougie in simulated difficult tracheal intubation: a manikin study. Anaesthesia 2006; 61(5):478–81.
[50] Ezri T, Szmuk P, Warters RD, et al. Difficult airway management practice patterns among anesthesiologists practicing in the United States: have we made any progress? J Clin Anesth 2003;15:418–22.
[51] Afilalo M, Guttman A, Stern E, et al. Fiberoptic intubation in the emergency department: a case series. J Emerg Med 1993;11(4):387–9.
[52] Delaney KA, Hessler R. Emergency flexible fiberoptic nasotracheal intubation: a report of 60 cases. Ann Emerg Med 1988;17(9):919–26.
[53] Mlinek EJ Jr, Clinton JE, Plummer D, et al. Fiberoptic intubation in the emergency department. Ann Emerg Med 1990;19(4):359–62.
[54] Borland LM, Casselbrant M. The Bullard laryngoscope. A new indirect oral laryngoscope (pediatric version). Anesth Analg 1990;70(1):105–8.
[55] Liem EB, Bjoraker DG, Gravenstein D. New options for airway management: intubating fibreoptic stylets. Br J Anaesth 2003;91(3):408–18.
[56] Sprung J, Weingarten T, Dilger J. The use of WuScope fiberoptic laryngoscopy for tracheal intubation in complex clinical situations. Anesthesiology 2003;98(1):263–5.
[57] Cohn AI, McGraw SR, King WH. Awake intubation of the adult trachea using the Bullard laryngoscope. Can J Anaesth 1995;42(3):246–8.

[58] Shulman GB, Connelly NR. A comparison of the Bullard Laryngoscope versus the flexible fiberoptic broncho scope during intubation in patients afforded inline stabilization. J Clin Anesth 2001;13(3):182–5.

[59] Lim TJ, Lim Y, Liu EH. Evaluation of ease of intubation with the GlideScope or Macintosh laryngoscope by anaesthetists in simulated easy and difficult laryngoscopy. Anaesthesia 2005;60(2):180–3.

[60] Cooper RM, Pacey JA, Bishop MJ, et al. Early clinical experience with a new videolaryngoscope (GlideScope) in 728 patients. Can J Anaesth 2005;52(2):191–8.

[61] Cooper RM. Complications associated with the use of the GlideScope videolaryngoscope. Can J Anaesth 2007;54(1):54–7.

[62] Lai HY, Chen IH, Chen A, et al. The use of the GlideScope for tracheal intubation in patients with ankylosing spondylitis. Br J Anaesth 2006;97(3):419–22.

[63] Brofeldt BT, Panacek EA, Richards JR. An easy cricothyrotomy approach: the rapid four-step technique. Acad Emerg Med 1996;3:1060–3.

[64] Bair AE, Panacek EA, Wisner DH, et al. Cricothyrotomy: a 5-year experience at one institution. J Emerg Med 2003;24(2):151–6.

[65] Erlandson MJ, Clinton JE, Ruiz E, et al. Cricothyrotomy in the emergency department revisited. J Emerg Med 1989;7:115–8.

[66] Holmes JF, Panacek EA, Sakles JC, et al. Comparison of 2 cricothyrotomy techniques: standard method versus rapid 4-step technique. Ann Emerg Med 1998;32(4):442–6.

[67] Schaumann N, Lorenz V, Schellongowski P, et al. Evaluation of Seldinger technique emergency cricothyroidotomy versus standard surgical cricothyroidotomy in 200 cadavers. Anesthesiology 2005;102:7–11.

[68] Abbrecht PH, Kyle RR, Reams WH, et al. Insertion forces and risk of complications during cricothyroid cannulation. J Emerg Med 1992;10:417–26.

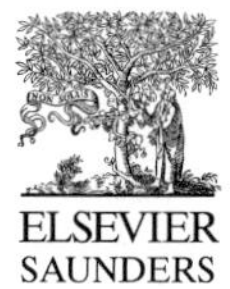

ELSEVIER
SAUNDERS

Emerg Med Clin N Am 25 (2007) 623–642

EMERGENCY
MEDICINE
CLINICS OF
NORTH AMERICA

Identification and Resuscitation of the Trauma Patient in Shock

Michael N. Cocchi, MD[a], Edward Kimlin, MD[a], Mark Walsh, MD[b], Michael W. Donnino, MD[c,d,e,*]

[a]*Department of Emergency Medicine, Harvard Affiliated Emergency Medicine Residency, Beth Israel Deaconess Medical Center, One Deaconess Road, West Campus Clinical Center, 2nd Floor, Boston, MA 02215, USA*

[b]*Indiana University School of Medicine—South Bend, South Bend, IN, USA*

[c]*Harvard School of Medicine, Boston, MA, USA*

[d]*Department of Emergency Medicine, Beth Israel Deaconess Medical Center, One Deaconess Road, West Clinical Center 2, Boston, MA 02215, USA*

[e]*Department of Medicine, Division of Pulmonary Critical Care, Beth Israel Deaconess Medical Center, Boston, MA, USA*

Trauma is a major source of morbidity and mortality in the United States and world-wide. When analyzed from a global perspective, the World Health Organization estimates that over 5 million people died of traumatic injury in the year 2000, accounting for 9% of global mortality and 12% of the global disease burden [1]. In the United States, traumatic injury is the fifth most frequent cause of death, with roughly 10% of the population suffering from some type of traumatic injury in any given year [2]. Although trauma impacts all age groups, it has an especially significant impact on the younger patient demographic, with roughly 50% of those who die being between 15 and 44 years of age [3].

Regardless of the mechanism of injury, hemorrhage is a leading cause of death following trauma [4–7]. Injury-induced hemorrhage accounts for the largest proportion of mortality within the first hour of trauma center care, causes 50% of injury-associated death within the first 24 hours of trauma care, and claims more lives than any other injury-induced pathology within the first 48 hours of care [7,8]. Moreover, hemorrhage-induced hypotension in trauma patients is predictive of greater than 50% mortality. Unlike more

* Corresponding author. Department of Emergency Medicine, Beth Israel Deaconess Medical Center, One Deaconess Road, West Clinical Center 2, Boston, MA 02215.

E-mail address: mdonnino@bidmc.harvard.edu (M.W. Donnino).

doi:10.1016/j.emc.2007.06.001 *emed.theclinics.com*

insidious processes, traumatic hemorrhagic shock kills quickly, with the bulk of its victims succumbing within the first few hours of emergency department arrival [9]. Though hemorrhage remains the most common etiology of trauma-related shock, other forms of shock such as obstructive, cardiogenic, or neurogenic may occur and need to be considered as well.

This article focuses on rapid diagnosis and treatment of the patient suffering from trauma-related shock, including early identification of patients at risk for occult hypoperfusion. Resuscitation strategies (delayed resuscitation, damage control resuscitation), end points of resuscitation, and the role of blood products and pro-coagulants for resuscitation are discussed.

Early identification of shock

One of the most crucial elements in determining the etiology of shock is to first recognize its presence. Overt hypotension clearly identifies the shocked patient; however, not all patients in shock initially exhibit hypotension. Shock is defined most simply as inadequate tissue perfusion. Particularly in the early stages of disease, determination of tissue hypoperfusion is oftentimes challenging, as the body will immediately engage in compensatory mechanisms designed to prevent cardiovascular collapse. For the clinician, recognizing this compensatory phase of shock is essential to early diagnosis and management (Table 1).

Most commonly, the etiology of shock in trauma is related to hypovolemia caused by uncontrolled hemorrhage. The Advanced Trauma Life Support guidelines illustrate the progressive phases in the development of shock by dividing degrees of hemorrhage into four classes. These classes have been essentially derived from expert opinion and do not necessarily apply to each individual, as physiology varies; however, the insidious progression from class I to class IV hemorrhagic shock is illustrated in Table 2.

Hypotension upon presentation represents decompensated shock and carries little ambiguity as to the perfusion status of the trauma patient. The mortality in patients with hemorrhagic shock presenting with hypotension exceeds 50% overall [9], and this figure is even higher in the elderly patient [10,11]. The definition of initial hypotension has arbitrarily been defined as below a systolic pressure of 90 mm Hg; however, recent investigators have challenged this parameter, reporting that a more appropriate cut point may be a systolic pressure of less than 109 mm Hg on initial presentation. Investigators based this potentially new cut point on data indicating that patients whose presentation systolic blood pressure (SBP) ranges from 91 mm Hg to 109 mm Hg have an increased mortality, compared with their counterparts with systolic pressures greater than 109 mm Hg [12]. The retrospective nature of this study renders this data preliminary at best, but serves as a careful reminder of the arbitrary nature of the 90 mm Hg cut point. Heart rate is a more sensitive indicator of inadequate

Table 1
Indicators of hypoperfusion in the trauma patient

Monitoring method	Indicators of hypoperfusion
Physical examination	• Cool, clammy skin • Change in mental status (anxiety, confusion, lethargy, obtundation, coma) • Decreased urine output • Prolonged capillary refill
Vital signs	• May be normal initially • Tachycardia, bradycardia • Hypotension • Tachypnea • Hypothermia • Shock index (heart rate/systolic blood pressure) > 0.9
Metabolic markers	• Metabolic acidosis • Increased lactate • Increased base deficit

perfusion than hypotension; however, this variable can also be deceptive at times. In a study by Victorino and colleagues [13], upwards of 35% of trauma patients with hypotension did not display tachycardia. Trauma patients without hypovolemia may display tachycardia because of fear and

Table 2
Classes of hemorrhage

Signs monitored on initial presentation[a]	Class I	Class II	Class III	Class IV
Blood loss (mL)	Up to 750	750–1500	1500–2000	>2000
Blood loss (% blood volume)	Up to 15%	15%–30%	30%–40%	>40%
Pulse rate	<100	>100	>120	>140
Blood pressure	Normal	Normal	Decreased	Decreased
Pulse pressure (mm Hg)	Normal or increased	Decreased	Decreased	Decreased
Respiratory rate	14–20	20–30	30–40	>35
Urine output (mL/hr)	>30	20–30	5–15	Negligible
CNS/Mental status	Slightly anxious	Mildly anxious	Anxious, confused	Confused, lethargic
Fluid replacement (3:1 rule)	Crystalloid	Crystalloid	Crystalloid and blood	Crystalloid and blood

The guidelines in Table 2 are based on the 3-for-1 rule. This rule derives from the empiric observation that most patients in hemorrhagic shock require as much as 300 mL of electrolyte solution for each 100 mL of blood loss. Applied blindly, these guidelines can result in excessive or inadequate fluid administration. For example, a patient with a crush injury to the extremity may have hypotension out of proportion to his or her blood loss and require fluids in excess of the 3:1 guidelines. In contrast, a patient whose ongoing blood loss is being replaced by blood transfusion requires less than 3:1. The use of bolus therapy with careful monitoring of the patient's response can moderate these extremes.

[a] For a 70-kg man.

From American College of Surgeons Committee on Trauma. Advanced trauma life support for doctors. 7th edition. Chicago (IL): American College of Surgeons; 2004; with permission.

pain, whereas those with hypovolemia may display "relative bradycardia" from paradoxically increased parasympathetic tone, age extreme, or medications (ie, beta blockers) [13,14].

The term "shock index" refers to the ratio of heart rate to SBP, and this variable may help identify hypoperfused patients with more subtle vital sign abnormalities. A shock index of greater than 0.9 has been found to be more sensitive than traditional vital sign analysis in identifying disease severity in a heterogeneous group of patients presenting to the emergency department [15]; however, a large retrospective study was unable to demonstrate an advantage of shock index over traditional vital sign analysis in trauma patients [16]. Prospective study of this variable in trauma patients is needed to determine if there is a role for this index beyond simple vital sign analysis. While the presence of vital sign abnormalities may indicate shock, the absence of these abnormalities does not completely exclude occult hypoperfusion in the traumatic patient [17].

Occult hypoperfusion

Occult hypoperfusion (inadequate organ and tissue perfusion in the presence of normal or relatively normal vital signs) can be identified through a careful physical examination plus an evaluation of metabolic markers of tissue hypoperfusion (see Table 1) [17]. Patients should be examined for physical manifestations of poor perfusion, such as cool and clammy skin, mental status changes, and decreased urine output. Metabolic markers of hypoperfusion include bicarbonate, base deficit, and lactic acidosis. With inadequate perfusion, cells will begin anaerobic metabolism and generate lactic acid as well as other acidic by-products. Several investigators have recently described the existence of occult hypoperfusion in the trauma patient. Brown and colleagues [14] studied 139 patients with penetrating abdominal trauma who had normal hemodynamics upon presentation and were taken to the operating room for laparatomy. Of the 139 patients studied, 82% (114) had less than 750 mL^3 of free intraperitoneal blood, 11% (15) had 750 to 1500 mL^3, and 7% (10) had more than 1500 mL^3 at laparotomy. Thus, despite seemingly reassuring vital signs, a number of these patients had a significant amount of intra-abdominal hemorrhage.

Parks and colleagues [18] recently further validated the clinically accepted concept that hypotension is a late sign of shock. In this study, researchers analyzed data from the National Trauma Data Bank and found that tissue hypoperfusion preceded overt hypotension in the majority of patients. Among the subjects reviewed, "mean and median systolic blood pressure did not decrease to less than 90 mm Hg until the base deficit was worse than −20, with mortality reaching 65%." These findings illustrate that significant pathology and hypoperfusion can be present in the normotensive patient, and that tissue hypoperfusion precedes hypotension in many patients. Occult hypoperfusion may be particularly concerning in the elderly as well, as Callaway and colleagues [19] report a mortality of 38% in normotensive elderly trauma patients with initial lactic acid levels of >4 mmol/dL. Thus, the use of lactic acid and base deficit can serve as metabolic markers of tissue hypoperfusion and should serve as adjuncts to a careful history and physical examination. Once shock is identified, either by overt vital sign abnormalities or through more subtle signs of tissue hypoperfusion, a search for the etiology and immediate measures to reverse hypoperfusion should begin.

Differential diagnosis of shock

Given that shock in the traumatically injured patient is generally a result of hypovolemia due to hemorrhage, the major focus of this article is on identifying and managing that entity; however, other possible etiologies can exist and need to be immediately considered (Box 1). The nonhemorrhagic causes of shock include obstructive, cardiogenic, distributive, and neurogenic. Differentiation of shock begins with the basic history and physical examination and can be supplemented with additional modalities, such as the bedside ultrasound, diagnostic peritoneal lavage, computed tomography, and explorative laparotomy.

Obstructive shock

Causes of trauma-induced obstructive shock include cardiac tamponade and tension pneumothorax. Chest trauma may cause cardiac tamponade or

Box 1. Differential diagnosis for trauma-related shock

- Obstructive shock
  - Cardiac tamponade,
  - Tension pneumothorax
  - Pulmonary thromboembolism[a]
- Cardiogenic shock
  - Cardiac contusion
  - Acute coronary syndrome[a]
- Distributive shock
  - Sepsis[b]
  - Adrenal insufficiency[b]
- Hypovolemic shock
  - Hemorrhage
- Neurogenic shock
  - Spinal cord injury

[a] Unlikely in acute trauma unless a precipitant to the trauma.
[b] Not observed in early trauma.

tension pneumothorax. Cardiac tamponade caused by penetrating or blunt injury may present with Beck's triad of hypotension, neck vein distention, and diminished heart tones [20]. However, the triad is often difficult to interpret in the trauma patient because hypovolemia may mask neck vein distention [21]. Furthermore, muffled heart tones are difficult to determine in the often noisy emergency department setting. Cardiac echocardiography has rapidly become an important modality for early and accurate diagnosis of tamponade. When available in the resuscitation room, echocardiography can reveal fluid in the pericardial sac and allow for rapid diagnosis and treatment [22,23]. In the setting of cardiac tamponade, collapse of the right atrium typically can be seen and aid in diagnosis. Note that the sensitivity of echocardiography is reduced in the presence of bilateral hemothoraces, a potential result of significant thoracic trauma [24]. Tension pneumothorax classically presents with diminished breath sounds on the side of the pnemothorax, hyperressonance to percussion, and tracheal deviation in the nonintubated patient. In the clinical setting, these classic findings can sometimes be deceiving, and clinical judgment and high clinical suspicion should ultimately guide the decision to immediately perform needle decompression and chest thoracostomy. When the patient is unstable, immediate needle decompression should be performed followed by chest tube thoracostomy. These interventions should be performed before radiologic confirmation, as a tension pneumothorax is a time-dependent, life-threatening lesion.

Cardiogenic shock

Cardiogenic shock would be a rare finding in the trauma patient but could occur from a significant cardiac contusion, a myocardial infarction resulting from the stress of the traumatic injury, or from myocardial ischemia as the inciting event leading to the trauma. Cardiac contusion, often referred to as blunt cardiac injury (BCI), is unlikely to occur as an isolated entity and is most often associated with other coaxial injuries [25]. While there are no established diagnostic criteria for BCI, clinicians concerned about this entity in patients with direct trauma to the chest should obtain a 12-lead electrocardiogram (ECG) upon arrival in the emergency department; echocardiography may be considered depending on the clinical scenario and hemodynamic status of the patient [21]. Several studies have examined the role of ECG and cardiac serum biomarkers (creatine phosphokinase-MB isoenzyme, troponin I) in the evaluation and disposition of patients with BCI. Wisner and colleagues [26] retrospectively reviewed data on 2252 blunt trauma patients admitted to their hospital and found that no patients who were hemodynamically stable on admission with a normal ECG had clinically significant complications. A meta-analysis of retrospective and prospective studies on BCI found that an abnormal ECG, and abnormal CK-MB isoenzymes, correlated with intervention-requiring complications, while patients with a normal ECG and CPK-MB levels did not develop clinically significant complications. In the prospective trials, 58 out of 2210 patients (2.6%) developed complications, while in the retrospective studies 112 out of 2471 patients (4.5%) developed complications related to BCI; the majority of complications were related to arrhythmias (76% and 77%, respectively) [27]. More recent studies in the trauma literature have addressed the value of cardiac troponin and have generally concluded that a normal ECG and normal troponin are reassuring for ruling out significant BCI [28–30]. However, the issues of length of telemetry monitoring and whether serial cardiac biomarkers need to be obtained and trended over time remain controversial.

In theory, the stress of a traumatic injury could result in myocardial infarction with resultant cardiogenic shock, though this would be very rare. Echocardiography, ECG, and cardiac enzymes would help in defining this particular entity. Finally, myocardial infarction may have lead to the traumatic injury and is and thus mislead the clinician. Shock out of proportion to the mechanism of injury or physical exam findings should raise suspicion for this etiology and is addressed specifically in a subsequent section, "Clinical mimicry of trauma-induced shock."

Treatment of cardiogenic shock from cardiac contusion is with intravenous fluids and inotropes, as needed. Some patients may require interventions, such as a cardiac balloon pump [31–33]. Early consultation with a cardiologist should be considered. Cardiogenic shock from an etiology such as a primary myocardial lesion is difficult to treat in the presence of traumatic injury, because modalities such as anticoagulation cannot be employed.

Neurogenic shock

Neurogenic shock is caused by an insult to the spinal cord, often at the cervical or high thoracic level, resulting in a loss of sympathetic tone and creating a state of peripheral dilatation with subsequent hypotension. Typically, bradycardia rather than tachycardia accompanies the hypotension. Even in cases with suspected spinal trauma, it is critical to exclude hemorrhagic or obstructive causes of shock, as these are more common and require immediate intervention. Treatment of neurogenic shock includes hemodynamic support with intravenous fluids as well as atropine, vasopressors, or inotropes as needed. The use of high-dose corticosteroids in this condition remains controversial and is beyond the scope of this article.

Clinical mimicry of trauma-induced shock

While the vast majority of trauma patients presenting with shock have an etiology related to the immediate trauma, a minority of patients may develop shock from another cause with resultant trauma. Clinicians should consider a nontraumatic etiology of shock when the physical examination and the mechanism of injury do not correlate with the presence of shock. For example, a patient in shock who was involved a single car crash without significant damage to the vehicle or significant bodily injury, should raise suspicion for a competing etiology. A 12-lead ECG or computed angiography of the chest may surprisingly reveal that the patient in a motor vehicle crash who loses consciousness has an acute myocardial infarction or a pulmonary embolism. Endocrinologic emergencies, such as diabetic ketoacidosis and myxedema coma, can result in trauma or actually be precipitated by trauma [34]. Rarely, anaphylactic shock caused by drug and latex allergy could develop in the resuscitation bay by unsuspected iatrogenic mechanisms [35,36]. While these scenarios remain rare, consideration should be given when the shock state is not consistent with the severity of trauma or the identification of traumatic injury.

Management of hemorrhagic shock

Sequential assessment of the airway, breathing, and circulation should rapidly identify nonhemorrhagic causes of shock requiring immediate intervention, such as tension pneumothorax or cardiac tamponade. Persistent hypotension or hypoperfusion from hemorrhagic shock requires simultaneous resuscitation and a definitive strategy to obtain hemostasis. The following sections will focus upon identifying the source of hemorrhage, resuscitation strategies, end points of resuscitation, and adjunctive measures for resuscitation and achieving hemostasis (blood products and procoagulants) for patients with hemorrhagic shock.

Identifying the source of hemorrhage

While in many cases the etiology of hemorrhage is easily identifiable, such as a penetrating gunshot to the abdomen, the origin of hemorrhage may be unknown. The focused assessment with sonography for trauma (FAST) examination can rapidly identify free fluid in the abdominal cavity indicative of hemorrhage. Fluid, or blood, can be visualized using four main windows: perihepatic, perisplenic, suprapubic, and pericardial. Sensitivity and specificity may depend on experience of the operator and amount of free fluid present, but generally fall in the range of 87% to 100% for nonradiologists (generally emergency medicine physicians and surgeons) evaluating blunt thoracoabdominal trauma patients [37–39]. Moreover, nonradiologists have been found to have equivalent accuracy to radiologists in evaluation of the FAST examination [40]. However, despite well-trained operators, small amounts of blood may not be detected by FAST; Branney and colleagues [41] prospectively determined that only 10% of observers were able to detect intraperitoneal fluid (infused by diagnostic peritoneal lavage) with fluid volumes of less than 400 mL.

For some patients, the source of hemorrhage will remain unclear after history, physical examination, and FAST examination. In those who are hemodynamically stable, computed tomography of the chest and abdomen can identify the source of bleeding. For the unstable patient, immediate transfer to the operating room for control of hemorrhage should be considered. Hemorrhage from the thoracic cavity or from within the peritoneum can be controlled with laparotomy; however, consideration should be given to other sources of occult hemorrhage before transport to the operating room. Specifically, a pelvic fracture with retroperitoneal hemorrhage can be the source of life-threatening hemorrhage and shock. The definitive therapy, in that case, may be angiography and embolization rather than operative intervention. A diagnostic peritoneal lavage (DPL) can be performed in the resuscitation room to determine whether or not intraperitoneal hemorrhage is present. With the advent of the FAST examination, the use of the DPL has decreased because intraperitoneal fluid is most often determined with ultrasound. However, DPL can be useful in the event that the FAST is negative or indeterminate, and the origin of hemorrhage remains unclear. In circumstances when pelvic or retroperitoneal hemorrhage is not suspected and the source of blood loss is from either the chest or abdomen, a DPL can be performed in the operating room before determining the choice of first incision (chest versus abdomen).

Resuscitation strategies

The guiding principle in management of shock is to restore tissue perfusion and control the source of the insult. Hemorrhagic shock poses the particular challenge of balancing the timing and kind of resuscitation in relation to the achievement of hemostasis. The traditional strategy of early resuscitation beginning in the field and continuing into the operating room has recently been challenged, specifically in penetrating trauma. A prospective trial by Bickell and colleagues [4] compared immediate versus delayed fluid resuscitation in hypotensive patients with penetrating torso injuries. The investigators reported that patients in whom fluids were restricted until arrival in the operating room had lower mortality, fewer postoperative complications, and shorter hospital length of stay. The proposed mechanism for the reported improved outcomes in the delayed resuscitation group stems from the concept that under-resuscitation allows for blood coagulation followed by "auto-resuscitation," such that blood pressure is restored. In a follow-up study, Dutton and colleagues [42] performed a prospective trial to compare resuscitation strategies and divided patients into either restrictive resuscitation (goal SBP greater than 80 mm Hg) versus liberal resuscitation (goal SBP greater than 100 mm Hg). They did not find any difference in mortality between groups but did find that hemorrhage took longer to control in the group with the liberal fluid strategy.

The overall strategy of delayed resuscitation remains controversial and the original Bickell study had several limitations. First, in the delayed group Bickell and colleagues [4] note that the initial systolic pressures were 59 mm Hg in the field, yet improved to 113 mm Hg in the preoperative setting. The increase in overall pressure in the group reflects several issues, including the fact that patients may have been hypotensive from tension pneumothorax or cardiac tamponade, rather than hypovolemia from on-going hemorrhagic shock. Once reversed, high-volume resuscitation was not necessary. Study investigators conceded that many of the patients examined were not in hemorrhagic shock, and they used the term "post-trauma hypotension" rather than hemorrhagic shock to describe them. In addition, in explaining the phenomena of increased blood pressure between the field and preoperative setting, study investigators noted that this group included "some with severe hypotension, who had died by this time." Perhaps this subgroup is the most concerning: could early resuscitation in these profoundly hypotensive patients have supported perfusion and allowed for the possibility of survival? Bickell and colleagues also report that a number of patients received fluid in the delayed resuscitation group (8%), though the remainder reportedly only received antibiotics and intravenous contrast. The 8% protocol violations, though small, raise the potential for bias and provision of fluid to those who may have truly needed it. Finally, the study was performed at a single center, focused on penetrating torso trauma only, and has yet to be reproduced. Despite the shortcomings, there may be some important concepts that can be derived from the Bickell study. Prior to achievement of hemostasis, high-volume resuscitation in the presence of relatively normal blood pressure could potentially be detrimental, and treatment of occult hypoperfusion may be more appropriate after hemostasis is obtained. However, recognition and identification of occult hypoperfusion is still essential and early operative intervention for on-going hemorrhage remains paramount.

In seeming contrast to Bickell's work, recent publications have reported on the concept of damage control resuscitation [43]. Damage control resuscitation refers to early field and emergency department high-volume resuscitation, predominately with blood and procoagulant blood products (ie, plasma, platelets, cryoprecipitate) rather than crystalloid. The concept of damage control resuscitation emerged from surgeons in the battlefields in Iraq and Afghanistan and reflects a strategy employed for the most profoundly wounded patients, such as those with anticipated massive transfusions. On the battlefield, approximately 7% of traumatically injured patients will require massive transfusion, in contrast to 1% in the civilian population. The focus of damage control resuscitation is to provide blood products and procoagulants rather than crystalloid to resuscitate the patient, as well as prevent the dilutional effects of crystalloid on coagulation and core temperature. The end points of resuscitation, proposed by the proponents of this approach, consist of metabolic goals (relief of lactic acidosis, normalization of base excess) in addition to such traditional goals as urine output and blood pressure normalization. A standard order set for damage control resuscitation consists of 6 units of packed red cells, 6 units of fresh frozen plasma, 12 units of platelets, and 10 units of cryoprecipitate to be infused as a pre-emptive modality during early resuscitation. Though surgeons in the field report better efficacy with this approach, little data has yet to be published, but promises to be forthcoming.

Combining the concepts of delayed resuscitation, damage control resuscitation, and traditional advanced trauma life support resuscitation strategies may be seemingly difficult, yet invoking the concept of therapy tailored to the individual may help guide clinical management. In hemorrhagic shock, the profoundly injured and profoundly hypotensive patient would seemingly not do well with a delayed resuscitation strategy. For this population, invoking a damage control resuscitation strategy, consisting of a high volume of blood products, in addition to emergent operative control may be life saving. For the less severely ill, such as those with occult hypoperfusion or transient hypotension, high-volume resuscitation before achievement of hemostasis may not be warranted. Definitive control of hemorrhage should be obtained immediately. After hemostasis is obtained, adequate resuscitation guided by the end points of resuscitation can be achieved. For those in the in-between category, the exact resuscitation strategy remains unclear; however, the authors would favor providing the necessary volume resuscitation to maintain adequate pressures to allow for safe delivery of the patient to the operating room. Again, after achievement of hemostasis, resuscitation strategies can continue based on the end points of resuscitation discussed in the next section.

The choice of fluid for initial resuscitation has also been the focus of much debate. The concept of damage control resuscitation mitigates the use of crystalloid in favor of blood products, stating that plasma may be the ultimate resuscitation fluid providing both volume and procoagulant properties. Crystalloid may rapidly and temporarily restore pressure and perfusion, but is limited by the dilutional effect and the inability of crystalloid to remain in the intravascular space. Differences between lactated ringers and normal saline are minimal and probably not clinically significant, particularly in the early resuscitation period. Compared to normal saline, lactated ringers are slightly hypotonic and could theoretically result in less capacity to remain intravascular. Conversely, normal saline contains 154 milliequivalents of chloride, and infusion of high quantities may result in a hyperchloremic, metabolic acidosis. The clinical significance of this induced acidosis remains unknown. Hypertonic solutions, such as hetastarch and albumin, have also been used and studied. The debate between crystalloid and colloids is extensive and a comprehensive review is beyond the scope of this article. However, there has yet to be a study to show an advantage of hypertonic or colloid solutions over crystalloid resuscitation.

A recent randomized, controlled trial with albumin in a heterogenous population failed to show any advantage over crystalloid [44]. Moreover, hetastarch may result in coagulopathy and renal damage, thus raising the possibility of harm for the patient in hemorrhagic shock. Thus, no clear advantage exists in the usage of hypertonic or colloid solutions as compared with crystalloid. Blood products and procoagulant colloids may serve as ideal fluid for those with severe hemorrhage, with the advantage of reversing coagulopathy, restoring hemoglobin, and avoiding dilutional coagulopathy. However, in patients with less severe hemorrhage, exposure to blood products may result in potentially unwanted effects on the immune system and risk for associated lung injury. Again, a proper assessment and balance based on the degree of shock and illness of the individual patient is required.

End points of resuscitation

The goal of resuscitation is to restore and maintain adequate tissue perfusion; however, determining when perfusion has been restored may be difficult. As discussed in the previous section, the exact timing for aggressive resuscitation and achievement of end points of resuscitation remains controversial and should be considered for each individual. The following section will discuss the various indicators or end points of resuscitation without regard to timing. Perhaps one of the most important distinctions that needs to be made by the clinician is the difference between perfusion and pressure. Oftentimes, pressure variables are used as surrogates for perfusion; however, this strategy can sometimes lead to erroneous assessment of adequate perfusion. Examples of pressure variables include blood pressure, central venous pressure, and pulmonary capillary wedge pressure. There is no perfect measurement of perfusion; however, indicators of perfusion include metabolic parameters (bicarbonate, base deficit, lactic acidosis), physical exam findings (cool, clammy skin), and urine output (reflecting low flow to the kidneys). Each of these end points of resuscitation has both advantages and limitations, and perhaps the best approach is to take all factors into account at the bedside of the individual patient.

Heart rate and blood pressure

As discussed in the section on identification of shock, overt vital sign abnormalities are the frontline in determination of the perfusion status of the trauma patient. Likewise, the restoration of blood pressure and heart rate to normal values serves as an important end point of resuscitation. However, as noted earlier, the normality or relative normality of vital signs does not necessarily equate to normal perfusion. Therefore, volume replacement should aim to restore blood pressure and pulse rate; after these ends have been achieved the clinician needs to evaluate the patient for any other indicators of ongoing tissue hypoperfusion.

Central venous pressure

Central venous pressure monitoring as a guide to resuscitation has been suggested in certain circumstances and is discussed in the current Advanced Trauma Life Support guidelines. However, use of this variable, particularly in the early resuscitation phase of the patient with hemorrhagic shock, may be fraught with pitfalls. Again, the following discussion assumes hemorrhagic shock and not other etiologies. If an accurately calibrated central venous pressure is initially very high, one would have to immediately consider such entities as pericardial tamponade or tension pneumothorax, conditions which should hopefully be diagnosed without the use or need of central venous pressure measurements.

Central venous pressure represents a pressure and not a perfusion variable. As such, an adequate central venous pressure can be present with poor perfusion; conversely a low central venous pressure can be present in patients with normal perfusion. Understanding this basic concept is essential to use of this variable. The normal central venous pressure range is 0 mm Hg to 6 mm Hg. This means that a central venous pressure in the patient with traumatic shock should be low, and this would not be unexpected in either the well- or hypoperfused patient. In contrast, many conditions can increase central venous pressure regardless of underlying volume status or perfusion. For example, patients with chronic obstructive pulmonary disease may have very high baseline central venous pressures. Patients receiving positive pressure ventilation, particularly those requiring positive-end expiratory pressure, will have increased central venous pressures, as will patients requiring any form of vasopressor therapy. Moreover, acidosis may result in central vascular vasoconstriction despite hypovolemia [45]. Not surprisingly, oftentimes central venous pressure calibrations are inaccurate or erroneously calculated. In essence, central venous pressure is an indirect measure of volume affected by other causes of pressure elevation, including erroneous calculation. In the initial stages of hemorrhagic shock, this variable should be used with caution. With very rare exception, patients in the early stages of hemorrhagic shock with persistent hypotension or hypoperfusion should be provided with volume resuscitation, regardless of central venous pressures. In the later stages of shock or in shock of a mixed etiology, central venous pressure could be used to help guide management, however interpretation should be taken into the context of patient characteristics, other hemodynamic variables, and external physiologic factors.

Urine output

Urine output remains an important, noninvasive end point of resuscitation in the patient with shock, and typically a urine output of less than 0.5 mL per kilogram per hour is considered inadequate in the shock state. Decreased perfusion to the kidneys results in decreased urine output and provides an excellent measure of resuscitation. However, this end point is limited in the early stage of trauma, as the evaluation of urine output requires the tincture of time. Also, other causes of decreased urine output exist, such as underlying renal disease (ie, end-stage renal disease) or acute tubular necrosis. In unclear cases, diagnostic and clinical measures should be employed to distinguish whether oliguria is flow related (ie, prerenal) versus nonflow related; however, these are beyond the scope of the current article. Finally, in some cases, normal or high urine outputs (particularly in the initial time period) can occur in the face of inadequate perfusion. Therefore, urine output, like all end points of resuscitation, needs to be taken in context of the overall clinical picture and in conjunction with other measures of resuscitation.

Lactate clearance and base deficit

Lactic acidosis may indicate tissue hypoperfusion even when vital signs are initially normal or relatively normal. In addition to allowing for identification of shock or hypoperfusion, lactic acid levels can also provide an end point of resuscitation and indicator of restored perfusion. Effective lactate clearance has been found to be associated with lower mortality levels in trauma, sepsis, and postcardiac arrest [46–48]. Therefore, effective lactate clearance in the patient with traumatic shock signifies a more favorable overall outcome in the long-term, and provides an end point of resuscitation in the short-term. Like all of the end points discussed, lactate clearance has shortcomings. For unclear reasons, some patients with significant hypoperfusion do not mount a high lactate level. Conversely, some conditions are associated with elevated lactic acid levels without associated tissue hypoperfusion; examples of these conditions include seizure activity, severe respiratory distress (work of breathing), certain medications (ie, anti-retrovirals, metformin, linazolid, albuterol), thiamine deficiency, carbon monoxide or cyanide toxicity, and diabetic ketoacidosis.

In addition to lactate clearance, base deficit may provide yet another metabolic end point of resuscitation. Arterial base deficit represents the degree of metabolic acidosis, calculated as how many milliequivalents of base would need to be added to a liter of blood to normalize the pH. A retrospective analysis of prospectively collected data on 100 trauma patients by Kincaid and colleagues [49], revealed that patients with persistently elevated base deficit had higher rates of multiple organ failure and death when compared with those with a low base deficit. Davis and colleagues [50] found the base deficit calculated on admission for trauma patients was predictive of need for early transfusion of blood products, as well as increased complications, including adult respiratory distress syndrome and multisystem organ failure. The most significant shortcoming of base deficit is that other diseases and physiologic states may alter base deficit without reflecting an alteration of perfusion; several examples of this include renal failure, chronic obstructive pulmonary disease, or acidosis from any of a number of additional nonperfusion related causes.

Lactate and base deficit can be used both in the initial resuscitation period, as well as during the subsequent inpatient hospitalization. A recent study by Martin and colleagues [51] compared simultaneously measured serum lactate levels and arterial base deficit levels in 1298 patients in the surgical intensive care unit, 79% of which were trauma patients, and found that in approximately one third of the cases there was disagreement between the two measures. Additionally, lactate was more predictive of morbidity and mortality than was base deficit among their study population.

Lactic acidosis and base deficit arguably remain the best metabolic markers of tissue hypoperfusion that we can measure and follow. As with any other laboratory test, these variables must be interpreted and incorporated with the entire clinical context when managing critically ill trauma patients.

Achieving hemostasis

Perhaps the most important aspect of the management of hemorrhagic shock is to obtain hemostasis. Obtaining hemostasis can be definitively achieved by proper identification of the source of hemorrhage and an immediate measure to control it. Operative therapy is required for uncontrolled thoracic or intraperitoneal hemorrhage, whereas angiography and cauterization is typically employed for retroperitoneal bleeding from a pelvic source. While active resuscitation and a move toward definitive hemostasis is being made, consideration can be given to adjuncts of hemostasis and resuscitation, such as blood products and procoagulants.

Blood and blood products in traumatic shock

Since World War I, human blood products have been the gold standard in large volume resuscitation efforts. However, the reliance on human blood products is limited by several factors, including availability, relatively short shelf life, and potential to transmit disease. Moreover, packed red blood cell units contain scant amounts of platelets and coagulation factors, thereby contributing to the dilutional element of hemorrhage-related coagulopathy, particularly when dosed in the absence of procoagulation adjuncts. At present, human red cell alternatives have been unsuccessful in matching the efficacy of human red cells in the setting of massive volume replacement [52].

Despite these shortcomings, transfusion of packed red cells remains the gold standard in resuscitation of the actively hemorrhaging patient. Though controversy exists as to when transfusion should be undertaken, most would agree that transfusion should be provided in ongoing hemorrhage if hemodynamic instability persists after approximately 2 L of crystalloid infusion. Hypoperfusion in the absence of hypotension should be considered a possible indication for transfusion as well. Ultimately, bedside clinical judgment will determine the need for transfusion. In critically ill hemorrhaging patients, a very low threshold for transfusion should be maintained.

To mitigate coagulopathy and assist in hemostasis, additional blood components should be considered when providing large volume resuscitation, including fresh frozen plasma (FFP), platelets, and fibrinogen concentrate or cryoprecipitate [2,53,54]. Definitive evidence regarding the optimal timing, dose, and combination of these agents remains elusive. Gonzalez and colleagues [54] performed a retrospective study evaluating the timing of FFP administration, and found that the severity of coagulopathy in trauma patients upon admission to the intensive care unit is associated with decreased survival. Based on these findings, the investigators suggest earlier use of FFP and argue that more aggressive use of FFP could improve mortality and reduce total in-hospital transfusion requirements. However, outcome data is limited and systematic review of known studies in this area failed to show significant improvement in blood saving or promotion of hemostasis [55]. However, only one of these studies was focused specifically on trauma resuscitation.

In addition to FFP, replacement of individual coagulation factors, such as factor VIIa, have been studied and used in the setting of traumatic hemorrhage over the past decade. Interest in factor VIIa for hemorrhagic shock surged following a case report from Israel, where an exsanguinating soldier who sustained a penetrating inferior vena cava tear failed traditional hemostatic efforts, only to be stabilized by two doses of factor VIIa [56]. Evidence supporting the use of factor VIIa is relatively sparse but perhaps encouraging, with retrospective and small prospective studies suggesting mitigation of coagulopathy and perhaps improved outcome [57–60]. Despite evidence of potential efficacy, large randomized controlled trials have yet to be performed and the universal application of factor VIIa remains unknown [61–64]. Future prospective trials will hopefully help to identify the value of factor VIIa in the treatment of traumatic hemorrhage.

Another proposed method of reversing the coagulopathy of trauma is the use of antifibrinolytic agents, such as aprotinin and tranexamic acid (TXA). These drugs are lysine analogs, substituting for lysine in plasminogen and thereby promoting fibrinolysis [65]. Both of these compounds have proven to significantly reduce perioperative bleeding and intraoperative transfusion requirements in a variety of surgical settings [66,67]. However, data in traumatic hemorrhage is limited and insufficient to provide any recommendations either for or against the use of these adjuncts [68]. A randomized, controlled trial of TXA in hemorrhagic shock is currently underway [69].

At this time, transfusion of FFP, cryoprecipitate, and platelets remain the traditional adjuncts in minimizing the coagulopathy associated with hemorrhagic shock. The optimal dosages and timing of administration remains unknown; however, we would support early administration of products to minimize coagulopathy. Other adjuncts, such as factor VIIa and antifibrinolytics, continue to be studied as outcome data remains lacking for these therapies.

Summary

Management of the critically ill trauma patient requires rapid identification and differentiation of the patient in shock. Overt shock with accompanying hypotension is not difficult to identify, though occult hypoperfusion (normal pressure in the presence of tissue hypoperfusion) may be subtle. Most often, patients with shock following trauma are suffering from ongoing hemorrhage, though other etiologies may be present. The initial examination should rapidly reveal nonhemorrhagic causes of shock. Once the etiology of shock is identified, definitive therapy should be initiated. Achievement of hemostasis and restoration of tissue perfusion remain paramount for the treatment of hemorrhagic shock. The timing and kind of resuscitation of hemorrhagic shock may vary depending on the severity of injury and patient physiology, though delivery of a viable patient to the operating room is the primary goal of the emergency physician. Delayed resuscitation in penetrating torso trauma remains controversial, and the potential application of this approach is discussed in detail in the main portion of this article. Damage control resuscitation, consisting of high volume blood products and procoagulants, may be lifesaving for the profoundly injured and profoundly hypotensive patient. Once hemostasis is achieved, resuscitation aimed at specific end points should be used. Each end point of tissue perfusion has advantages and disadvantages, and the optimal resuscitation strategy should take all parameters into account in context of the individual patient. The rapid identification, differentiation, resuscitation, and achievement of hemostasis will ultimately lead to optimal outcome in the management of the patient with traumatic shock.

References

[1] Sauaia A, Moore FA, Moore EE, et al. Epidemiology of trauma deaths: a reassessment. J Trauma 1995;38(2):185–93.

[2] Spahn DR, Rossaint R. Coagulopathy and blood component transfusion in trauma. Br J Anaesth 2005;95(2):130–9.

[3] Gando S, Tedo I, Kubota M. Posttrauma coagulation and fibrinolysis. Crit Care Med 1992; 20(5):594–600.

[4] Bickell WH, Wall MJ Jr, Pepe PE, et al. Immediate versus delayed fluid resuscitation for hypotensive patients with penetrating torso injuries. N Engl J Med 1994;331(17):1105–9.

[5] Hardaway RM 3rd. The significance of coagulative and thrombotic changes after injury. J Trauma 1970;10(4):354–7.

[6] Miller RD, Robbins TO, Tong MJ, et al. Coagulation defects associated with massive blood transfusions. Ann Surg 1971;174(5):794–801.

[7] Kauvar DS, Lefering R, Wade CE. Impact of hemorrhage on trauma outcome: an overview of epidemiology, clinical presentations, and therapeutic considerations. J Trauma 2006; 60(6 Suppl):S3–11.

[8] Risberg B, Medegard A, Heideman M, et al. Early activation of humoral proteolytic systems in patients with multiple trauma. Crit Care Med 1986;14(11):917–25.

[9] Heckbert SR, Vedder NB, Hoffman W, et al. Outcome after hemorrhagic shock in trauma patients. J Trauma 1998;45(3):545–9.

[10] Knudson MM, Lieberman J, Morris JA Jr. Mortality factors in geriatric blunt trauma patients. Arch Surg 1994;129(4):448–53.
[11] Horst HM, Obeid FN, Sorensen VJ. Factors influencing survival of elderly trauma patients. Crit Care Med 1986;14(8):681–4.
[12] Edelman DA, White MT, Tyburski JG, et al. Post-traumatic hypotension: should systolic blood pressure of 90–109 mm Hg be included? Shock 2007;27(2):134–8.
[13] Victorino GP, Battistella FD, Wisner DH. Does tachycardia correlate with hypotension after trauma? J Am Coll Surg 2003;196(5):679–84.
[14] Brown CV, Velmahos GC, Neville AL, et al. Hemodynamically "stable" patients with peritonitis after penetrating abdominal trauma: identifying those who are bleeding. Arch Surg 2005;140(8):767–72.
[15] Rady MY, Smithline HA, Blake H, et al. A comparison of the shock index and conventional vital signs to identify acute, critical illness in the emergency department. Ann Emerg Med 1994;24(4):685–90.
[16] King RW, Plewa MC, Buderer NM, et al. Shock index as a marker for significant injury in trauma patients. Acad Emerg Med 1996;3(11):1041–5.
[17] Blow O, Magliore L, Claridge JA, et al. The golden hour and the silver day: detection and correction of occult hypoperfusion within 24 hours improves outcome from major trauma. J Trauma 1999;47(5):964–9.
[18] Parks JK, Elliott AC, Gentilello LM, et al. Systemic hypotension is a late marker of shock after trauma: a validation study of advanced trauma life support principles in a large national sample. Am J Surg 2006;192(6):727–31.
[19] Callaway D, Rosen C, Baker C, et al. Lactic acidosis predicts mortality in normotensive elderly patients with traumatic injury. Acad Emerg Med 2007;14(S152).
[20] Spodick DH. Acute cardiac tamponade. N Engl J Med 2003;349(7):684–90.
[21] Pretre R, Chilcott M. Blunt trauma to the heart and great vessels. N Engl J Med 1997;336(9):626–32.
[22] Ciccone TJ, Grossman SA. Cardiac ultrasound. Emerg Med Clin North Am 2004;22(3):621–40.
[23] Patel AN, Brennig C, Cotner J, et al. Successful diagnosis of penetrating cardiac injury using surgeon-performed sonography. Ann Thorac Surg 2003;76(6):2043–6 [discussion: 2046–7].
[24] Meredith JW, Hoth JJ. Thoracic trauma: when and how to intervene. Surg Clin North Am 2007;87(1):95–118, vii.
[25] Cachecho R, Grindlinger GA, Lee VW. The clinical significance of myocardial contusion. J Trauma 1992;33(1):68–71 [discussion: 71–3].
[26] Wisner DH, Reed WH, Riddick RS. Suspected myocardial contusion. Triage and indications for monitoring. Ann Surg 1990;212(1):82–6.
[27] Maenza RL, Seaberg D, D'Amico F. A meta-analysis of blunt cardiac trauma: ending myocardial confusion. Am J Emerg Med 1996;14(3):237–41.
[28] Salim A, Velmahos GC, Jindal A, et al. Clinically significant blunt cardiac trauma: role of serum troponin levels combined with electrocardiographic findings. J Trauma 2001;50(2):237–43.
[29] Velmahos GC, Karaiskakis M, Salim A, et al. Normal electrocardiography and serum troponin I levels preclude the presence of clinically significant blunt cardiac injury. J Trauma 2003;54(1):45–50 [discussion: 50–1].
[30] Collins JN, Cole FJ, Weireter LJ, et al. The usefulness of serum troponin levels in evaluating cardiac injury. Am Surg 2001;67(9):821–5 [discussion: 825–6].
[31] Demas C, Flancbaum L, Scott G, et al. The intra-aortic balloon pump as an adjunctive therapy for severe myocardial contusion. Am J Emerg Med 1987;5(6):499–502.
[32] Holanda MS, Dominguez MJ, Lopez-Espadas F, et al. Cardiac contusion following blunt chest trauma. Eur J Emerg Med 2006;13(6):373–6.

[33] Penney DJ, Bannon PG, Parr MJ. Intra-aortic balloon counterpulsation for cardiogenic shock due to cardiac contusion in an elderly trauma patient. Resuscitation 2002;55(3): 337–40.
[34] Wartofsky L. Myxedema coma. Endocrinol Metab Clin North Am 2006;35(4):687–98, vii–viii.
[35] Pryor JP, Vonfricken K, Seibel R, et al. Anaphylactic shock from a latex allergy in a patient with spinal trauma. J Trauma 2001;50(5):927–30.
[36] Stewart AG, Ewan PW. The incidence, aetiology and management of anaphylaxis presenting to an accident and emergency department. QJM 1996;89(11):859–64.
[37] Rothlin MA, Naf R, Amgwerd M, et al. Ultrasound in blunt abdominal and thoracic trauma. J Trauma 1993;34(4):488–95.
[38] Brooks A, Davies B, Smethhurst M, et al. Prospective evaluation of non-radiologist performed emergency abdominal ultrasound for haemoperitoneum. Emerg Med J 2004; 21(5):e5.
[39] Goletti O, Ghiselli G, Lippolis PV, et al. The role of ultrasonography in blunt abdominal trauma: results in 250 consecutive cases. J Trauma 1994;36(2):178–81.
[40] Buzzas GR, Kern SJ, Smith RS, et al. A comparison of sonographic examinations for trauma performed by surgeons and radiologists. J Trauma 1998;44(4):604–6 [discussion: 607–8].
[41] Branney SW, Wolfe RE, Moore EE, et al. Quantitative sensitivity of ultrasound in detecting free intraperitoneal fluid. J Trauma 1995;39(2):375–80.
[42] Dutton RP, Mackenzie CF, Scalea TM. Hypotensive resuscitation during active hemorrhage: impact on in-hospital mortality. J Trauma 2002;52(6):1141–6.
[43] Holcomb JB, Jenkins D, Rhee P, et al. Damage control resuscitation: directly addressing the early coagulopathy of trauma. J Trauma 2007;62(2):307–10.
[44] The SAFE Study investigators. A comparison of albumin and saline for fluid resuscitation in the intensive care unit. N Engl J Med 2004;350:2247–56.
[45] Pinto-Plata VM, Pozo-Parilli JC, Baum-Agay A, et al. Effect of blood pH on pulmonary artery pressure, left atrial pressure and fluid filtration rate in isolated rabbit lung. Rev Esp Fisiol 1995;51(3):117–23.
[46] Husain FA, Martin MJ, Mullenix PS, et al. Serum lactate and base deficit as predictors of mortality and morbidity. Am J Surg 2003;185(5):485–91.
[47] Abramson D, Scalea TM, Hitchcock R, et al. Lactate clearance and survival following injury. J Trauma 1993;35(4):584–8, [discussion: 588–9].
[48] Nguyen HB, Rivers EP, Knoblich BP, et al. Early lactate clearance is associated with improved outcome in severe sepsis and septic shock. Crit Care Med 2004;32(8):1637–42.
[49] Kincaid EH, Miller PR, Meredith JW, et al. Elevated arterial base deficit in trauma patients: a marker of impaired oxygen utilization. J Am Coll Surg 1998;187(4):384–92.
[50] Davis JW, Parks SN, Kaups KL, et al. Admission base deficit predicts transfusion requirements and risk of complications. J Trauma 1996;41(5):769–74.
[51] Martin MJ, FitzSullivan E, Salim A, et al. Discordance between lactate and base deficit in the surgical intensive care unit: which one do you trust? Am J Surg 2006;191(5):625–30.
[52] Heier HE, Bugge W, Hjelmeland K, et al. Transfusion vs. alternative treatment modalities in acute bleeding: a systematic review. Acta Anaesthesiol Scand 2006;50(8):920–31.
[53] MacLeod JB, Lynn M, McKenney MG, et al. Early coagulopathy predicts mortality in trauma. J Trauma 2003;55(1):39–44.
[54] Gonzalez EA, Moore FA, Holcomb JB, et al. Fresh frozen plasma should be given earlier to patients requiring massive transfusion. J Trauma 2007;62(1):112–9.
[55] Stanworth SJ, Brunskill SJ, Hyde CJ, et al. Is fresh frozen plasma clinically effective? A systematic review of randomized controlled trials. Br J Haematol 2004;126(1):139–52.
[56] Kenet G, Walden R, Eldad A, et al. Treatment of traumatic bleeding with recombinant factor VIIa. Lancet 1999;354(9193):1879.

[57] Geeraedts LM Jr, Kamphuisen PW, Kaasjager HA, et al. The role of recombinant factor VIIa in the treatment of life-threatening haemorrhage in blunt trauma. Injury 2005;36(4): 495–500.

[58] Dutton RP, McCunn M, Hyder M, et al. Factor VIIa for correction of traumatic coagulopathy. J Trauma 2004;57(4):709–18 [discussion: 718–9].

[59] Rizoli SB, Boffard KD, Riou B, et al. Recombinant activated factor VII as an adjunctive therapy for bleeding control in severe trauma patients with coagulopathy: subgroup analysis from two randomized trials. Crit Care 2006;10(6):R178.

[60] Rizoli SB, Nascimento B Jr, Osman F, et al. Recombinant activated coagulation factor VII and bleeding trauma patients. J Trauma 2006;61(6):1419–25.

[61] Vincent JL, Rossaint R, Riou B, et al. [Recommendations on the use of recombinant activated factor VII as an adjunctive treatment for massive bleeding. A European perspective]. Crit Care 2006;10(4):R120.

[62] Ganguly S, Spengel K, Tilzer LL, et al. Recombinant factor VIIa: unregulated continuous use in patients with bleeding and coagulopathy does not alter mortality and outcome. Clin Lab Haematol 2006;28(5):309–12.

[63] Vincent JL, Rossaint R, Riou B, et al. Recommendations on the use of recombinant activated factor VII as an adjunctive treatment for massive bleeding—a European perspective. Crit Care 2006;10(4):R120.

[64] Mohr AM, Holcomb JB, Dutton RP, et al. Recombinant activated factor VIIa and hemostasis in critical care: a focus on trauma. Crit Care 2005;9(Suppl 5):S37–42.

[65] Porte RJ, Leebeek FW. Pharmacological strategies to decrease transfusion requirements in patients undergoing surgery. Drugs 2002;62(15):2193–211.

[66] Gai MY, Wu LF, Su QF, et al. Clinical observation of blood loss reduced by tranexamic acid during and after caesarian section: a multi-center, randomized trial. Eur J Obstet Gynecol Reprod Biol 2004;112(2):154–7.

[67] Levi M, Cromheecke ME, de Jonge E, et al. Phrmacological strategies to decrease excessive blood loss in cardiac surgery: a meta-analysis of clinically relevant endpoints. Lancet 1999; 354(9194):1940–7.

[68] Coats T, Roberts I, Shakur H. Antifibrinolytic drugs for acute traumatic injury. Cochrane Database Syst Rev 2004;4:CD004896.

[69] Dyer O. Trial of drug for trauma patients includes victims of Iraqi violence. BMJ 2006; 332(7552):1234.

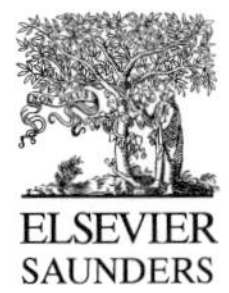

ELSEVIER
SAUNDERS

Emerg Med Clin N Am 25 (2007) 643–654

EMERGENCY
MEDICINE
CLINICS OF
NORTH AMERICA

Optimal Trauma Outcome: Trauma System Design and the Trauma Team

Vincent J. Markovchick, MD, FAAEM[a,b,*], Ernest E. Moore, MD, FACS[c,d]

[a] *Emergency Medical Services, Denver Health, 777 Bannock Street, MC 0108, Denver, CO 80204, USA*

[b] *Division of Emergency Medicine, Department of Surgery, University of Colorado Health Sciences Center, 777 Bannock Street, Denver, CO 80204, USA*

[c] *Surgery and Trauma Service, Denver Health, 777 Bannock Street, MC 0206, Denver, CO 80204, USA*

[d] *Department of Surgery, Denver Health, 777 Bannock Street, Denver, CO 80204, USA*

Trauma system design

Trauma is the number one killer of Americans under age 34, and optimal care of trauma patients is best provided when there is a well-functioning, comprehensive system of trauma care. Results of a recent poll indicate that 61% of the American public is unaware that injury is the leading cause of death for those ages 1 to 34. Only eight states currently have fully functioning trauma systems [1]. A recent meta-analysis of 14 published articles evaluating the impact of implementing trauma systems found a 15% reduction in mortality in favor of the presence of a trauma system [2]. Trauma system development in the United States has evolved over the past 35 years, and the organization taking the lead on trauma system development, review, and verification has been the American College of Surgeons Committee on Trauma (ACS/COT). The ACS/COT trauma center classification scheme has assisted communities in trauma system development [3]. The goal of a mature trauma system is to match the needs of the injured patients to the capabilities of the trauma receiving facility, thus maximizing the chances for the best possible outcome.

A national survey conducted in 2002 by the United States Department of Health Resources and Services Administration (HRSA) revealed that most

* Corresponding author. Emergency Medical Services, Denver Health, 777 Bannock Street, MC 0108, Denver, CO 80204.

E-mail address: vince.markovchick@dhha.org (V.J. Markovchick).

0733-8627/07/$ - see front matter
doi:10.1016/j.emc.2007.07.002

Table 1
State assessment of West criteria

State	Authority	Designation	Standards	Survey	Limit	Protocols	Monitor
Alabama	No	No	NA[a]	NA	NA	NA	NA
Alaska	Yes	Yes (1996)	Yes	Yes	No	No	Yes
Arizona	No	No	NA	NA	NA	NA	NA
Arkansas	Yes	Yes (2002)	Yes	Yes	No	No	Yes
California	Yes	Yes (1980)	Yes	Varies	Yes	Yes	Yes
Colorado	Yes	Yes (1998)	Yes	Yes	No	Yes	Yes
Connecticut	Yes	Yes (1995)	Yes	Yes	No	Yes	Yes
Delaware	Yes	Yes (1998)	Yes	Yes	No	Yes	Yes
Florida	Yes	Yes (1985)	Yes	Yes	No	Yes	No
Georgia	Yes	Yes (1981)	Yes	Yes	No	No	No
Hawaii	Yes	Yes (1995)	Yes	Yes	No	Yes	No
Idaho	No	No	NA	NA	NA	NA	NA
Illinois	Yes	Yes (1988)	Yes	Yes	Yes	Yes	Yes
Indiana	No	No	NA	NA	NA	NA	NA
Iowa	Yes	Yes (2001)	Yes	Yes	No	Yes	Yes
Kansas	Yes	No[b]	NA	NA	NA	NA	NA
Kentucky	No	No	NA	NA	NA	NA	NA
Louisiana	Yes	Yes (1989)	Yes	Yes	No	No	No
Maine	Yes	Yes (1998)	Yes	Yes	No	Yes	Yes
Maryland	Yes	Yes (1978)	Yes	Yes	Yes	Yes	Yes
Massachusetts	Yes	No[b]	NA	NA	NA	NA	NA
Michigan	No	No	NA	NA	NA	NA	NA
Minnesota	No	No	NA	NA	NA	NA	NA
Mississippi	Yes	Yes (2000)	Yes	Yes	No	Yes	Yes
Missouri	Yes	Yes (1987)	Yes	Yes	No	No	No
Montana	Yes	No[b]	NA	NA	NA	NA	NA
Nebraska	No[b]	No	NA	NA	NA	NA	NA
Nevada	Yes	Yes (1988)	Yes	Yes	No	Yes	No
New Hampshire	Yes	Yes (1997)	Yes	No[b]	No	Yes	No

New Jersey	Yes	Yes (1981)	Yes	Yes	Yes	Yes	Yes
New Mexico	Yes	Yes (1986)	Yes	Yes	Yes	Yes	Yes
New York	Yes	Yes (1990)	Yes	Yes	Yes	Yes	Yes
North Carolina	Yes	Yes (1982)	Yes	Yes	No	No	No
North Dakota	Yes	Yes (1993)	Yes	Yes	No	Yes	No
Ohio	Yes	No[b]	NA	NA	NA	NA	NA
Oklahoma	Yes	Yes (2001)	Yes	Yes	No	Yes	Yes
Oregon	Yes	Yes (1987)	Yes	Yes	Yes	Yes	Yes
Pennsylvania	Yes	Yes (1986)	Yes	Yes	No	Yes	Yes
Rhode Island	No	No	NA	NA	NA	NA	NA
South Carolina	Yes	Yes (1980)	Yes	Yes	No	Yes	No
South Dakota	No	No	NA	NA	NA	NA	NA
Tennessee	Yes	Yes (1988)	Yes	Yes	No	Yes	No
Texas	Yes	Yes (1993)	Yes	Yes	No	Yes	Yes
Utah	Yes	Yes (1985)	Yes	Yes	No	No	Yes
Vermont	No	No	NA	NA	NA	NA	NA
Virginia	Yes	Yes (1981)	Yes	Yes	No	Yes	Yes
Washington	Yes	Yes (1993)	Yes	Yes	Yes	Yes	Yes
West Virginia	Yes	Yes (1985)	Yes	Yes	No	No	Yes
Wisconsin	No	No	NA	NA	NA	NA	NA
Wyoming	Yes	Yes (2001)	Yes	Yes	No	No	Yes
Total yes	38	34	34	32	8	25	23

[a] not applicable.
[b] In process.
From U.S. Department of Health and Human Services, Health Resources and Services Administration. Trauma—EMS Systems Program, August 2003.

states have passed enabling legislation for trauma center development and initiated a formal process for trauma center designation. At that time, however, the number of states that had an active trauma center designation process was 34 (Table 1). Some states used ACS criteria and others developed their own criteria. The trend over time has been for states to develop their own criteria or use a combination of ACS and state criteria, taking into consideration regional resources and political realities. In a landmark paper in 1998, West and colleagues [4] emphasized that it is critical to limit the number of designated trauma centers based on community need. Regrettably, this HRSA survey indicated that of the 34 states with enabling legislation for trauma center development, only eight limited the number of trauma centers based on community needs (Table 2). This major flaw is undoubtedly due to financial interests of competing health care systems.

It is clear that in some communities there is an "arms race" with designations of large numbers of level 1, 2, and 3 trauma centers. The result of this over-designation is that the numbers of patients cared for who have severe trauma is suboptimal in some institutions. For example, some designated level 2 or 3 trauma centers with no in-house surgeon coverage occasionally have difficulty with a timely response from the on-call trauma surgeon. To maintain the skills of the staff of a level 1 trauma center, at least 650 patients who have an Injury Severity Score greater than 15 per year should be seen [5]. Many studies of multiple procedures, such as coronary bypass surgery and organ transplant, have revealed that optimal results occur in centers that do large numbers of procedures versus centers that do smaller numbers of procedures. The same concept is true for trauma. Physicians, nurses, and ancillary support personnel who care for severe trauma on a regular basis acquire and maintain valuable skills. Those physicians, nurses, and ancillary support personnel who care for severe trauma on an occasional basis are put in a somewhat compromised position, and there also is the potential for suboptimal patient outcome in such situations. Therefore, an objective needs assessment should be performed in all communities in regard to how many and what level trauma centers are necessary, and the number of trauma centers should be limited so that the valuable resources and expense of trauma care can be kept to a minimum while at the same time ensuring optimum outcome. The goal should be to have the best trauma outcomes at the lowest possible costs.

The trauma team

In the early 1970s, with the advent of trauma system development and the specialty recognition of trauma surgery, surgeons on the ACS/COT were legitimately concerned about the care rendered to trauma patients arriving in emergency departments (EDs). At that time, EDs were staffed by non–emergency medicine, residency trained, non–board certified physicians who often had no training beyond postgraduate year 1 or internship year after medical school or who had residency training in nonsurgical specialties. With the recognition of emergency medicine as a specialty in 1979 and the steadily increasing number of emergency medicine residency training programs, the quality of care rendered by emergency physicians in EDs across the country has improved enormously. Emergency medicine is one of the most competitive specialties in medicine. This has resulted in a dramatic increase in the quality not only of trauma care but also overall care rendered in EDs.

At the same time, the interest in trauma surgery as a specialty has begun to wane. In recent years, fewer surgery residents have expressed an interest in trauma surgery as a career and, as a result, there is a looming shortage of qualified trauma surgeons to staff designated trauma centers. Because there always will be a need for trauma surgeons to be present on, or shortly after, arrival of certain major trauma patients, emergency physicians and their trauma surgeon colleagues must work together to formulate rational protocols to optimize the valuable and scarce resource of the trauma surgeons and minimize their unnecessary urgent responses to EDs. The goal should be to have a trauma surgeon present on arrival for those patients who have a high likelihood of going to an operating room immediately for limb- or life-threatening injuries.

In all editions of the ACS/COT manual, a primary issue has been the mandatory presence of a surgeon on arrival of trauma patients. This has been based on the assumption that only a trauma surgeon is skilled in the initial management of an injured patient, although continuity of care also has been suggested. With the evolution of emergency medicine as a specialty, the increasing number of high-quality, well-trained emergency medicine graduates, and advances in ultrasound and CT technology, the role of emergency physicians and trauma surgeons in EDs should be re-evaluated. Emergency physicians now are well trained and well qualified in emergent, acute airway management and in the performance of life-saving emergency diagnostic and therapeutic procedures in EDs, such as thoracic and abdominal ultrasound examinations, decompression of tension pneumothoraces, performance of cricothyroidotomy, and, in rare instances, ED thoracotomy. A recent article by Green highlights the need to rethink mandating a trauma surgeon be present on arrival of a significant number of trauma patients transported to EDs in level 1 trauma centers [6]. Green appropriately emphasizes, "The two historical factors that originally prompted this requirement, frequent exploratory laparotomies and emergency physicians without trauma training, no longer exist in most modern trauma centers." Green observes that it is not "professionally satisfying to require the general surgeon to emergently interrupt their other duties to attend patients unlikely to require their urgent intervention." He contends further that research has not confirmed improvement in patient outcome attributable to early surgeon involvement and notes that surgeons are not present routinely during the resuscitative phase of trauma care in Canada and Europe. Finally,

Table 2
Characteristics of trauma centers

State	Limit on number of trauma centers	Limit on duration of initial designation (in years)	Periodic reverification occurs	Limit on duration of redesignation (in years)	Formal contracts with trauma centers present	Designation standards for pediatric hospitals	Designation standards for burn hospitals
Alabama	NA[a]	NA	NA	NA	NA	NA	NA
Alaska	No	Yes (3)	Yes	Yes (3)	No	Yes	Yes
Arizona	NA	NA	NA	NA	NA	NA	NA
Arkansas	No	Yes (3)	Yes	Yes (3)	No	No[b]	Yes
California	Yes	Yes (3)	Yes	Yes (3)	Yes	Yes	Yes
Colorado	No	Yes (3)	Yes	Yes (3)	No	Yes	Yes
Connecticut	No	Yes (3)	Yes	Yes (3)	No	Yes	No
Delaware	No	Yes (3)	Yes	Yes (3)	Yes	Yes	No
Florida	No	Yes (7)	Yes	Yes (7)	Yes	Yes	Yes
Georgia	No	Yes (3)	No[b]	Yes (3)	No	Yes	Yes
Hawaii	No	No	No	No	No	Yes	Yes
Idaho	NA	NA	NA	NA	NA	NA	NA
Illinois	Yes	Yes (2)	Yes	Yes (2)	No	No[b]	No
Indiana	NA	NA	NA	NA	NA	NA	NA
Iowa	No	Yes (4)	Yes	Yes (3)	No	No	No
Kansas	NA	Yes (3)	No	Yes (3)	No	Yes	Yes
Kentucky	NA	Yes (3)	Yes	Yes (3)	Yes	Yes	Yes
Louisiana	No	Unknown	No[b]	Unknown	No[b]	Yes	Yes
Maine	No	Yes (3)	No[b]	Yes (3)	No	No	No
Maryland	Yes	Yes (5)	Yes	Yes (5)	Yes	Yes	Yes
Massachusetts	NA	Yes (3)	Yes	Yes (3)	Unknown	Yes	Unknown
Michigan	NA	NA	NA	NA	NA	NA	NA
Minnesota	NA	NA	NA	NA	NA	NA	NA
Mississippi	No	Yes (15 mo)	Yes	Yes (3)	No	Yes	No
Missouri	No	Yes (5)	Yes	Yes (5)	Yes	Yes	No
Montana	NA	Yes (3)	No[b]	Yes (3)	No[b]	No	No
Nebraska	NA	Yes (3)	Yes	Yes (3)	No	Yes	Yes

Nevada	No	Yes (3)	Yes	Yes (3)	No	No	No
New Hampshire	No	No Limit	No	No Limit	No	Yes	No
New Jersey	Yes	Yes (3)	Yes	Yes (3)	Yes	Yes	Yes
New Mexico	Yes	Yes (3)	Yes	Yes (3)	Yes	No	No
New York	Yes	No Limit	Yes	No Limit	Yes	Yes	Yes
North Carolina	No	Yes (3)	Yes	Yes (4)	No	No	No
North Dakota	No	Yes (3)	Yes	Yes (3)	Yes	No	No
Ohio	NA	Yes (3)	No[b]	Yes (3)	No	Yes	No
Oklahoma	No	No Limit	Yes	No Limit	Yes	Yes	Yes
Oregon	Yes	Yes (3)	Yes	Yes (3)	No	Yes	No
Pennsylvania	No	Yes (1)	Yes	Yes (2)	Yes	Yes	Yes
Rhode Island	NA	Yes (3)	Yes	Yes (3)	No	Unknown	Unknown
South Carolina	No	Yes (5)	Yes	Yes (5)	No	No	No
South Dakota	NA	NA	NA	NA	NA	NA	NA
Tennessee	No	Yes (5)	Yes	Yes (5)	No	Yes	No
Texas	No	Yes (3)	Yes	Yes (3)	Yes	No	No
Utah	No	Yes (3)	Yes	Yes (3)	No	Yes	No
Vermont	—	Yes (3)	Yes	Yes (3)	No	No	No
Virginia	No	Yes (2)	Yes	Yes (3)	No	No	No
Washington	Yes	Yes (3)	Yes	Yes (3)	Yes	Yes	Yes
West Virginia	No	No	No[b]	No	No[b]	No	Yes
Wisconsin	NA	NA	NA	NA	NA	NA	NA
Wyoming	No	Yes (3)	Yes	Yes (3)	No	No	No
Total yes	8	36	33	36	14	26	18
Total no	26	2	9	2	27	15	22
Total unknown	NA	1	NA	1	1	1	2

[a] not applicable.
[b] In process.
From U.S. Department of Health and Human Services, Health Resources and Services Administration. Trauma—EMS Systems Program, August 2003.

Green suggests, constructively, that individual trauma centers should be permitted the flexibility to design their specific trauma activation and alert criteria based on outcome research in their center. A subsequent editorial by Moore presents a surgeon's perspective [7]. Moore concurs that "it is time to reassess when the surgeon must be present in the Emergency Department (ED) for trauma evaluations and management" but argues that the strategic question is when a surgeon should assume the responsibility for a patient who has potential significant injuries in the ED, not if a surgeon should be involved in the ED phase of trauma care. It is a fact that in legitimate level 1 trauma centers there are patients for whom the earliest possible attendance by a surgeon is life saving. For example, patients who are exsanguinating secondary to penetrating wounds of major vessels in the neck, chest, or abdomen, such as the subclavian artery and pulmonary hilar, heart, and major abdominal and pelvic vessels, can be saved only by immediate surgical intervention in an operating room.

On the contrary, there is little surgeons can provide urgently that experienced emergency physicians cannot accomplish for patients arriving in an ED who have isolated respiratory compromise or altered mental status [8]. Moore acknowledges further that a rebellion among trauma surgeons throughout the United States is emerging because of diminishing operative procedures and increasing unsavory obligations; conspicuous in the latter are onerous nocturnal fire alarms in EDs without purpose [9]. The challenge of expanding operative procedures for trauma surgeons is being pursued through the new specialty of acute care surgery [10], but the issue of unrewarding duties of trauma surgery largely has been ignored [8]. Success with acute care surgery will depend on efficient and effective use of time outside operating rooms. Moore also cautions that trauma outcomes research is challenging because it is difficult to define comparable study groups. Anatomic scoring (eg, the Injury Severity Score) inherently is flawed and, without a physiologic component, is inadequate to judge quality of care. Further, trauma-related mortality of unselected study populations is an insensitive barometer because the data overwhelmingly are diluted with patients who will survive irrespective of initial treatment. Consequently, surrogate markers may be more appropriate study endpoints. For example, time to an operating room from ED presentation for patients who have active torso hemorrhage is a defendable benchmark. Delayed intervention resulting in protracted shock or blood transfusion may have profound adverse effects on short- and long-term patient recovery. Unfortunately, preventable deaths caused by persistent splenic hemorrhage continue despite megadetector CT scanners. Other examples of critical and potentially lifesaving interventions include the time from ED arrival to administrations of β-blockade for patients who have a thoracic aortic injury and placement of an epidural catheter for elderly patients who have multiple rib fractures.

Even in states that have trauma systems, many hospitals in small to medium-sized cities and virtually all rural hospitals do not have the resources or staff to be a level 1, 2, or, in some cases, even a level 3 center. Virtually all of the institutions, however, have functioning EDs. Therefore, a significant number of severely injured patients are not cared for initially in a designated trauma center. In these institutions, the only physician present and providing the initial care for patients is an emergency medicine physician. Therefore, it is imperative that emergency medicine specialists be well trained in initial evaluation, resuscitation, and stabilization of critically injured patients. To this end, all training programs should enable emergency medicine residents to have the opportunity to direct major resuscitations, perform procedures necessary for the resuscitation and stabilization of patients, and be aware of which patients need to be transferred to a trauma center for a higher level care. All hospitals that are not designated trauma centers should have transfer agreements with centers that provide a higher level of trauma care, in particular the unique resources of a level 1 trauma center.

In hospitals that are designated trauma centers, there must be a close working relationship between the emergency medicine specialist and the trauma surgeons. To facilitate this, there must be protocols in place for the initial triage and resuscitation of major trauma patients. These protocols should be formulated in a collaborative fashion between emergency medicine and trauma surgery. Trauma care, perhaps more than any other area of medicine, truly is a team effort that is a continuum from roadside through rehabilitation. Optimal care of trauma patients involves practitioners in multiple disciplines who are well trained and must work together in a collaborative fashion. Care of seriously injured patients begins in a prehospital arena with well-trained emergency medical technicians (EMTs) responding who can perform extrication and rapid transport to an appropriate receiving hospital ED. To this end, Basic Trauma Life Support certifications and EMT-paramedic courses provide excellent skills for EMTs to manage injured patients in a prehospital arena.

Prehospital destination protocols should be delineated clearly to identify patients who would benefit most from transport to a level 1 trauma center. Physiologic and anatomic parameters (Table 3) are most reliable in identifying these patients most likely to benefit from care at a level 1 trauma center. Reliance on mechanism of injury alone results in over-triage of patients to level 1 or 2 centers. Other criteria that are used include mechanism of injury and special needs, such as a burn or limb replantation center. From a patient care perspective, ambulances should bypass other EDs or lower-level trauma centers for the select small number of patients who are severely injured.

On arrival in an ED, a trauma team should consist of well-trained and qualified emergency physicians and trauma surgeons and nurses and technicians trained adequately in trauma care, including radiology, special diagnostic imaging, laboratory, and blood bank. An operating room with a qualified anesthesiologist must be available immediately as should key surgical subspecialists, including neurosurgeons and orthopedic surgeons.

Table 3
Prehospital triage criteria for transport to a level 1 trauma center

Children (ages 0–12 or <5 ft in height)	Adult
1. Intubation or	1. Intubation or
2. Respiratory distress or	2. SBP <90 mm Hg or
3. Capillary refill > 2 s or blood pressure abnormal or age (<70 + 2 × age) or	3. Respiratory rate <10 or >29 with distress or
4. GCS motor score ≤ 5	4. GCS motor score ≤ 5
Anatomy (any one of the below)	
1. Penetrating injuries—head, neck, torso, pelvis	
2. Flail chest	
3. Bilateral femur fractures	
4. Unstable pelvis or suspected significant pelvic fracture	
5. Paralysis or evidence of spinal cord injury	
6. Amputation above the wrist or ankle	
7. Significant burns	
8. Unreactive or unequal pupils	

Trauma care extends well beyond EDs with care in an operating room, surgical ICU, surgical inpatient units, and subsequent rehabilitation services.

Current ACS/COT trauma system requirements for level 1, 2, and 3 state that ideally a surgeon should be present in an ED on arrival for all major resuscitations in these designated trauma centers. If a surgeon is not present on arrival, one must be present within 15 minutes of a patient's arrival. The ACS/COT current "major criteria" for which this surgical presence is mandated include (1) confirmed hypotension (systolic blood pressure [SBP] 90 mm Hg); (2) respiratory compromise requiring intubation; (3) penetrating gunshot wound to the neck, chest, abdomen, or pelvis; (4) a Glasgow Coma Scale (GCS) score of less than 8 attributed to trauma; and (5) discretion of an emergency physician. Individual trauma centers can extend the criteria for which the trauma team is activated, and often this includes injury mechanism. There is financial incentive for institutions to over-triage and increase the number of trauma team responses, because they can charge a significant additional fee for the presence of the trauma team personnel on arrival of patients.

The current recommendations by the ACS/COT should be reconsidered with the advances in the training and capabilities of emergency physicians. For example, the mandate that a surgeon be present on arrival of a patient simply because a patient has a GCS score of less than 8 or has been intubated in the field is shown in recent studies to be unwarranted. A study from Denver Health demonstrates that, with the exception of patients who have sustained stab wounds to the torso, trauma patients who have some degree of respiratory compromise or who have been intubated in

Box 1. Modified criteria for trauma activation

1. Blunt trauma with SBP less than 90 mm Hg or comparable level of hypotension in a child
2. Penetrating injury
   A. Injury to neck or torso with SBP less than 90 mm Hg or comparable level of hypotension in a child
   B. Gunshot wounds penetrating the torso or
   C. Stab wounds to the torso that require endotracheal intubation
3. Mechanically unstable pelvic injury (open or obvious by physical examination)
4. Respiratory compromise, obstruction, or intubation with presumed thoracic, abdominal, or pelvic injury
5. GCS score less than 8 with presumed thoracic, abdominal, or pelvic injury
6. Amputation proximal to the ankle or wrist
7. Transfer patients from other facilities receiving blood to maintain vital signs or
8. Suspicion that patient likely will require urgent operative intervention

the field do not need a surgeon present on the arrival in the ED [8]. In addition, the majority of trauma patients who have a GCS score of less than 8 have either an abnormal mental status secondary to isolated head trauma or metabolic or toxicologic reasons. Therefore, the authors have modified the criteria at Denver Health for trauma activation and have developed the following protocol (Box 1).

These protocols are a dynamic document and will be revised in the future based on the critical evaluation of trauma outcome data from the authors' trauma registry and continuous quality improvement (CQI) processes.

In summary, optimal trauma care is a team effort from roadside through rehabilitation. Close collegial collaboration between emergency medicine specialists and trauma surgeons is essential. All efforts and protocols for trauma care should be based on objective CQI outcome data. The ultimate goal should be to make the most efficient use of resources that result in the best possible outcome for the trauma patient.

References

[1] Champion HR, Mabee MS, Meredith JW. The state of US trauma systems: public perceptions versus reality—implications for US response to terrorism and mass casualty events. Am Coll Surg 2006;951–61.

[2] Celso B, Tepas B, Langland-Orbon B, et al. A systematic review and meta-analysis comparing outcome of severely injured patients treated in trauma centers following the establishment of trauma systems. J Trauma 2006;60:371–8.

[3] Committee on Trauma. American College of Surgeons resources for optimal care of the injured patient. Chicago: American College of Surgeons; 2006. p. 19.

[4] West JG, Williams MJ, Trunkey DD, et al. Trauma systems: current status—future challenges. JAMA, 1099(259):3597–600.

[5] Nathens AB, Jurkovich FH, Maier RV, et al. Relationship between trauma center volume and outcomes. JAMA 2001;285:1164–71.

[6] Green SM. Is there evidence to support the need for routine surgeon presence on trauma patient arrival? Ann Emerg Med 2006;47(5):405–11.

[7] Moore EE. Role of the acute care surgeon in the emergency department management of trauma. Ann Emerg Med 2006;47(5):413–4.

[8] Ciesla DJ, Moore EE, Moore JB, et al. Intubation alone does not mandate trauma surgeon presence on patient arrival to the emergency department. J Trauma 2004;56:937–42.

[9] Esposito TJ, Rotondo M, Barie PS, et al. Making the case for paradigm shift in trauma surgery. J Am Coll Surg 2006;202:655–7.

[10] The Committee to Develop the Reorganized Specialty of Trauma, Surgical Critical Care and Emergency Surgery. Acute care surgery: trauma, critical care, and emergency surgery. J Trauma 2005;58:614–6.

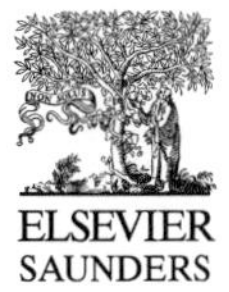
ELSEVIER
SAUNDERS

EMERGENCY MEDICINE CLINICS OF NORTH AMERICA

Emerg Med Clin N Am 25 (2007) 655–678

Traumatic Brain Injury

William Heegaard, MD, MPH*,
Michelle Biros, MD, MS

Department of Emergency Medicine, Hennepin County Medical Center, University of Minnesota Medical School, 701 Park Avenue S, Minneapolis, MN 55415, USA

Traumatic brain injury (TBI) refers to the potential for significant injury to the brain parenchyma following head trauma. This article covers pertinent principles, management approaches, and current controversies in severe, moderate, and minor TBI. Controversies covered include hypertonic saline (HTS) for increased intracranial pressure (ICP), prehospital intubation of patients who have experienced TBI, and the use of recombinant factor VIIa (rFVIIa).

Traumatic head injury has plagued humankind since the beginning of civilization. The writings of Hippocrates refer to trephination [1], and early writings on the practice of neurosurgery describe the management of head trauma. Although the most common mechanism for TBI has changed since antiquity from assaults to motor vehicle–associated injuries, TBI remains the single largest cause of trauma morbidity and accounts for nearly one third of all trauma deaths (Fig. 1) [2–4].

An estimated 1.1 million patients are evaluated each year in emergency departments for acute TBI [3]. TBI occurs most often in young people, with a peak incidence at 15 to 24 years of age [4]. Smaller peaks occur in children younger than 5 years of age and in individuals older than 85 years [4]. Child abuse is common in children younger than 4 years of age who present with severe to moderate TBI (Fig. 2) [5].

TBI is commonly categorized by means of the Glasgow Coma Scale (GCS) [6] as severe (GCS $\leq$ 8), moderate (GCS 9–13), and minor (GCS 14–15). Severe TBI accounts for approximately 10% of all cases, whereas moderate TBI accounts for another 10%; the remaining 80% are classified as minor [4].

* Corresponding author.
E-mail address: emdoc@yahoo.com (W. Heegaard).

doi:10.1016/j.emc.2007.07.001

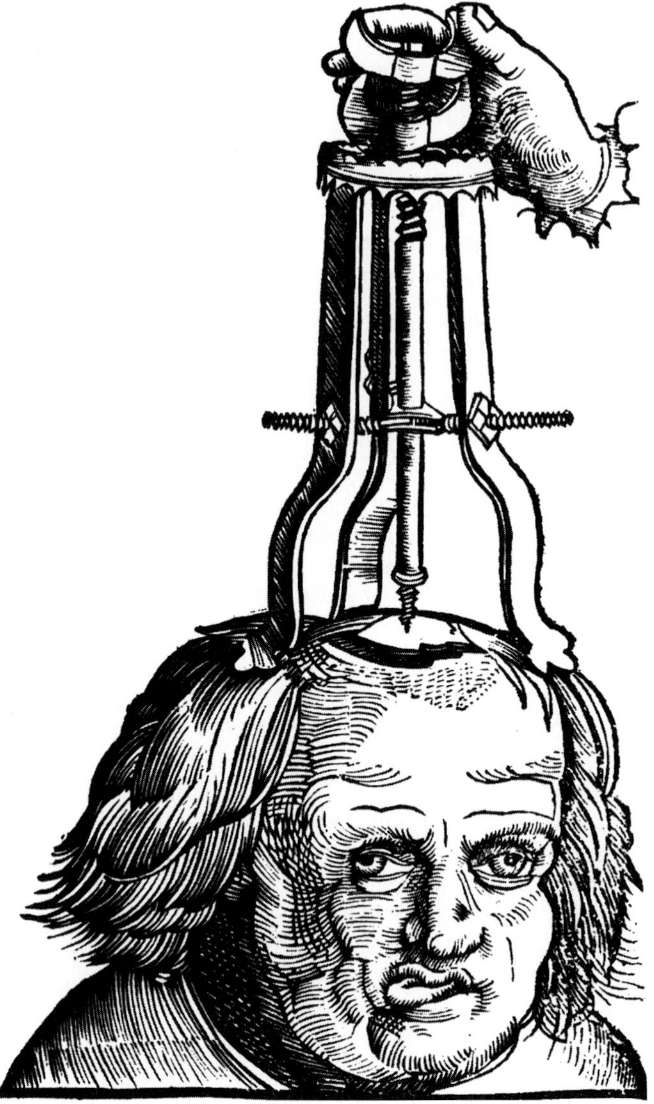

Fig. 1. Von Gersdorff. Feldtbuch der Wundartzney. Strossberg, J Schott, 1517. Illustration showing the method of elevating depressed skull fractures. Right third and twelfth nerve palsies and left facial weakness are present. (*From* Von Gersdorf, Hans. Feldbuch der Wundartzney, 1527. Wellcome Library, London.)

Because the emergency physician (EP) must manage patients who have head injuries of differing clinical severity caused by a variety of mechanisms, it is essential for clinicians to have a firm understanding of all categories of TBI.

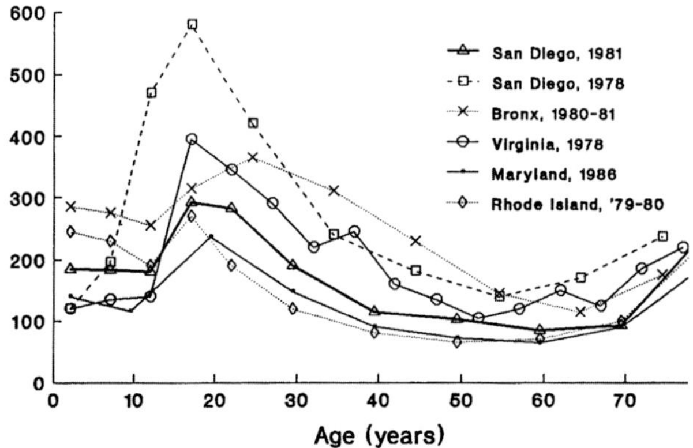

Fig. 2. Age-specific brain injury incidence rates per 100,000 populations, selected United States studies (*From* Kraus J, McArthur D. Epidemiology of head injury. In: Cooper P, Golfinos J, editors. Head injury. 4th edition. New York: McGraw-Hill; 2000. p. 11; with perrmission).

Physiology and pathophysiology of traumatic brain injury

A full discussion of the pathophysiology of TBI is beyond the scope of this article; however, major aspects of the physiology and pathophysiology of TBI must be understood because they form the basis of our clinical management. TBI is a dynamic process; a diagram of the contributing factors and cascading pathophysiologic events associated with TBI are shown in Fig. 3. For a more detailed description of brain physiology and pathophysiology following TBI, the reader is referred to several references [7–9].

The brain is a semisolid structure that weighs about 1400 g (3 lb) and occupies about 80% of the cranial vault [10]. It uses approximately 20% of the entire oxygen volume consumed by the body. To support this high metabolic rate, the brain receives approximately 15% of total cardiac demand.

A key concept in normal brain functioning is the maintenance of adequate cerebral perfusion pressure (CPP), which is defined as the difference between the mean arterial pressure (MAP) and the ICP. CPP is calculated by subtracting the ICP from the MAP and serves as a rough estimate of cerebral blood flow (CBF). Changes in CPP after TBI are correlated with clinical outcome. In the normal brain, CBF is maintained at constant levels when the MAP is 60 to 150 mm Hg. Cerebral vessels maintain the desirable CBF through their ability to constrict and dilate depending on changing physiologic conditions [11]. This is referred to as autoregulation. When a traumatic injury occurs, autoregulation and CBF often are disrupted. Hypertension, alkalosis, and hypocarbia result in cerebral vasoconstriction; hypotension, acidosis, and hypercarbia cause cerebral vasodilation.

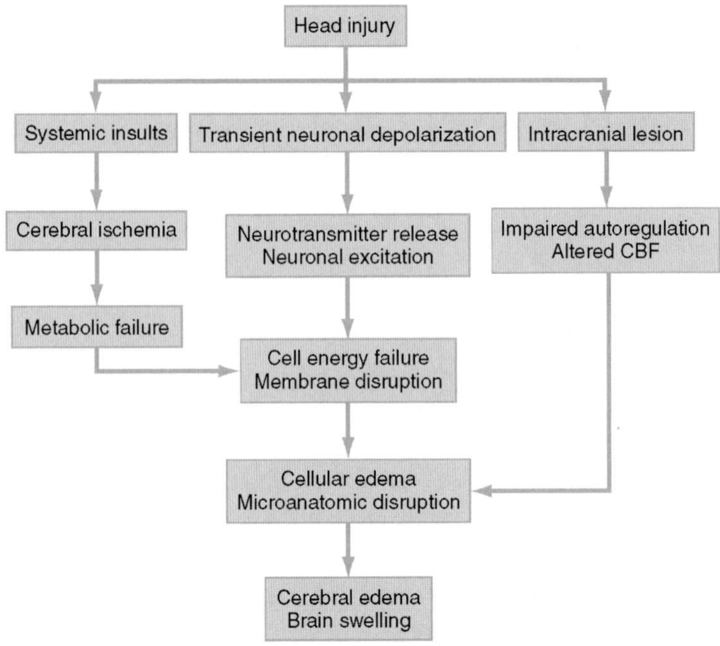

Fig. 3. Contributing events in the pathophysiology of secondary brain injury. CBF, cerebral blood flow.

The importance of cerebral vasoactivity and its relationship to systemic PCO_2 and partial pressure of oxygen (PaO) has been known for some time. This relationship acts as the foundation for the use of hyperventilation in the acute setting to control presumed increased ICP after severe head injury. Because PCO_2 decreases with hyperventilation, cerebral vasoconstriction usually occurs. This vasoconstriction results in decreased parenchymal blood volume, which, in turn, may buffer the effects of increasing edema or an expanding hematoma within the rigid cranial vault; however, a significant reduction in systemic PCO_2 levels caused by prolonged hyperventilation can result in severe vasoconstriction at the adjacent or penumbra regions of injured brain tissue, causing brain ischemia and cell death [12–14]. For these reasons and because of the risk for reperfusion injury, the use of prophylactic hyperventilation and prolonged hyperventilation in the ICU is not recommended (Fig. 4) [14].

ICP is related directly to the volume of intracranial contents, including blood, cerebrospinal fluid (CSF), and brain parenchyma. This relationship is explained by the Monro-Kellie doctrine [15,16]. In the United States, the use of ICP monitoring and control has become standard in cases of moderate and severe TBI, despite the lack of prospective controlled research studies showing clear efficacy as an individual patient treatment modality. The role of ICP monitoring in the initial emergency department (ED)

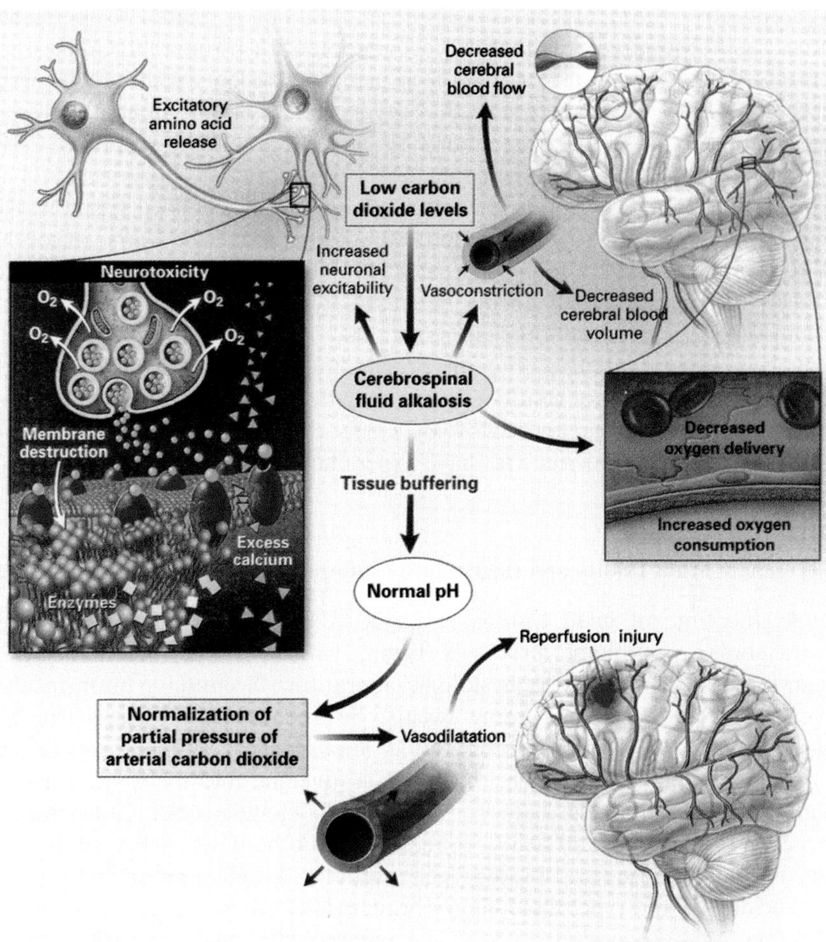

Fig. 4. Neurologic effects of hypocapnia. Systemic hypocapnia results in cerebrospinal fluid alkalosis, which decreases CBF, cerebral oxygen delivery, and, to a lesser extent, cerebral blood volume. The reduction in ICP may be lifesaving in patients in whom the pressure is severely elevated; however, hypocapnia-induced brain ischemia may occur because of vasoconstriction (impairing cerebral perfusion), reduced oxygen release from hemoglobin, and increased neuronal excitability, with the possible release of excitotoxins, such as glutamate. Over time, cerebrospinal fluid pH and, hence, CBF, gradually return to normal. Subsequent normalization of the partial pressure of arterial carbon dioxide can result in cerebral hyperemia, causing reperfusion injury to previously ischemic brain regions. (*From* Laffey JG, Kavanagh BP. Hypocapnia. N Engl J Med 2002;347:44; with permission. Copyright © 2002, Massachusetts Medical Society.)

resuscitation of patients who have experienced a severe or moderate TBI remains unclear. Methods to reduce elevated ICP in the acute setting include brief hyperventilation, the use of osmotic and diuretic agents, and CSF drainage.

Congestive brain swelling occurs after TBI and is related to increased intracranial blood volume that can occur soon after trauma [9]. Congestive brain swelling is especially common in pediatric patients who have experienced TBI. Most experts believe that the increased blood volume is caused by vasodilatation, which is a response by the brain to maintain optimal CBF in the face of damaged brain tissue.

Cerebral edema is due to an absolute increase in cerebral tissue water content. Diffuse cerebral edema can occur at any time in the course of severe TBI. Two types of cerebral edema occur in the setting of trauma: vasogenic and cytotoxic. Vasogenic edema is caused by transvascular leakage from compromised tight endothelial junctions of blood–brain barrier [9]. Vasogenic edema often accumulates preferentially in the white matter. Intracellular processes that result in brain cell death cause cytotoxic edema. Recent work suggests that cytotoxic cerebral edema is the predominant form of edema in patients who have experienced TBI [17].

Secondary brain insults and their relationship to outcome

At the time of head trauma, a series of destructive intracellular and extracellular pathologic processes begin, which include neurochemical, neuroanatomic, and neurophysiologic alterations. Secondary brain insults contribute to these devastating events. Secondary brain insults can be categorized as systemic or intracranial. Examples of systemic secondary brain insults include hypotension, hypoxia, anemia, and hyper- and hypocapnia. Intracranial secondary brain insults include severe intracranial hypertension, extra-axial lesions (that compress otherwise unaffected tissue), seizures (that cause focal brain hypermetabolism), and cerebral edema.

The degree and type of secondary brain insults are major determinants in the final neurologic outcome of the patient who has experienced TBI. Preexisting factors, such as the patient's age and trauma-related systemic events, also impact secondary brain insults. A primary goal in the emergency care of the patient who has experienced a head injury is prevention or reduction of systemic conditions that are known to worsen outcome after TBI. Several investigational agents are under study in ongoing head injury clinical treatment trials and may alter the destructive processes of secondary brain injury [18].

Certain systemic secondary brain insults clearly can worsen patient outcome. Hypotension and hypoxia contribute significantly to secondary brain injury and have been associated with worsening morbidity and mortality following TBI [19]. As many as 35% of patients who have experienced TBI are estimated to suffer from hypotension (blood pressure $<$ 90 mm Hg) at some point in their clinical course [19]. Hypotension reduces cerebral perfusion, worsens cerebral ischemia, and nearly doubles the mortality from TBI [19,20]. Hypoxia (P $<$ 60 mm Hg) occurs often in the patient who has experienced TBI [21]; when its occurrence is documented, the overall mortality of severe head injury doubles [19,22].

Data from the Traumatic Coma Data Bank showing the devastating effects of systemic insults on the outcome of TBI are given in Tables 1 and 2.

Minor head trauma

Minor head trauma is defined as isolated head injury producing a GCS score of 14 to 15 [23]. It is the most common degree of head injury in patients who present to EDs for evaluation. Most episodes of minor head trauma occur in the context of sports and other recreational activities.

By the time most patients with minor head trauma present to the ED, they are asymptomatic. When symptoms are present, headache is the most common complaint; however, nausea and emesis are common. Patients occasionally describe experiencing disorientation, confusion, or amnesia; these symptoms usually are brief and transient and may occur immediately or shortly after the injury. In adult patients, these symptoms often are believed to suggest the presence of intracranial lesions, but data supporting this supposition are sparse.

After a complete neurologic and mental status examination, additional diagnostic workup and subsequent management hinges on risk stratification in patients with minor head trauma. Roughly, 3% of all patients with minor head trauma sustain a sudden, unexpected neurologic deterioration; less than 1% have surgically significant lesions [24]. A goal of many research studies has been to determine which patients who have experienced a minor head trauma are at risk for an intracranial lesion and, therefore, require acute neuroimaging. The results of these studies have been conflicting, likely because different methods, definitions, and outcomes have been used. For example, although some studies have shown that adult patients who

Table 1
Data from the Medical College of Virginia (1982): outcome by secondary insult at time of arrival at hospital for nonmutually exclusive insults

			Outcome percentage		
Secondary insults	Patients (N)	Percentage of total patients	Good or moderate	Severe or vegetative	Dead
Total cases	225	100	56	10	34
Neither	120	53	64	12	24
Hypoxia	78	35	41	9	50
Hypotension	34	15	35	12	53

Hypoxia = $PaO_2 < 60$ mm Hg; hypotension = Systolic blood pressure < 95 mm Hg.

Data from Miller JD, Becker DP. Secondary insults to the injured brain. J R Coll Surg Edinb 1982;27:292.

Table 2
Traumatic Coma Database data: outcome by secondary insult at time of arrival at Traumatic Coma Database hospital ER for non-mutually exclusive insults

			Outcome (%)		
Secondary insult	Patients (N)	Percentage of total patients	Good or moderate	Severe or vegetative	Dead
Total cases	699[a]	100.0	42.9	20.5	36.6
Neither	456	65.2	51.1	21.9	27.0
Hypoxia	130	18.6	29.2	20.8	50.0
Hypotension	165	23.6	19.4	15.8	64.8
Both	52	7.4	5.8	19.2	75.0

Hypoxia = $PaO_2 < 60$ mm Hg; hypotension = Systolic blood pressure < 90 mm Hg.

[a] The total number of patients is 699 instead of 717 because of missing admission data on blood pressure or arterial blood gas values in 18 patients.

From Chesnut RM, Marshall LF, Klauber MR, et al. The role of secondary brain injury in determining outcome from severe head injury. J Trauma 1993;34(2):584; with permission.

experienced a minor head trauma and had a presenting GCS score of 15 and a history of a loss of consciousness (LOC) may be at increased risk for an intracranial lesion, the negative predictive value of LOC for the presence of TBI has not been determined [23]. Other authorities suggested that the duration of LOC in patients who have experience a minor head injury correlated directly with the occurrence of an intracranial injury, but this has not been determined in well-done studies [25]. Although high-risk minor head trauma criteria have been proposed to guide the decision to obtain neuroimaging, the less controversial approach for the EP is to consider who does not need neuroimaging. Box 1 provides criteria of degrees of risk for patients with minor head injury.

Neuroimaging in patients who have minor head injuries

A key management decision for EPs is whether a head CT scan should be obtained on patients who have sustained minor head trauma. Many neurosurgical studies advocate for CT scanning of all patients who have sustained a minor head trauma who give a history of LOC or amnesia for the traumatic event [25,26]; however, these studies undoubtedly suffer from selection bias, because neurosurgical consultation probably occurs only for a select, more injured population. Other authorities recommend in-hospital or prolonged ED observation to allow rapid identification of those few patients who have experienced a minor head trauma who suddenly deteriorate. Prolonged ED observation may have merit in some circumstances, such as in intoxicated patients who have sustained a minor head injury and who need to obtain sobriety before they can be evaluated fully for a delayed complication of minor head trauma. In these patients, a CT scan may be unnecessary if ED resources are available that allow meticulous

Box 1. Risk stratification in patients with minor head trauma

High risk
- Focal neurologic findings
- Asymmetric pupils
- Skull fracture on clinical examination
- Multiple trauma
- Serious, painful, distracting injuries
- External signs of trauma above the clavicles
- Initial GCS score of 14 or 15
- Loss of consciousness
- Posttraumatic confusion/anemia
- Progressively worsening headache
- Vomiting
- Posttraumatic seizure
- History of bleeding disorder/anticoagulation
- Recent ingestion of intoxicants
- Unreliable/unknown history of injury
- Previous neurologic diagnosis
- Previous epilepsy
- Suspected child abuse
- Age older than 60 years or younger than 2 years

Medium risk
- Initial GCS score of 15
- Brief LOC
- Posttraumatic amnesia
- Vomiting
- Headache
- Intoxication

Low risk
- Currently asymptomatic
- No other injuries
- No focality on examination
- Normal pupils
- No change in consciousness
- Intact orientation/memory
- Initial GCS score of 15
- Accurate history
- Trivial mechanism
- Injury more than 24 hours ago
- No or mild headache
- No vomiting
- No preexisting high-risk factors

From Marx J, Hockberger R, Walls R, et al, editors. Rosen's emergency medicine: concepts and clinical practice. 6th edition. Mosby; 2006;349–82; with permission.

observation and reevaluation with serial examinations. Some experts advocate CT scanning and observation [25], but most do not believe that this is necessary because the risk for intracranial lesions and delayed complications is minimal in these otherwise low-risk patients who have minor head trauma. From a practical standpoint, EPs generally use selective scanning or observation, based on the risk assessment of the patient who has sustained a minor head trauma. Neuroimaging usually is not indicated for nonintoxicated, low-risk patients [23]. Those with moderate risk probably should undergo CT scanning or prolonged observation. High-risk criteria for adult patients who have sustained a minor head trauma that correlate with an increased likelihood of intracranial lesions include headache, vomiting, age older than 60 years, drug or alcohol intoxication, short-term memory deficits, external signs of trauma above the clavicles, and posttraumatic seizures [27,28]. Other presumed high-risk criteria are listed in Box 1. CT scanning should be considered strongly in patients with these high-risk findings.

In most adult patients, skull radiographs are not recommended if the patient is deemed to require neuroimaging; CT scanning is the preferred study and will yield information about the skull and the brain. Rarely, skull radiographs may be useful in patients who cannot undergo a head CT scan (eg, CT not immediately available). Radiographs may reveal a skull fracture, pneumocephalus, fluid (presumed to be blood) in the sinuses, or penetrating foreign bodies [29]. These findings may assist in the decision to transfer the patient to a center capable of more advanced neurotrauma management. External physical signs of head trauma by themselves do not predict TBI in patients who have sustained a minor head trauma, but the risk is increased substantially if a skull fracture is present [23]; however, the absence of clinical or radiographic findings of a fracture does not rule out TBI.

When an isolated skull fracture is found by clinical or radiographic examination, it usually is a linear fracture, which has limited clinical significance in adults. The presence of a basilar skull fracture substantially increases the risk for intracranial lesions associated with minor head trauma [20]. When a skull fracture is suspected based on the clinical examination, the most efficient management strategy is to consider a CT scan without obtaining plain radiographs.

Disposition

Most low-risk patients who have sustained a minor head injury can be discharged safely from the ED after a normal examination, but competent observation of 4 to 6 hours is advised [4]. Patients with moderate or high-risk minor head trauma who are discharged from the ED should have an appropriate early follow-up arranged. All patients should be educated on the signs and symptoms of delayed complications of head injury. In addition, they should have access to a telephone and should be monitored in the acute posttrauma period by a responsible, sober adult. If these requirements cannot be met or if there are any concerns about the safety of the discharged patient with minor head injury, a brief inpatient observation period (ie, 12 to 24 hours) is advisable.

A second ED visit by the patient who has sustained a minor head injury is common because of the persistence of symptoms or the development of new concerns. A careful neurologic examination must be performed to determine the presence of delayed complications of minor head injury. There are few data to support a repeat CT scan in the presence of a nonfocal neurologic examination if a first scan at the time of the initial presentation was normal. Referral to a neurologist is warranted for these patients.

Concussions

A concussion is a transient brief interruption of neurologic function after minor head trauma, with or without an LOC, usually as a result of acceleration-deceleration forces to the head [30]. Although anyone can sustain a concussion, it is most often a consequence of a sports-related minor head injury. At least 300,000 sports-related concussions are reported yearly to the Centers for Disease Control and Prevention, and as many as 8% of United States high school and college football players sustain concussions each football season [31]. The most common complaints after concussion are headache, confusion, and amnesia; the neurologic examination is nonfocal. Patients will be amnestic for the traumatic event, and duration of the amnestic period suggests the severity of the sustained injury. In young children, acute symptoms of concussion often include restlessness, lethargy, confusion, or irritability. The consequences of the impact can persist for several days. A recent study of concussed football players showed acute symptoms lasting at least 5 days, cognitive impairments lasting up to 7 days, and balance deficits for up to 5 days after concussion. Although 91% were back to their preinjury baseline by 1 week, some had problems for as long as 3 months after injury [31].

Various theories have been proposed to explain the physical and functional signs and symptoms following a concussion. These include shearing or stretching of white matter fibers, temporary neuronal dysfunction, transient alterations in levels of neurotransmitters, or temporary changes in CBF and oxygen use. A convulsive theory also has been suggested [32]. Regardless of the underlying pathophysiology, it has been shown that levels of specific neurotransmitters remain elevated after head injury, and a hypermetabolic state may persist in the brain for several days to weeks postinjury [33,34]. Although this may not be of immediate concern when examining the ED patient who has a concussion, it may factor into the decision to allow an athlete to return to play after an episode of minor head injury. The second impact syndrome (SIS) has been described in a small number of athletes who sustain a second concussion before being completely asymptomatic from the first [35]. Shortly after the second impact, the patient experiences a rapid, usually fatal, neurologic decline. The existence and frequency of the SIS are controversial, but the potential for this serious problem affects subsequent management decisions. The proposed pathophysiology of the SIS involves prolonged neurochemical disruptions and altered autoregulatory mechanisms after a first concussion that make the brain particularly vulnerable to reinjury. With a second impact, the already abnormal neurophysiology is triggered to promote rapid and extensive brain swelling and subsequent herniation after a seemingly minor second impact occurring within 5 to 7 days after the first concussion [35]. Many pediatric and sports medicine professional organizations have developed recommendations for return to play after a sports-related concussion. No single set of guidelines has been accepted universally, but all are predicated on the concern for a period of neurologic vulnerability following impact. Most advise that players who have sustained a concussion should not return to play for at least 1 week after they have become asymptomatic. If the player experienced LOC or prolonged posttraumatic amnesia at the time of concussion, most authorities recommend that the patient should not return to sports until he or she has been symptom-free for at least 1 month [36].

Vague symptoms, such as headaches, sensory sensitivity, memory or concentration difficulties, irritability, sleep disturbances, or depression, may persistent for prolonged periods after a concussion. These constitute the postconcussive syndrome (PCS). For many years, it was believed that the PCS was psychosomatic, but functional imaging and sophisticated neuropsychometric testing have documented abnormalities, confirming a pathophysiologic basis for PCS [37]. Patients who suffer with a headache, nausea, or dizziness immediately after concussion seem to have an increased likelihood of having PCS.

Disposition of patients with concussion

With regard to neuroimaging and disposition, the management decisions faced by the EP for patients with concussion are identical to those for patients with minor head injury. In addition, the EP may be encouraged by coaches, eager parents, and the concussed athletes themselves to allow return to play. From the ED standpoint, patients with a sports-related concussion probably should not be allowed to return to play from the ED even if they are symptom-free; if still symptom-free 1 week after the impact, their primary care physician may clear them to return to play. Subsequently, all concussed patients may suffer from PCS, regardless of a benign examination on ED presentation, and it is advisable to suggest scheduled primary care follow-up for reassessment if PCS occurs.

Update on the management of severe and moderate traumatic brain injury

Moderate traumatic brain injury: clinical features and acute management

Patients with moderate TBI have a GCS score of 9 to 13. Their clinical presentation can vary widely. Patients may have had LOC, a brief posttraumatic seizure, and be confused, but most patients can follow commands on arrival to the ED. Facial and other systematic trauma often is present. Patients may complain of a worsening headache and nausea. Focal neurologic deficits may be present.

The EP needs to be especially aware of one specific presentation of moderate TBI: the "talk-and-deteriorate" patient. The talk-and-deteriorate patient is able to talk initially, but deteriorates to a GCS score consistent with severe TBI within 48 hours [38]. Approximately 75% of talk-and-deteriorate patients have an extra-axial hematoma, either subdural or epidural. If the extra-axial hematomas are detected early and treated rapidly, these patients have excellent clinical outcomes; however, if the talk-and-deteriorate patient presents initially with a GCS score of nine or greater and later deteriorates to having a GCS score of 8 or less, they have a worse outcome than those who presented originally with severe TBI (GCS score < 8) [38]. The key to the successful management of talk-and-deteriorate patients, as well as patients who have sustained moderate TBI in general, involves close clinical observation for subtle mental status changes or focal neurologic findings, liberal use of CT scanning, and early neurosurgical intervention. If a patient presenting with moderate TBI deteriorates in an ED in which no neurosurgeon is available and develops findings consistent with herniation syndrome, immediate intervention with brief hyperventilation and osmotic therapy should be initiated. If this does not halt or reverse the neurologic decline, consideration should be given for ED trephination and hematoma evacuation before emergency medical services (EMS) transfer to a trauma center for definitive care [39].

Disposition

All patients with moderate TBI should undergo CT scanning and be admitted for observation, even with an apparently normal CT scan. Most patients who have sustained moderate TBI improve significantly over several days [40,41]. Neurologic checks should be performed frequently during their in-house observation. If the patient's condition does not improve, a repeat CT scan should be performed within 12 to 24 hours.

Severe traumatic brain injury: clinical features and acute management

Most authorities define severe TBI as a patient who presents acutely with a GCS score of 8 or less. Furthermore, any intracranial contusion, hematoma, or brain laceration falls within the category of severe TBI.

Approximately 10% of all patients who have sustained TBI and who arrive at the ED alive have severe TBI [3,4]. Several factors, such as pupillary responsiveness, patient age, associated medical conditions, initial motor examination, and the presence of prolonged secondary brain or systemic insult affect the patient's prognosis [22,42,43]. It is estimated that 25% of all patients who sustain severe TBI eventually have lesions that require neurosurgical intervention [22]. The mortality of adult patients who sustain severe TBI is approximately 60% [3,4]; the mortality for children who sustain severe TBI is lower [42]. Most adult survivors of severe TBI suffer from severe disability. Children older than 1 year of age have improved neurologic outcomes following severe TBI when compared with adults [42,44].

Cushing's reflex or Cushing's phenomenon is an acute clinical entity that may occur during the ED resuscitation of the patient who has sustained severe TBI. This phenomenon includes three clinical signs: severe progressive hypertension, bradycardia, and diminished or irregular respiratory effort. Cushing's reflex is associated with significant increases in ICP and impending herniation syndrome. The full triad of clinical signs is seen in only one third of cases of life-threatening increased ICP [40]. The presence of Cushing's phenomenon should prompt immediate aggressive ICP management, including hyperventilation and maximal osmotic therapy.

The acute ED management of severe head injury is directed at reducing secondary injuries and expediting a definitive diagnosis and management strategy.

A stepwise approach is described below.

Management of airway

Patients who have sustained a severe head injury require airway management. Rapid sequence intubation (RSI) is effective and the preferred method for securing the airway, especially if patients who have sustained TBI are combative or agitated.

Treat hypotension

Hypotension is a terminal event in TBI, and patients who are hypotensive solely from TBI likely will have clinical evidence of herniation. Therefore, unless a patient who has sustained severe TBI is herniating, hypotension must be considered to be from another source. Systemic hypotension severely worsens outcome in patients who have experienced severe TBI [19]; aggressive fluid resuscitation should be initiated to achieve a systolic blood pressure greater than 90 mm Hg. Fluids and blood products will not increase ICP in a hypotensive patient who has sustained TBI. As many as 60% of patients with severe head injury have sustained multiple trauma [43], and vigilance must be maintained to search for other systematic injuries that may be responsible for observed hypotension.

Acute short-term hyperventilation

Acute hyperventilation is a life-saving intervention that can prevent or delay herniation in the patient who has experienced a severe TBI. The goal is to reduce the P_{CO_2} to the range of 30 to 35 mm Hg. Hyperventilation will reduce ICP by causing cerebral vasoconstriction; the onset of effect is within 30 second [40]. Hyperventilation decreases the ICP by about 25% in most patients; if the patient does not respond to this acute intervention rapidly, the prognosis for survival generally is poor. Prolonged hyperventilation is not recommended because it may cause profound vasoconstriction and ischemia. Prophylactic hyperventilation also is not recommended. Hyperventilation should be viewed as a short-term life-saving intervention and should be used in the ED only when a patient who has sustained severe TBI experiences a neurologic decline or demonstrates signs consistent with herniation.

Consider an osmotic agent

If the patient is not responding to intubation and acute hyperventilation and there is significant concern for a space-occupying extra-axial hematoma or immediate herniation, the use of osmotic diuretics, such as mannitol or HTS, should be considered. With deepening coma, pupil inequality, or other deterioration of the neurologic examination, osmotic agents may be lifesaving. The Brain Trauma Foundation and the European Brain Injury Consortium recommend mannitol as the osmotic drug of choice [45]; however, many institutions and leading experts in TBI are using HTS as an alternative to mannitol. The dose for mannitol is 0.25 to 1 g/kg. Mannitol reduces cerebral edema by creating an osmotic gradient that promotes fluid transfer from the tissues into the vascular space. The osmotic effects occur within minutes and peak about 60 minutes after bolus administration. The ICP-lowering effects of a single bolus of mannitol may last for 6 to 8 hours [46,47].

HTS at concentrations ranging from 3.1% to 23% have been used to treat patients who have sustained TBI and have elevated ICPs [45]. HTS causes plasma volume expansion, reduction of vasospasm, and diminished posttraumatic inflammatory response. HTS seems to be most beneficial in pediatric TBI and cerebral edema [45]; data in adults are sparse and not conclusive.

Seizure prophylaxis

Posttraumatic seizures occur in as many as 12% of all patients sustaining blunt head trauma and 50% of those with penetrating head injury [19]. Posttraumatic seizures do not predict epilepsy, but early seizures can worsen secondary brain injury by causing hypoxia, hypercarbia, the release of excitatory neurotransmitters, and increased ICP. The prophylactic use of antiepileptic drugs in acute TBI was reported to reduce the risk for early seizures by 66% [48]; however, early seizure prophylaxis does not prevent late posttraumatic seizures. The goal of emergency antiepileptic therapy is to prevent additional insult caused by seizures to the damaged brain [48,49].

Benzodiazepines are rapid-acting, first-line anticonvulsants. Lorazepam (0.05 to 0.15 mg/kg intravenously [IV], every 5 minutes up to a total of 4 mg) is most effective at aborting status epilepticus [50]. An alternative is diazepam (0.1 mg/kg, up to 5 mg IV, every 5 minutes up to a total of 20 mg). For long-term anticonvulsant activity, phenytoin (13 to 18 mg/kg IV) or fosphenytoin (13 to 18 phenytoin equivalents/kg) can be given.

Neuroimaging and early neurosurgical involvement

In the ED, a noncontrast CT scan of the head is the imaging modality of choice for patients with TBI [51]. A head CT will determine if acute traumatic lesions are present and direct subsequent management. In addition to intracranial and extra-axial lesions, skull fractures, including basilar fractures, can be detected with the bone windows of the CT. Plain skull radiographs generally are not indicated for patients who have sustained moderate or severe TBI.

Common extra-axial hematomas

Epidural hematoma

Epidural hematomas (EDHs) predominately are a result of a direct mechanical force that results in a skull fracture. Most often, this fracture occurs across the middle meningeal artery or a dural sinus. The temporoparietal region is the most likely site for an EDH. EDH is primarily a disease of the young and accounts for 0.5% to 1% of all patients who have experienced TBI [40]. Most often unilateral, the deterioration of a patient who has an EDH from arterial bleeding can be rapid and dramatic. EDHs are rare in elders and children younger than 2 years because of the close attachment of the dura to the skull in both patient populations.

Although many clinicians associate an EDH with a subsequent "lucid interval," this classic presentation only occurs approximately 30% of the time [52]. The development of symptoms and signs of EDH are entirely dependent on how quickly the EDH is developing within the cranial vault. The radiographic findings of EDH on noncontrast head CT scans include a biconvex or lenticular hyperdense lesion. Margins are sharp, and the hematoma frequently compresses the brain parenchyma toward the midline. The most common site of EDH is the temporal-parietal region (Fig. 5).

Recent studies have investigated the indications for immediate operative intervention for EDHs. Epidurals greater than 30 cm^3 in volume should be evacuated surgically, regardless of the patient's GCS score. Furthermore, it is strongly recommended that comatose patients with an acute EDH and anisocoria on papillary examination undergo surgical evacuation as soon as possible [53].

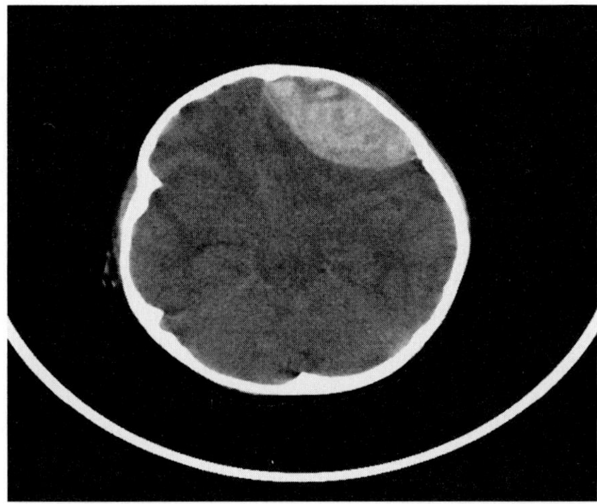

Fig. 5. Noncontrast head CT showing a large mixed-density EDH located in the left frontal hemisphere.

Subdural hematoma

Subdural hematomas (SDHs) are caused frequently by acceleration-deceleration injuries, such as a motor vehicle accident or a fall onto a hard surface. The clinical presentation of an SDH can vary, depending on the patient's age, the presence of multisystem injuries, or the presence of altered mental status from a nontraumatic cause (eg, alcohol or drug intoxication). The blood clot of an SDH forms between dura mater and brain. Because of the constant and slow increase in pressure as the SHD expands, it often causes extensive parenchyma tissue injury surrounding the site of the clot.

SDHs are much more common than EDHs and are present in between 12% and 29% of patients who have sustained a severe TBI [54]. SDH is common in elder patients, most often as the result of a fall.

Most patients with an SDH present with a GCS score less than 8. Approximately 12% to 38% of patients will have a lucid period at some point in their presentation [55,56]. The overall mortality of patients who have an SDH and require surgical intervention is between 40% and 60% [54]. Because of associated brain injury caused by the SDH, the delay in clinical signs and symptoms, and the more advanced mean age of the at-risk population, the mortality associated with SDH is much higher than that associated with EDH.

In children, the presence of an SDH should prompt consideration of child abuse. Many types of injury can produce SDH in children, but the infant who is shaken repeatedly and forcibly is especially susceptible. On examination, the infant may have a bulging fontanelle or an enlarged head circumference. A careful history may elicit long-standing constitutional symptoms, such as failure to thrive or lethargy.

On CT, SDHs appear hyperdense and hug the convexity of the brain with a crescent shape. They often extend beyond the suture lines, which is in contrast to EDH. Associated intraparenchymal lesions also are common (Fig. 6).

Current consensus guidelines [54] recommend that acute SDHs with a thickness greater than 10 mm or a midline shift of more than 5 mm on CT should be evacuated surgically, regardless of the patient's GCS score. Research indicates that the longer the time between clinical worsening and operative treatment, the worse the patient's clinical outcome [54,57]; in these cases, surgical evacuation should be performed as soon as possible.

Controversies in severe and moderate traumatic brain injury

Prehospital intubations and traumatic brain injury

Controversy exists regarding prehospital intubations in patients with severe and moderate head injuries. It is unclear if field intubations truly improve neurologic outcome or survival. Unsuccessful attempts at field intubations may add to out-of-hospital time and increase the risk for aspiration or hypoxia.

It has long been a tenet in prehospital care that patients who have sustained a severe head injury need necessary airway interventions to prevent hypoxia. Hypoxia and hypotension have been found to worsen patient outcome in TBI [19,58]. In 1997, Winchell and Hoyt [59] showed that patients who had sustained severe head injuries and who were intubated in the prehospital setting had an improved survival compared with those

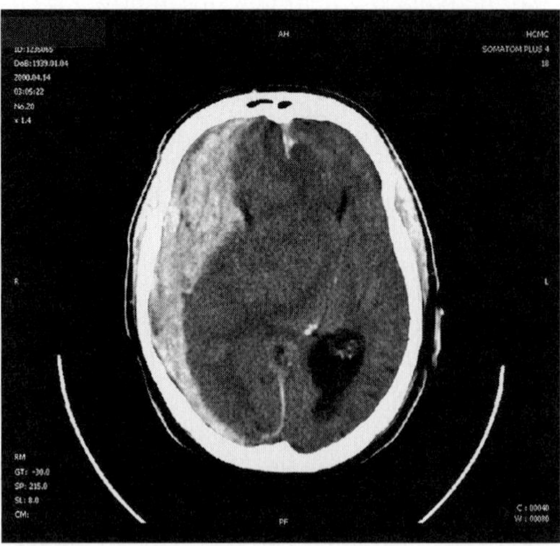

Fig. 6. Large mixed-density right-sided SDH with significant midline shift. The obliteration of the lateral ventricle also has occurred.

who were not intubated; however, since that time, research by Davis and colleagues [60,61] out of San Diego and Wang and colleagues [62] at the University of Pittsburgh challenged the routine practice of prehospital intubation of patients who had experienced TBI. Davis and colleagues [21,60,61,63–66] have published several papers on prehospital intubation as part of the San Diego paramedic RSI trial. These trials included patients who had severe head injuries. Using a matched historical control research design [67], they found a significant increase in mortality and morbidity in patients who sustained severe head injuries and underwent prehospital RSI. Potential explanations included frequent hypoxic episodes with associated bradycardia, unintentional hyperventilation, and prolonged scene times for those undergoing prehospital RSI.

Wang and colleagues [62], using Pennsylvania trauma registry data, found a fourfold increase in mortality in patients who sustained TBI with ground ambulance intubation compared with ED intubation. Curiously, their research found flight clinician intubation of severe head injury was associated with decreased mortality and improved neurologic outcome. This last finding may indicate that the higher airway management training requirements of air medical programs have a positive impact on the clinical outcome of patients with severe head injuries.

Several important concerns have been raised regarding these studies. First, Davis's research group was working with a large paramedic service that received RSI training only once during the course of the study. Second, Davis and colleagues' research was done with paramedics performing RSI. Most EMS in the United States do not use neuromuscular blocking agents to facilitate endotracheal intubation. Last, Wang and colleagues' research used a static measure of trauma, the abbreviated injury scale score, to categorize TBI and used a nonvalidated neurologic outcome measure. Regardless of these concerns, the research by Davis and colleagues [60,66,67] and Wang and colleagues [62] should prompt medical directors of EMS to reevaluate current clinical care protocols and training techniques.

A definitive answer on the value of prehospital intubation for patients who have sustained severe TBI is unavailable at this time. More research is needed and will occur in this key area of emergency care. Although hypoxia has been shown to worsen outcome after severe TBI, the research presented above does not give a clear picture of the best field management of the airway of the patient who has experienced a head injury. Clearly, when an airway is at risk, intubation should occur. When this is done for patients who have sustained TBI, however, it is essential to consider those factors that are suspected to worsen outcome: frequent hypoxic episodes during intubation, with or without concurrent bradycardia; unintentional hyperventilation of intubated patients; prolonged scene times because of the time demands of the intubation process; and persistent hypotension, likely from other injuries that go unattended while the airway management occurs.

Hypertonic saline

The continual pursuit of improving outcomes in severe and moderate TBI has resulted in renewed interest in HTS for control of ICP. Mannitol has been the mainstay for control of elevated ICP in the acute severe head injury for decades. Despite mannitol being considered a standard, little comparative data exist on mannitol and other ICP lowering medications [68]. A recent Cochrane database review [68] concluded that high-dose mannitol may be more beneficial than conventional-dose mannitol in the acute management of severe TBI. The Brain Trauma Foundation and the European Brain Injury Consortium recommend mannitol as the osmotic drug of choice [45].

An ideal osmotic agent to be used in TBI should be nontoxic with minimal systemic side effects, yet exert a strong transendothelial osmotic gradient. Mannitol has many of these characteristics. Its benefits are derived from three factors: cardiac output is increased, resulting in better CPP and cerebral oxygenation; diuresis and dehydration occur secondary to an increased osmotic load; and CSF production is decreased. Its limitations include hyperosmolality, occasional hypotension from excessive osmotic diuresis, and concern that mannitol crystals accumulate in cerebral tissue and can cause subsequent rebound intracranial hypertension.

HTS has been used for severe TBI since 1919 [69]. Human and animal studies have demonstrated that HTS can reduce ICP significantly [70–72]. HTS is being used increasingly in clinical practice, with reported improved control of intracranial hypertension [45,70,72,73]; however, fewer than 300 patients have been enrolled in all clinical trials that have used HTS [45]. Much of the clinical research on HTS involves children. Few patients have been studied using a prospective, randomized, control study design. Complicating the interpretation of these findings is a variation in protocols regarding HTS concentration and administration when used to reduce ICP in patients who have experienced TBI.

The most encouraging clinical data come from the pediatric patients who have sustained TBI. Most institutions that have adopted HTS as a first-line therapy for intracranial hypertension use a continuous infusion of 3% normal saline [74]. Potential adverse events that have been associated with HTS include renal failure, central pontine myelinoysis, and rebound ICP elevation [45].

The clinical studies using HTS for acute resuscitation of severe TBI are vexing. Early research by Vassar and colleagues [75] and Wade and colleagues [76–82], using a post hoc analysis of trauma data, seemed promising for HTS and TBI. Recent work by Cooper and colleagues [70] showed no improvement in ICP and CPP with HTS versus lactated Ringer's in hypotensive patients who had a head injury. Morbidity and mortality outcome data were equal in both groups. The investigators concluded that there was no advantage for the prehospital use of HTS compared with Ringer's lactate solution [70].

In summary, animal and human data clearly show that HTS expeditiously decreases intercranial pressures. Case studies in pediatric patients in the ICU support the use of HTS as an osmotic agent, without an increase in complications. Current human clinical data are inconclusive with regard to primary patient outcome measures, such as reduced morbidity and mortality. Many centers seem to be using HTS as a therapeutic adjunct alternative to mannitol while awaiting more definitive data.

Recombinant factor VIIa

Considerable interest has developed over the use of rFVIIa in intracerebral and extra-axial hemorrhages. rFVIIa is a hemostatic agent that originally was developed to treat bleeding in hemophiliacs. A single, appropriate dose of rVIIa for a 70-kg individual can exceed $4500 [83]. The total cost can approach $20,000, depending on the treatment protocol. Use of rVIIa should be individualized and made in concert with an institution's treatment protocol.

References

[1] Hippocratic writings. In: Lloyd GER, editor. London: Penguin Group; 1978.
[2] Sosin D, Sniezek J, Waxweiler R. Trends in death associated with traumatic brain injury, 1979–1992. JAMA 1995;273:1778–80.
[3] Jager TE, Weiss HB, Coben JH, et al. Traumatic brain injuries evaluated in U.S. emergency departments, 1992–1994. Acad Emerg Med 2000;7(2):134–40.
[4] Kraus J, McArthur D. Epidemiology of brain injury. In: Cooper P, Golfinos J, editors. Head injury. 4th edition. New York: McGraw-Hill Publishers; 2000. p. 1–26.
[5] Greenwald BD, Burnett DM, Miller MA. Congenital and acquired brain injury. 1. Brain injury: epidemiology and pathophysiology. Arch Phys Med Rehabil 2003;84(3 Suppl 1):S3–7.
[6] Teasdale G, Jennett B. Assessment of coma and impaired consciousness. A practical scale. Lancet 1974;2(7872):81–4.
[7] Chesnut RM. The management of severe traumatic brain injury. Emerg Med Clin North Am 1997;15(3):581–604.
[8] Heegaard W, Biros M. Head injury. In: Marx J, Hockberger R, Walls R, editors. Rosen's emergency medicine. 6th edition. Philadelphia: Mosby Elsevier; 2006. p. 349–82.
[9] Graham D, Gennarelli T. Pathology of brain damage after head injury. In: Cooper P, Golfinos J, editors. Head injury. 4th edition. New York: McGraw-Hill; 2000. p. 133–54.
[10] Rockswold G. Head injury. In: Tintanelli J, editor. Emergency medicine. New York: McGraw-Hill; 1996. p. 913–21.
[11] Zwienenberg M, Muizellar J. Vascular aspects of severe head injury. In: Miller L, Hayes R, editors. Head trauma: basic, preclinical and clinical directions. 1st edition. New York: Wiley-Liss; 2001. p. 303–26.
[12] Reivech M. Arterial Pco_2 and cerebral hemodynamics. Am J Physiol 1964;206:25.
[13] Laffey JG, Kavanagh BP. Hypocapnia. N Engl J Med 2002;347(1):43–53.
[14] Muizelaar JP, Marmarou A, Ward JD, et al. Adverse effects of prolonged hyperventilation in patients with severe head injury: a randomized clinical trial. J Neurosurg 1991;75(5): 731–9.
[15] Kellie G. An account of the appearances observed in the dissection of two of the three individuals presumed to have perished in the storm of the third, and his bodies were discovered in

the vicinity of Leith on the morning of the 4th November 1821 with some reflections on the pathology of the brain. Trans Med Chir Sci (Edinburgh) 1824;1:84–169.
[16] Monro A. Observation on the structure and function of the nervous system. Edinburgh (Scotland): Creek and Johnson; 1783.
[17] Marmarou A, Signoretti S, Fatouros PP, et al. Predominance of cellular edema in traumatic brain swelling in patients with severe head injuries. J Neurosurg 2006;104(5): 720–30.
[18] Cernak I. Recent advances in neuroprotection for treating traumatic brain injury. Expert Opin Investig Drugs 2006;15(11):1371–81.
[19] Bullock MR, Chesnut RM, Clifton GL, et al. The Brain Foundation and American Association of Neurological Surgeons. Guidelines for the management of severe traumatic brain injury. J Neurotrauma 2000;17:471–8.
[20] Wilberger J. Emergency care and initial evaluation. In: Cooper R, Golfino J, editors. Head injury. New York: McGraw-Hill Publishers; 2000. p. 63–132.
[21] Davis DP, Ochs M, Hoyt DB, et al. Paramedic-administered neuromuscular blockade improves prehospital intubation success in severely head-injured patients. J Trauma 2003; 55(4):713–9.
[22] Cruz J. Severe acute brain trauma. In: Cruz J, editor. Neurologic and neurosurgical emergencies. Philadelphia: Saunders; 1998. p. 405–36.
[23] Servadei F, Teasdale G, Merry G. Defining acute mild head injury in adults: a proposal based on prognostic factors, diagnosis, and management. J Neurotrauma 2001;18(7):657–64.
[24] Narayan R. Closed head injury. In: Rengachary SS, Ellenbogen RG, editors. Principles of neurosurgery. London: Wolfe; 1994. p. 235–92.
[25] Ingebrigtsen T, Romner B. Routine early CT-scan is cost saving after minor head injury. Acta Neurol Scand 1996;93(2–3):207–10.
[26] Arienta C, Caroli M, Balbi S. Management of head-injured patients in the emergency department: a practical protocol. Surg Neurol 1997;48(3):213–9.
[27] Haydel MJ, Preston CA, Mills TJ, et al. Indications for computed tomography in patients with minor head injury. N Engl J Med 2000;343(2):100–5.
[28] Stiell IG, Wells GA, Vandemheen K, et al. The Canadian CT Head Rule for patients with minor head injury. Lancet 2001;357(9266):1391–6.
[29] MacLaren RE, Ghoorahoo HI, Kirby NG. Skull X-ray after head injury: the recommendations of the Royal College of Surgeons Working Party report in practice. Arch Emerg Med 1993;10(3):138–44.
[30] Sports-related recurrent brain injuries–United States. MMWR Morb Mortal Wkly Rep 1997;46(10):224–7.
[31] McCrea M, Guskiewicz KM, Marshall SW, et al. Acute effects and recovery time following concussion in collegiate football players: the NCAA Concussion Study. JAMA 2003; 290(19):2556–63.
[32] Shaw N. The neurophysiology of concussion: progress in neurobiology. Philadelphia: Elsevier; 2002.
[33] Bergsneider M, Hovda DA, Lee SM, et al. Dissociation of cerebral glucose metabolism and level of consciousness during the period of metabolic depression following human traumatic brain injury. J Neurotrauma 2000;17(5):389–401.
[34] Chen SH, Kareken DA, Fastenau PS, et al. A study of persistent post-concussion symptoms in mild head trauma using positron emission tomography. J Neurol Neurosurg Psychiatr 2003;74(3):326–32.
[35] McCrory P. Does second impact syndrome exist? Clin J Sport Med 2001;11(3):144–9.
[36] Harmon KG. Assessment and management of concussion in sports. Am Fam Physician 1999;60(3):887–92, 894.
[37] De Kruijk JR, Leffers P, Menheere PP, et al. Prediction of post-traumatic complaints after mild traumatic brain injury: early symptoms and biochemical markers. J Neurol Neurosurg Psychiatr 2002;73(6):727–32.

[38] Rockswold GL, Pheley PJ. Patients who talk and deteriorate. Ann Emerg Med 1993;22(6): 1004–7.
[39] Mahoney BD, Rockswold GL, Ruiz E, et al. Emergency twist drill trephination. Neurosurgery 1981;8(5):551–4.
[40] Greenberg M. Handbook of neurosurgery. Lakeland (FL): Greenberg Graphics; 1997.
[41] Colohan AR, Oyesiku NM. Moderate head injury: an overview. J Neurotrauma 1992;(9 Suppl 1):S259–64.
[42] Feickert HJ, Drommer S, Heyer R. Severe head injury in children: impact of risk factors on outcome. J Trauma 1999;47(1):33–8.
[43] Siegel JH. The effect of associated injuries, blood loss, and oxygen debt on death and disability in blunt traumatic brain injury: the need for early physiologic predictors of severity. J Neurotrauma 1995;12(4):579–90.
[44] Weiner H, Weinberg J. Head injury in the pediatric age group. In: Cooper P, Golfinos J, editors. Head injury. 4th edition. New York: McGraw-Hill; 2000. p. 419–56.
[45] White H, Cook D, Venkatesh B. The use of hypertonic saline for treating intracranial hypertension after traumatic brain injury. Anesth Analg 2006;102(6):1836–46.
[46] Gaab MR, Hollerhage HG, Walter GF, et al. Brain edema, autoregulation, and calcium antagonism. An experimental study with nimodipine. Adv Neurol 1990;52:391–400.
[47] Gaab MR, Seegers K, Smedema RJ, et al. A comparative analysis of THAM (Tris-buffer) in traumatic brain oedema. Acta Neurochir Suppl (Wien) 1990;51:320–3.
[48] Schierhout G, Roberts I. Anti-epileptic drugs for preventing seizures following acute traumatic brain injury. Cochrane Database Syst Rev 2001;4:CD000173.
[49] Chang BS, Lowenstein DH. Practice parameter: antiepileptic drug prophylaxis in severe traumatic brain injury: report of the Quality Standards Subcommittee of the American Academy of Neurology. Neurology 2003;60(1):10–6.
[50] Treiman DM, Meyers PD, Walton NY, et al. A comparison of four treatments for generalized convulsive status epilepticus. Veterans Affairs Status Epilepticus Cooperative Study Group. N Engl J Med 1998;339(12):792–8.
[51] Britt P, Heiserman J. Imaging evaluation. In: Cooper R, Golfino J, editors. Head injury. New York: McGraw-Hill; 2000. p. 27–62.
[52] Chiles B, Cooper P. Extra-axial hematomas. In: Loftus C, editor. Neurosurgical emergencies. Park Ridge (IL): AANS; 1994. p. 73–100.
[53] Bullock MR, Chesnut R, Ghajar J, et al. Surgical management of acute epidural hematomas. Neurosurgery 2006;58(Suppl 3):S7–15 [discussion: Si–iv].
[54] Bullock MR, Chesnut R, Ghajar J, et al. Surgical management of acute subdural hematomas. Neurosurgery 2006;58(Suppl 3):S16–24 [discussion: Si-iv].
[55] Wilberger JE Jr, Harris M, Diamond DL. Acute subdural hematoma: morbidity and mortality related to timing of operative intervention. J Trauma 1990;30(6):733–6.
[56] Wilberger JE Jr, Harris M, Diamond DL. Acute subdural hematoma: morbidity, mortality, and operative timing. J Neurosurg 1991;74(2):212–8.
[57] Seelig JM, Becker DP, Miller JD, et al. Traumatic acute subdural hematoma: major mortality reduction in comatose patients treated within four hours. N Engl J Med 1981;304(25): 1511–8.
[58] Chesnut RM, Marshall LF, Klauber MR, et al. The role of secondary brain injury in determining outcome from severe head injury. J Trauma 1993;34(2):216–22.
[59] Winchell RJ, Hoyt DB. Endotracheal intubation in the field improves survival in patients with severe head injury. Trauma Research and Education Foundation of San Diego. Arch Surg 1997;132(6):592–7.
[60] Davis DP, Peay J, Sise MJ, et al. The impact of prehospital endotracheal intubation on outcome in moderate to severe traumatic brain injury. J Trauma 2005;58(5):933–9.
[61] Davis DP, Vadeboncoeur TF, Ochs M, et al. The association between field Glasgow Coma Scale score and outcome in patients undergoing paramedic rapid sequence intubation. J Emerg Med 2005;29(4):391–7.

[62] Wang HE, Peitzman AB, Cassidy LD, et al. Out-of-hospital endotracheal intubation and outcome after traumatic brain injury. Ann Emerg Med 2004;44(5):439–50.
[63] Davis DP, Kimbro TA, Vilke GM. The use of midazolam for prehospital rapid-sequence intubation may be associated with a dose-related increase in hypotension. Prehosp Emerg Care 2001;5(2):163–8.
[64] Davis DP, Peay J, Serrano JA, et al. The impact of aeromedical response to patients with moderate to severe traumatic brain injury. Ann Emerg Med 2005;46(2):115–22.
[65] Davis DP, Serrano JA, Vilke GM, et al. The predictive value of field versus arrival Glasgow Coma Scale score and TRISS calculations in moderate-to-severe traumatic brain injury. J Trauma 2006;60(5):985–90.
[66] Davis DP, Stern J, Sise MJ, et al. A follow-up analysis of factors associated with head-injury mortality after paramedic rapid sequence intubation. J Trauma 2005;59(2):486–90.
[67] Davis DP, Hoyt DB, Ochs M, et al. The effect of paramedic rapid sequence intubation on outcome in patients with severe traumatic brain injury. J Trauma 2003;54(3):444–53.
[68] Wakai A, Roberts I, Schierhout G. Mannitol for acute traumatic brain injury. Cochrane Database Syst Rev 2005;4:CD001049.
[69] Weed L, McKibben P. Experimental alteration of brain bulk. Am J Physiol 1919;48:531–58.
[70] Cooper DJ, Myles PS, McDermott FT, et al. Prehospital hypertonic saline resuscitation of patients with hypotension and severe traumatic brain injury: a randomized controlled trial. JAMA 2004;291(11):1350–7.
[71] Peterson B, Khanna S, Fisher B, et al. Prolonged hypernatremia controls elevated intracranial pressure in head-injured pediatric patients. Crit Care Med 2000;28(4):1136–43.
[72] Vialet R, Albanese J, Thomachot L, et al. Isovolume hypertonic solutes (sodium chloride or mannitol) in the treatment of refractory posttraumatic intracranial hypertension: 2 mL/kg 7.5% saline is more effective than 2 mL/kg 20% mannitol. Crit Care Med 2003;31(6):1683–7.
[73] Bell SE, Hlatky R. Update in the treatment of traumatic brain injury. Curr Treat Options Neurol 2006;8(2):167–75.
[74] Adelson PD, Bratton SL, Carney NA, et al. Guidelines for the acute medical management of severe traumatic brain injury in infants, children, and adolescents. Chapter 11. Use of hyperosmolar therapy in the management of severe pediatric traumatic brain injury. Pediatr Crit Care Med 2003;4(Suppl 3):S40–4.
[75] Vassar MJ, Perry CA, Gannaway WL, et al. 7.5% sodium chloride/dextran for resuscitation of trauma patients undergoing helicopter transport. Arch Surg 1991;126(9):1065–72.
[76] Wade CE, Grady JJ, Kramer GC, et al. Individual patient cohort analysis of the efficacy of hypertonic saline/dextran in patients with traumatic brain injury and hypotension. J Trauma 1997;42(Suppl 5):S61–5.
[77] Boffard KD, Riou B, Warren B, et al. Recombinant factor VIIa as adjunctive therapy for bleeding control in severely injured trauma patients: two parallel randomized, placebo-controlled, double-blind clinical trials. J Trauma 2005;59(1):8–15 [discussion: 15–8].
[78] Dutton RP, Hess JR, Scalea TM. Recombinant factor VIIa for control of hemorrhage: early experience in critically ill trauma patients. J Clin Anesth 2003;15(3):184–8.
[79] Kenet G, Walden R, Eldad A, et al. Treatment of traumatic bleeding with recombinant factor VIIa. Lancet 1999;354(9193):1879.
[80] Mayer SA. Recombinant activated factor VII for acute intracerebral hemorrhage. Stroke 2007;38(Suppl 2):763–7.
[81] Stein DM, Dutton RP, O'Connor J, et al. Determinants of futility of administration of recombinant factor VIIa in trauma. J Trauma 2005;59(3):609–15.
[82] Thomas GO, Dutton RP, Hemlock B, et al. Thromboembolic complications associated with factor VIIa administration. J Trauma 2007;62(3):564–9.
[83] Levi M, Peters M, Buller HR. Efficacy and safety of recombinant factor VIIa for treatment of severe bleeding: a systematic review. Crit Care Med 2005;33(4):883–90.

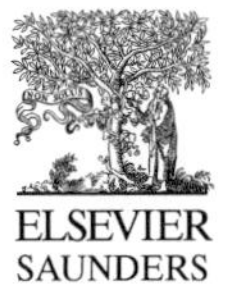

ELSEVIER
SAUNDERS

Emerg Med Clin N Am 25 (2007) 679–694

EMERGENCY
MEDICINE
CLINICS OF
NORTH AMERICA

Evaluation and Management of Neck Trauma

Niels K. Rathlev, MD*, Ron Medzon, MD, Mark E. Bracken, MD

Department of Emergency Medicine, Boston Medical Center, Boston University School of Medicine, One Boston Medical Center Place, Boston, MA 02118, USA

Blunt and penetrating trauma to the neck can result in life-threatening injuries that demand immediate attention and intervention on the part of the emergency physician and trauma surgeon. This article provides a literature-based update of the evaluation and management of injuries to aerodigestive and vascular organs of the neck. A brief review of cervical spine injuries related to penetrating neck trauma is also included. Airway injuries challenge even the most skilled practitioners; familiarity with multiple approaches to securing a definitive airway is required because success is not guaranteed with any single technique. Esophageal injuries often present in subtle fashion initially, but more than a 24-hour delay in diagnosis is associated with a marked increase in mortality. In total, 7% of injuries to critical structures of the neck involve major arterial vascular structures, including the subclavian and internal, external, and common carotid arteries [1]. Arterial injuries are a major source of morbidity and mortality for these patients. Currently, spinal cord injuries and thrombosis of the common and internal carotid arteries account for 50% of all deaths attributable to blunt and penetrating neck trauma.

Aerodigestive injuries

Epidemiology

Penetrating injuries to the airway and digestive tract are primarily caused by gunshot wounds and stab wounds. Wounds requiring operative repair are extremely rare. In one series of 12,789 consecutive trauma patients

* Corresponding author.
E-mail address: nrathlev@bu.edu (N.K. Rathlev).

doi:10.1016/j.emc.2007.06.006

over an 8-year period, only 12 (0.09%) patients had aerodigestive injuries [2]. Other studies place the injury rate closer to 5%. It is therefore difficult to conduct large-scale studies to determine optimal diagnostic and management decisions, and the existing literature reflects this.

Blunt trauma composes only about 5% of all neck trauma [3]. Aerodigestive injuries are rare but potentially life threatening and require a high index of suspicion to diagnose and treat properly. During a 9-year period (1988–1996) at one level 1 trauma center, 12,789 trauma patients were seen in the emergency department, of whom only 16 (0.13%) had tracheobronchial injuries [2]. Airway occlusion is the most immediately recognizable and rapidly fatal injury, but many other injuries to the aerodigestive tract present more insidiously and prove no less fatal.

The most common mechanism causing blunt trauma to the neck is the motor vehicle collision [4]. These injuries typically result from rapid acceleration and deceleration, or direct blow of the anterior neck on the steering column or dashboard crushing the trachea at the cricoid ring and compressing the esophagus against the cervical vertebrae. They can also occur from increased intrathecal pressure against a closed glottis from improper seat belt use [3].

Strangulation results from hanging, ligature suffocation, manual choking, and excessive manipulation. The usual mechanism of death in hangings occurs from pressure on the jugular veins, preventing venous return from the brain and backing blood up in the brain, resulting in a loss of consciousness. The now unconscious patient falls with all of his weight against the ligature, compressing the trachea and restricting airflow to the lungs. Irreversible asphyxiation follows in minutes [5]. Choke holds, no longer promoted in police training, typically generate greater force and injure by carotid artery occlusion or carotid body reflex. Clothesline injuries occur in sports (football tackle, martial arts), all-terrain vehicles, motorcycles, and snowmobiles. Direct blows by fists, feet, and other blunt weapons, and excessive cervical manipulation account for the remainder [6,7].

Clinical presentation

Any history that the patient is able to communicate about the mechanism of injury should be elicited. If the patient arrives by emergency medical services they should have information, as may friends or family who come with the patient. Clinical symptoms range from patients who have no symptoms to those who have life-threatening airway compromise or profound shock.

Penetrating injuries to the airway may present with dyspnea, hoarseness, and cough. Conversely, progressive airway obstruction from an external source, such as an expanding hematoma, often presents with abnormal respiratory patterns, stridor, dysphonia, tachypnea, or cyanosis. In 1985, Kelly and colleagues published a 20-year study that examined 106 consecutive patients who had neck trauma (100 penetrating and 6 blunt); all 80 patients who had tracheal injuries had signs of airway compromise in the emergency department. These signs included tachypnea, dyspnea, cyanosis, subcutaneous emphysema, and an abnormal respiratory pattern. Hemoptysis was an unreliable sign of serious injury and patients who had major vascular or tracheal injuries rarely survived [8]. Other investigators have found that breathing difficulties may not be present initially. Other presenting features include voice alteration, stridor, drooling, cervical subcutaneous emphysema, or crepitation, dyspnea, and distortion of the anatomy of anterior neck, including loss of normal landmarks, asymmetry, flattened thyroid prominence, and tracheal deviation [9].

The evaluation of blunt neck trauma begins with the airway. Greene [10] evaluated the clinical signs of laryngeal fracture according to anatomic location. Injuries above the glottis presented with cervical emphysema, progressive airway obstruction, palpable thyroid cartilage disruption, dysphagia, and hoarseness. Although injuries located below the glottis were not associated with swallowing difficulties and did not have early signs of airway compromise, they did present with hemoptysis and persistent air leak from the endotracheal tube in intubated patients [10].

Early detection of penetrating esophageal injuries remains difficult. The average delay to diagnosis from time of injury is usually many hours when using a selective approach, and the resultant morbidity and mortality are significant [11,12]. Although more than 90% of patients survive if the injury is detected within 24 hours, the survival rate drops precipitously after this time, usually from infectious complications, such as mediastinitis. Clinical findings of dysphagia, odynophagia, drooling, and hematemesis are approximately 80% sensitive for injury [10]. Clinical signs of esophageal injury are infrequently present, although crepitus in the neck or a sucking neck wound may be found on physical examination. Subcutaneous emphysema may be seen on plain radiographs.

Blunt esophageal injuries are uncommon. Dysphagia, blood in oral gastric and nasogastric aspirate, and crepitus are all sign of blunt esophageal rupture. In some cases there may be no initial signs of significant injury. This phenomenon is particularly relevant in the elderly population. Keogh and colleagues [13] describe two cases in which minor neck trauma caused significant airway compromise from delayed neck hematomas. Both patients were anticoagulated with warfarin.

Diagnostic evaluation

Penetrating injuries

Stable patients are approached from a selective set of criteria that are outlined in detail in Fig. 1. Lateral neck plain films and chest radiographs are useful initial tests. Subcutaneous emphysema is often the most common presenting sign in significant injury to the aerodigestive tracts [14]. In patients who have airway disruption, the surgical anatomy of the rupture creates

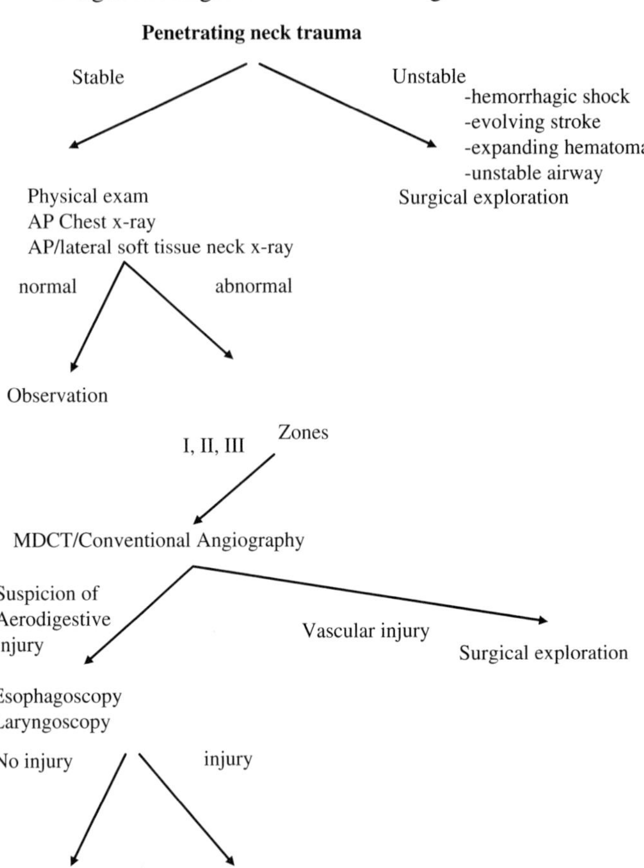

Fig. 1. Diagnostic algorithm for penetrating neck trauma.

predictable patterns of air leak on plain films. Patients who have laryngeal transection may have gross, deep, and superficial cervicofacial emphysema, whereas patients who have tracheal rupture often present with massive mediastinal and deep cervical emphysema without pneumothorax [15].

The improvement in speed and resolution of images by multidetector computed tomography (MDCT), including the 16-row multiplanar reconstructions, has had a significant impact on the adoption of selective management of penetrating neck injuries. CT can accurately identify extrapulmonary air, directly visualize tracheal wall disruption and signs of transtracheal balloon herniation in intubated patients, and locate extratracheal endotracheal tube position [16]. In cadaveric intubations with tracheal disruption, CT images closely match those compared with matched live cases, and equally good results comparing CT images to bronchoscopic images confirm the accuracy of CT. The reconstructions also help the surgeon to choose the optimal surgical approach. These studies also note that it takes an extreme amount of pressure to rupture the tracheal rings in cadavers, suggesting it would be unlikely for routine endotracheal balloon inflation during intubation to cause additional airway compromise in penetrating neck injuries [17,18].

Stable patients who have suspected airway injury should be evaluated with a combination of careful physical examination, plain films, CT, and bronchoscopy, depending on the institutional approach. Although three-dimensional (3D) reconstructive CT is extremely good at identifying and locating tracheal injuries, bronchoscopy must still be considered the gold standard test.

Barium swallow, flexible endoscopy, and rigid endoscopy all have sensitivities approaching 90%. In one study the combination of rigid endoscope and barium swallow found 100% of esophageal injuries [19]. MDCT may demonstrate free air in the neck caused by esophageal perforation or rupture (Fig. 2); however, this diagnostic modality cannot presently be considered a gold standard because large-scale studies have not been performed to measure its sensitivity for this potentially catastrophic entity. The combination of a barium swallow and endoscopy must be pursued if a high suspicion for esophageal perforation persists despite a negative MDCT.

Blunt injuries

Fig. 3 presents an approach for the diagnostic evaluation of blunt injuries. Imaging of the patient who has a blunt neck injury has evolved with the advent of high-resolution CT. Although lateral soft tissue neck

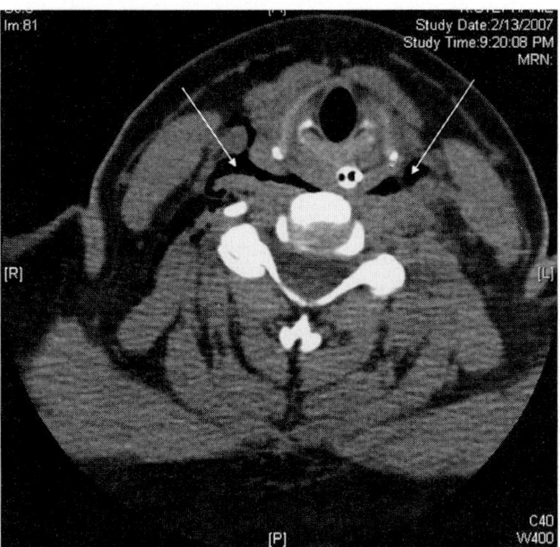

Fig. 2. Multidetector CT of the neck reveals free air adjacent to the esophagus secondary to a traumatic perforation (*arrows*).

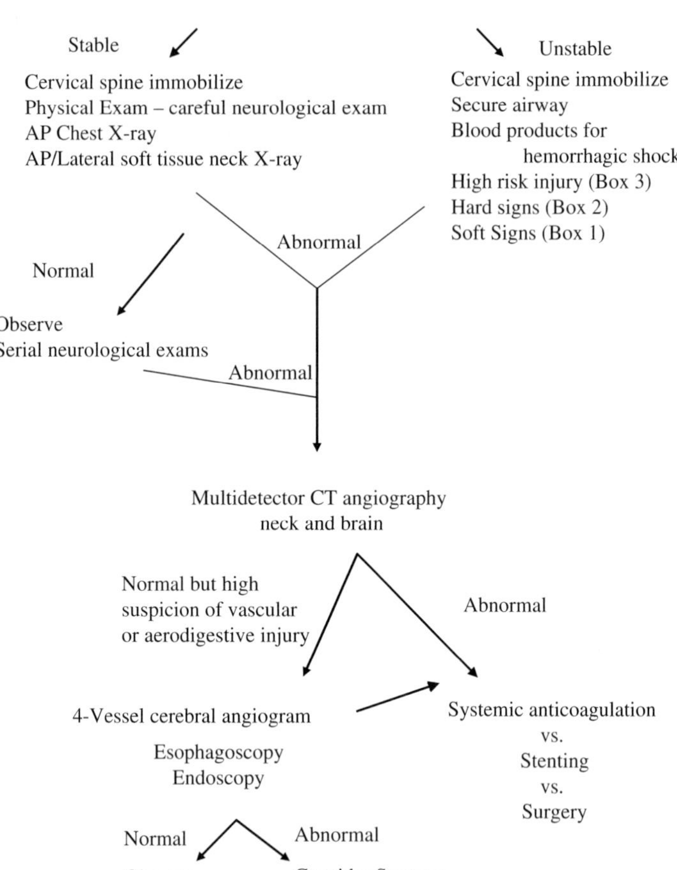

Fig. 3. Blunt neck trauma: vascular and aerodigestive injuries.

radiographs are rarely used exclusively to rule out aerodigestive injuries, significant injuries can be diagnosed reliably [15]. A chest radiograph remains a mainstay of the initial trauma workup in assessing for pneumothorax, hemothorax, and pneumomediastinum.

CT scanning is the initial imaging modality of choice in the hemodynamically stable patient and is used to guide selective operative management. Chen and colleagues [16] found that CT accurately diagnosed tracheal rupture with deep cervical air in intubated cadavers. Moriwaki studied 3-D reconstructed CT for diagnosing tracheal injury site. 3-D CT accurately identified the site of injury, as confirmed by bronchoscopy [17]. In conjunction with CT, panendoscopy ensures complete evaluation of aerodigestive injuries.

Schaefer and Brown [20] developed a classification system for laryngeal injuries based on a combination of CT scanning and endoscopy (Table 1).

Fiberoptic nasopharyngoscopy for a preliminary assessment of the extent of trauma and evaluation of vocal cord function, direct laryngoscopy for a detailed view of the larynx, bronchoscopy to examine the subglottic larynx, and esophagoscopy for evaluation of esophageal mucosa are all recommended in the workup of blunt neck trauma patients who have signs of injury. Additionally, barium swallow has been studied for esophageal injuries. Weigelt and colleagues [19] looked at 118 stable patients who had cervical trauma and compared barium swallow with endoscopy. All 10 esophageal injuries were identified when the two modalities were combined. water-soluble radiocontrast agent has replaced barium, but a swallow study alone does not rule out pharyngoesophageal leak. Before embarking on endoscopy, airway patency should be assessed and secured.

Management

Early and rapid airway assessment followed by definitive airway protection is the key to neck trauma management. The airway must be secured, and any hemorrhage must be staunched and replaced with blood products. These principles apply to penetrating and blunt neck injury. Most patients who have blunt neck trauma are wearing cervical spine collars that complicate the intubation. In-line cervical traction is a safe method for stabilizing the cervical spine during intubation. The optimal technique for intubating a patient who has penetrating neck injuries is by direct laryngoscopy, although it has not been studied at length. It is not clear when a patient should be observed expectantly for impending airway compromise or when the patient should be intubated to avoid a situation in which the anatomy becomes so distorted as to make the procedure more difficult or impossible leading to an emergent surgical airway. These remain clinical

Table 1
Management of laryngeal trauma

Group	Symptoms	Signs	Management
1	Minor airway symptoms	Minor hematoma, no fracture	Observation, humidified O_2
2	Airway compromise	Edema, mucosal disruption	Tracheostomy, direct laryngoscopy, esophagoscopy
3	Airway compromise	Massive edema, exposed cartilage, vocal cord immobility	Tracheostomy, exploration/repair
4	Airway compromise	Massive edema, exposed cartilage	Tracheostomy, exploration/repair, stent required

judgments. Clearly any patient in shock, with hypoxia, or with clear airway compromise needs immediate intubation.

It is safe to use rapid sequence intubation using a short-acting paralytic along with an induction agent. In the most recent series in the literature, 100% of 39 patients were successfully intubated using succinylcholine. In total, 12 patients underwent fiberoptic intubation by otolaryngology clinicians with 3 failures. Interestingly, those 3 patients were subsequently successfully intubated using rapid sequence intubation [21]. This example underscores the vital importance of the clinician using the technique with which he is most comfortable during emergent airway management. If the airway can be visualized through the traumatic wound because of tracheal disruption, it may be possible to intubate the trachea directly through the wound. A single case report describes the use of the gum elastic bougie to facilitate the intubation of a patient who had a self-induced deep slash wound to zone II and complete tracheal transection. When blind intubation failed, the bougie was used to intubate the trachea, the tracheal rings caused the typical clicking to confirm the bougie's location, and the endotracheal tube was successfully placed into the trachea over the bougie [22].

There are numerous alternative intubation methods if direct laryngoscopy fails or cannot be used. Flexible fiberoptic endoscopes can be used for orotracheal and nasotracheal intubations. These techniques require patient preparation with topical anesthetics and often intravenous sedation, and are therefore time consuming and depend on the experience of the operator. Newer rigid fiberoptic endoscopes and videolaryngoscope blades may aid in finding the vocal cords for intubation, although all of the fiberoptic methods are difficult to use in the presence of bleeding or heavy secretions.

Blind nasotracheal intubation historically has been discouraged because of a perceived high failure rate and potential for complications. A recent study of 40 patients intubated prehospital demonstrated a 90% success rate with a similar mortality rate to matched patients who were orotracheally intubated [23]. It is reasonable to consider this a technique in the prehospital setting where emergency orotracheal intubation is not possible. A surgical airway may be used as a last resort. Cricothyrotomy, or occasionally tracheostomy, is the required procedure because of altered anatomy. There is a risk that the operator could open an otherwise stable hematoma while incising through fascial planes and obscure the operative field along with causing significant hemorrhage.

The wound should be examined with care for degree of penetration, although probing is discouraged because it may inadvertently open a hematoma that was otherwise not actively bleeding. Patients who have progressive subcutaneous or mediastinal emphysema, severe dyspnea requiring intubation, difficulty in mechanical ventilation, uncontrolled hemorrhage, or patients who have an air leak from their chest tubes should all be directed to the operating room for definitive surgical management [24].

Penetrating injuries to the cervical spine

There are no reports of unstable cervical spine injuries in penetrating neck trauma by stab wounds. It is a rare individual who may possess the strength and ferocity to fracture the vertebral column during such an attack, let alone to create an unstable fracture. Gunshot wounds to the neck would need to fracture the cervical vertebrae in two columns to create an unstable fracture. The bullet must traverse the spinal cord to cause this injury, and the patient presents with neurologic signs. A 14-year study of patients sustaining gunshot wounds to the face and neck showed that all patients who had unstable cervical spine fractures also presented with neurologic signs [25]. In this study, 3 awake and neurologically intact individuals presented with gunshot wounds to the face resulting in stable cervical spine fractures A prior series found no cervical spine injuries in 174 patients who had gunshot wounds to the head [26]. Based on these results, immediate urgent treatment of the penetrating neck wound should take precedence over concerns for the cervical spine, including removing a cervical collar to gain access to the injury. All patients who have gunshot wounds to the neck and face should subsequently have a CT of the bony cervical spine to look for occult fractures, and once the injury has been addressed the collar should be replaced until radiography definitively shows there is no fracture.

Direct laryngoscopy using a Macintosh or Miller laryngoscope blade causes minimal movement of the cervical spine in healthy patients positioned on a rigid board (10–11 degrees of movement) before intubation [27]. Patients who need to be intubated can be safely managed with in-line traction and care to keep movement of the neck to a minimum during the procedure.

Vascular injuries

Epidemiology

Most penetrating neck injuries are caused by knives and low-energy gunshot wounds. Fortunately, these weapons impart a low level of kinetic energy to tissues compared with military rifles and shotguns. The mortality rate from these injuries is approximately 2% to 6%. The victims are primarily young men who have injuries sustained as a result of interpersonal violence.

Significant vascular injuries of the neck occur in approximately 1% to 3% of all major blunt trauma victims [28–31]. High-speed motor vehicle accidents cause most of these injuries [32]. Other mechanisms include motorcycle crashes, pedestrians struck by motor vehicles, falls, assaults, and hangings and near-hangings [33]. Although these injuries are rare, the morbidity and mortality rates are significantly higher than for penetrating trauma. The overall mortality related to blunt injuries is 20% to 30%; in addition, 37% to 58% of patients develop permanent neurologic deficits attributable to central nervous system ischemia [34].

In blunt trauma, injury to the cervical arteries is likely caused by rapid deceleration associated with hyperflexion, hyperextension, and rotation. Vascular structures are stretched over the cervical spine and shearing forces create intimal tears in the vessel wall [35]. Both blunt and penetrating vascular injuries result in the formation of pseudoaneurysm, dissection, arteriovenous fistula, complete transection, and thrombus formation with occlusion attributable to disruption of atherosclerotic plaque. Stroke in these patients is believed to be caused by occlusive thromboembolus. Compromise of collateral flow is presumably responsible for worse outcomes in patients who have atherosclerotic vascular disease [36].

Clinical presentation

The challenge for the emergency physician is to detect subtle but significant injuries that require intervention. This pertains specifically to patients who have no immediate indication for operative intervention because of airway compromise or hemodynamic instability. The presence of "hard signs" (Box 1) on physical examination indicates a high risk for vascular injury. Pulse deficit is not a sensitive indicator of significant injury because the pulses may be normal with nonocclusive injuries, such as an intimal flap or pseudoaneurysm, that nonetheless require surgical intervention. A bruit or thrill is pathognomonic of a traumatic arteriovenous fistula that typically needs surgical repair. "Soft" signs are less predictive of vascular injury and these are listed in Box 2. Central nervous system ischemia is considered a soft sign. A primary neurologic injury presents as an immediate deficit, whereas a neurologic injury caused by ischemia typically becomes evident over the course of minutes to hours. Proximity to a major vascular structure is not considered a high-risk feature in the absence of hard signs.

Blunt vascular injuries involving the carotid or the vertebral arteries are rare and the clinical presentation is often subtle and nonspecific. McKevitt documented that 60% of blunt cervical injuries were unsuspected at initial evaluation, and symptoms often were masked by concomitant head or thoracic injuries in multiple blunt trauma victims [36]. If identified and treated early, the likelihood of permanent devastating neurologic dysfunction is

Box 1. Hard signs of vascular injury

Bruit or thrill
Expanding or pulsatile hematoma
Pulsatile or severe hemorrhage
Pulse deficit

Box 2. Soft signs of vascular injury

Hypotension and shock
Stable, nonpulsatile hematoma
Central or peripheral nervous system ischemia
Proximity to a major vascular structure

decreased. The recognition of symptoms is typically delayed, and almost 25% of patients first develop signs and symptoms 24 hours postinjury. Often, the initial manifestation of a blunt vascular injury is an acute ischemic stroke attributable to a thromboembolic event.

The classic presentation is a neurologically intact victim who subsequently develops hemiparesis after a high-speed motor vehicle crash. There are no reliable clinical means with which to diagnose blunt carotid injury before development of neurologic deficits or stroke [37]. The vast majority of patients manifest neurologic deficits at the time of diagnosis of blunt carotid injury [28]. Definitive diagnostic testing should be pursued for patients who demonstrate any of the high-risk features listed in Box 3. With this approach, 72% of all blunt vascular injuries can be identified before the onset of neurologic deficits [34]. The incidence of blunt vascular injury in patients who have an ecchymosis from the shoulder seat belt is three times higher than the incidence in blunt trauma victims in general [31].

Vertebral artery injuries are associated closely with cervical spine injuries [33]. Some 33% of cervical spine fractures are associated with a vertebral artery injury after excluding simple spinous process fractures. Fractures involving the transverse foramen are present in 78% of these patients, whereas subluxation is associated with most of the remaining injuries. At

Box 3. High-risk criteria to for blunt cerebrovascular injuries

Severe hyperextension or flexion and rotation of neck
Significant soft tissue injury or large hematoma of the anterior neck
Cervical spine fracture
Seat belt sign across the neck
Massive epistaxis attributable to a carotid-cavernous sinus fistula,
Bruit or thrill
Stroke or transient ischemic attack
Unexplained neurologic abnormalities
Basilar skull fracture involving the petrous bone

least one of these bony injuries is present in 92% of patients who have vertebral artery injury. Bilateral injuries occur in approximately 15% of all patients [28,34]. Concurrent injuries are common; McKevitt and colleagues [36] found that almost 95% of patients who had blunt vascular injuries of the neck had a concomitant major thoracic injury or a Glasgow Coma Scale score less than 8.

Diagnostic evaluation

Conventional four-vessel cerebral angiogram remains the reference standard for evaluating the carotid and the vertebral arteries with a sensitivity in excess of 99%. It provides accurate assessment of the vessels with respect to the presence of dissection, pseudoaneurysm, occlusion, and transection. Rarely do injuries missed by angiography require repair and a normal study is highly predictive of survival from vessel injury [38,39]. Conversely, angiography is invasive, expensive, and resource intensive, and involves mobilizing interventional radiology. The complication rate is approximately 1%, usually involving the catheter insertion site or reactions to the intravenous contrast. Biffl and colleagues [35] developed a classification system for blunt carotid artery injuries based on the angiographic findings (Table 2). The system is successfully used to guide further management.

MDCT angiography has evolved as a sensitive, readily available, and less invasive diagnostic technique tool for the purpose of assessing patients at risk. In series of penetrating neck injuries, the sensitivity of MDCT angiography is 90% to 100% compared with conventional angiography and surgical exploration [40,41]. Most patients who meet screening criteria for blunt vascular injury currently undergo MDCT scanning for other reasons. Adding this technique to clinical evaluation reportedly increased the rate of identification of injuries by a factor of three, decreased the mean time to

Table 2
Denver grading scale for blunt carotid artery injury

Grade	Angiographic findings	Prognosis	Treatment
I	Vessel wall irregularity or dissection with <25% of luminal diameter	Good, 7% progress	Systemic anticoagulation controversial
II	Raised intimal flap, thrombus, dissection, or hematomas >25% of luminal diameter	Fair with treatment, 70% progress	Systemic anticoagulation
III	Pseudoaneurysm	Require intervention	Surgery or stenting
IV	Total vessel occlusion	Outcome assured at the time of diagnosis	Systemic anticoagulation
V	Transection	Very poor, high mortality	Surgery

Data from Biffl WL, Moore EE, Offner PJ, et al. Blunt carotid arterial injuries: implications of a new grading scale. J Trauma 1999;47:845–53.

diagnosis and decreased the rate of permanent neurologic sequelae from carotid arterial injuries [34]. In comparison with conventional angiography, MDCT angiography has a sensitivity of 68% and a specificity of 67%. MDCT angiography missed 55% of grade I injuries, 14% of grade II injuries, and 13% of grade III Injuries (see Table 2) [42]. The modality missed 53% of carotid injuries and 47% of vertebral injuries; approximately one third of the missed injuries were significant lesions, causing stroke in carotid distribution territory. Higher resolution, 64-slice technology will likely improve the sensitivity and specificity of MDCT angiography. The modality is limited by artifacts from metallic fragments and occasionally by abundant soft tissue air. In such cases, conventional angiography is required for optimal assessment.

Magnetic resonance angiography has shown some promise in assessing the presence for blunt vascular injury in patients who are hemodynamically stable and can undergo the procedure. Biffl and colleagues [43] demonstrated a sensitivity of 75% and specificity of 67%, magnetic resonance angiography compared with conventional angiography. Because of a marginal improvement in sensitivity over MDCT angiography, lack of routine availability and applicability to the acutely injured patient, magnetic resonance angiography is unlikely to become a routine screening tool for blunt vascular injuries of the neck.

Duplex ultrasonography is noninvasive, convenient, and low cost, but the sensitivity for vascular injury is highly operator dependent. In the hands of experienced technicians, the sensitivity of duplex ultrasound versus conventional angiography as the reference standard is 90% to 95% for injuries requiring intervention [44]. Duplex ultrasonography can miss nonocclusive injuries with preserved flow, such as intimal flaps and pseudoaneurysms. The technique is also limited by the ability to evaluate only the common carotid and external carotid arteries. Most injuries involve the internal carotid artery, which is not evaluated well by ultrasound.

Management

Definitive treatment is determined by the angiographic grading of vascular injury. In general, surgical repair is preferred over ligation except in the case of coma without antegrade flow. These cases are associated with a high risk for converting an ischemic to a hemorrhagic brain injury, uncontrollable hemorrhage, and inability to place a temporary shunt. Primary repair is preferred over graft placement when possible.

Surgical intervention for blunt injuries is an option for accessible lesions and includes resection, thrombectomy, and ligation of lesions involving the common or external carotid. Unfortunately, most blunt injuries involve the internal carotid artery, which is less accessible. Anticoagulation therapy has been instituted to reduce morbidity and mortality related to specific grades of injury to the carotid or vertebral arteries [33]. The grading system for these lesions proposed by Biffl and colleagues group these lesions into categories based on size, outcome, and treatment options for each (see Table 2). The rate of subsequent stroke in patients who were initially asymptomatic has been decreased by as much as 75% when systemic anticoagulation was instituted. These studies must be interpreted with caution, because a control group was not included. Some patients were also excluded because of coexisting traumatic injuries. Antiplatelet therapy has been used when concurrent injuries present a contraindication to systemic anticoagulation. Anticoagulation therapy also has proved to be beneficial in patients who have vertebral artery injuries. When treated with anticoagulation using heparin, aspirin, or aspirin and clopidogrel, neurologically intact patients who have early detection of blunt vertebral artery injury had a 0% incidence of stroke [34]. Other studies have similarly found that anticoagulation decreases the rate of neurologic morbidity in posterior circulation stroke [33].

Percutaneous angioplasty with stent placement after follow-up angiography has been used for the treatment of persistent blunt carotid injuries [45,46]. This intervention has raised concern regarding the danger of iatrogenic stroke and has yet to obtain wide acceptance [47,48]. Currently, it seems that the risks exceed the benefits, especially for carotid artery lesions.

Summary

Early airway management is crucial to successful management of severe penetrating and blunt neck injuries. Orotracheal intubation is the initial method of choice; however, no single method is successful 100% of the time. It is therefore crucial that practitioners are skilled in several different approaches to airway management, including providing a surgical airway. In patients who do not have obvious indications for operative intervention initially, evaluation for hard signs of vascular injury should be pursued. Hard signs include bruit, thrill, expanding or pulsatile hematoma, pulsatile or severe hemorrhage, pulse deficit, and central nervous system ischemia. A high degree of suspicion should be maintained for esophageal injury; unfortunately, radiographs do not exclude esophageal injury and triple endoscopy is the optimal diagnostic method for the evaluation of aerodigestive injury. The reference standard for vascular injury is conventional angiography. MDCT angiography is a noninvasive, less expensive, and more convenient alternative that is rapidly becoming the diagnostic tool of choice in the evaluation of cervical vascular injury caused by penetrating and blunt trauma.

References

[1] Carducci B, Lowe RA, Dalsey W. Penetrating neck trauma: consensus and controversies. Ann Emerg Med 1986;15:208–15.

[2] Huh J, Milliken JC, Chen JC. Management of tracheobronchial injuries following blunt and penetrating trauma. Am Surg 1997;63(10):896–9.

[3] Levy D. Neck Trauma, Emedicine. Available at: www.emedicine.com/emerg/topic331.htm. Accessed June 19, 2006:1–11.

[4] Britt LD, Peyser MB. Chapter 22: Trauma. 5th edition. 2004. p. 445–58.

[5] Hawley D. Violence: recognition, management, and prevention. A review of 300 attempted strangulation cases Part III: injuries in fatal cases. J Emerg Med 2001;21(3):317–22.

[6] Bernat RA. Combined laryngotracheal separation and esophageal injury following blunt neck trauma. Facial Plast Surg 2005;21(3):187–90.

[7] Shweikh AM, Nadkarni AB. Laryngotracheal separation with pneumopericardium after blunt trauma to the neck. Emerg Med J 2001;18:410–1.

[8] Kelly JP, Webb WR, Moulder PV, et al. Management of airway trauma. I: Tracheobronchial injuries. Ann Thorac Surg 1985;40(6):551–5.

[9] Goudy SL, Miller FB, Bumpous JM. Neck crepitance: evaluation and management of suspected upper aerodigestive tract injury. Laryngoscope 2002;112:791–5.

[10] Greene R, Stark P. Trauma of the larynx and trachea. Radiol Clin North Am 1978;16(2):309.

[11] Asensio JA, Berne J, Demetriades D, et al. Penetrating esophageal injuries: time interval of safety for preoperative evaluation—how long is safe? J Trauma 1997;43(2):319–24.

[12] Demetriades D, Theodorou E, Cornwell E, et al. Evaluation of penetrating injuries of the neck: prospective study of 223 patients. World J Surg 1997;21(1):41–8.

[13] Keogh IJ. Critical airway compromise caused by neck hematoma. Clin Otolaryngol 2002;27: 244–5.

[14] Gomez-Caro AA, Ausin HP, Moradiellos Diez FJ. Medical and surgical management of noniatrogenic traumatic tracheobronchial injuries. Arch Bronconeumol 2005;41(5):249–54.

[15] Spencer JA, Rogers CE, Westaby S. Clinico-radiological correlates in rupture of the major airways. Clin Radiol 1991;43(6):371–6.

[16] Chen JD, Shanmuganathan K, Mirvis SE, et al. Using CT to diagnose tracheal rupture. AJR 2001;176(5):1273–80.

[17] Moriwaki Y, Sugiyama M, Matsuda G, et al. Usefulness of the 3-dimensionally reconstructed computed tomography imaging for diagnosis of the site of tracheal injury (3D-tracheography). World J Surg 2005;29(1):102–5.

[18] Scaglione M, Romano S, Pinto A. Acute tracheobronchial injuries: impact of imaging on diagnosis and management implications. Eur J Radiol 2006;59(3):336–43.

[19] Weigelt JA, Thal ER, Snyder WH 3rd. Diagnosis of penetrating cervical esophageal injuries. Am J Surg 1987;154(6):619–22.

[20] Schaefer SD, Brown OE. Selective application of CT in the management of laryngeal trauma. Laryngoscope 1983;93:1473–5.

[21] Mandavia D, Qualls S, Rokos I. Emergency airway management in penetrating neck injury. Ann Emerg Med 2000;35(3):221–5.

[22] Scott JM, Lopez PP, Pierre E. Use of a gum elastic bougie (GEB) in a zone II penetrating neck trauma: a case report. J Emerg Med 2004;26(3):353–4.

[23] Weitzel N, Kendall J, Pons P. Blind nasotracheal intubation for patients with penetrating neck trauma. J Trauma 2004;56(5):1097–101.

[24] Gomez-Caro A, Ausin P, Moradiellos FJ. Role of conservative medical management of tracheobronchial injuries. J Trauma 2006;61(6):1426–34 [discussion: 1434–5].

[25] Medzon R, Rothenhaus T, Bono CM, et al. Stability of the cervical spine after gunshot wounds to the head and neck. Spine 2005;30(20):2274–9.

[26] Lanoix R, Gupta R, Leak L, et al. C-spine injury associated with gunshot wounds to the head: retrospective study and literature review. J Trauma 2000;49(5):860–3.

[27] Hastings RH, Duong H, Burton DW, et al. Cervical spine movements during laryngoscopy with the Bullard, Macintosh, and Miller laryngoscopes. Anesthesiology 1995;82(4):859–69.

[28] Fabian TC, Patton Jr. JH, Croce MA, et al. Blunt carotid injury: importance of early diagnosis and anticoagulant 1996;223:513–25.

[29] Kerwin AJ, Bynoe RP, Murray J, et al. Screening for blunt carotid and vertebral artery injuries is justified. J Trauma 2001;51:308–14.

[30] Biffl WL, Moore EE, Ryu RK, et al. The unrecognized epidemic of blunt carotid arterial injuries: early diagnosis improves neurologic outcome. Ann Surg 1998;228:462–70.
[31] Rozycki GS, Tremblay L, Feliciano DV, et al. A prospective study for the detection of vascular injury in adult and pediatric patients with cervicothoracic seat belt signs. J Trauma 2002;52:618–24.
[32] Biffl WL, Moore EE, Offner PJ, et al. Optimizing screening for blunt cerebrovascular injuries. Am J Surg 1999;178:517–22.
[33] Biffl WL, Moore EE, Elliott JP, et al. The devastating potential of blunt vertebral artery injuries. Ann Surg 2000;231:672–81.
[34] Miller PR, Fabian TC, Croce MA, et al. Screening for blunt cerebrovascular injuries: analysis of diagnostic modalities and outcomes. Ann Surg 2002;236:386–95.
[35] Biffl WL, Moore EE, Offner PJ, et al. Blunt carotid arterial injuries: implications of a new grading scale. J Trauma 1999;47:845–53.
[36] McKevitt EC, Kirkpatrick AW, Vertesi L, et al. Blunt vascular neck injuries: diagnosis and outcomes of extracranial vessel injury. J Trauma 2002;53:472–6.
[37] Carrillo EH, Osborne DL, Spain DA, et al. Blunt carotid artery injuries: difficulties with the diagnosis prior to neurologic event. J Trauma 1999;46:1120–5.
[38] Snyder WH, Thal ER, Bridges RA, et al. The validity of normal arteriograms in penetrating trauma. Arch Surg 1978;113:424–6.
[39] Rathlev NK. Penetrating neck trauma: mandatory versus selective exploration. J Emerg Med 1990;8:75–8.
[40] LeBlang SD, Nunez DB, Rivas LA, et al. Helical computed tomographic angiography in penetrating neck trauma. Emerg Radiol 1997;4:200–6.
[41] Munera F, Soto JA, Palacio D, et al. Diagnosis of arterial injuries caused by penetrating trauma to the neck: comparison of helical CT angiography and conventional angiography. Radiology 2000;216:356–62.
[42] Rogers FB, Baker EF, Osler TM, et al. Computed tomographic angiography as a screening modality for blunt cervical arterial injuries: preliminary results. J Trauma 1999;46:380–5.
[43] Biffl WL, Ray CE Jr, Moore EE, et al. Noninvasive diagnosis of blunt cerebrovascular injuries: a preliminary report. J Trauma 2002;53:850–6.
[44] Kuzniec S, Kauffman P, Molnar LJ, et al. Diagnosis of limb and neck arterial trauma using duplex ultrasonography. Cardiovasc Surg 1998;6:358–66.
[45] Kerby JD, May AK, Gomez CR, et al. Treatment of bilateral blunt carotid injury using percutaneous angioplasty and stenting: case report and review of the literature. J Trauma 2000; 49:784–7.
[46] Shames ML, Davis JW, Evans AJ. Endoluminal stent placement for the treatment of traumatic carotid artery pseudo aneurysm: case report and review of the literature. J Trauma 1999;46:724–6.
[47] Biffl WL, Moore EE, Ray C, et al. Emergent stenting of acute blunt carotid artery injuries: a cautionary note. J Trauma 2001;50:969–71.
[48] Baker WE, Servais El, Burke PA, et al. Blunt carotid injury. Curr Treat Options Cardiovasc Med 2006;8(2):167–73.

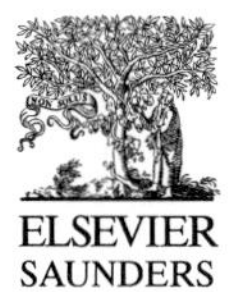
ELSEVIER
SAUNDERS

EMERGENCY
MEDICINE
CLINICS OF
NORTH AMERICA

Emerg Med Clin N Am 25 (2007) 695–711

Diagnostic Dilemmas and Current Controversies in Blunt Chest Trauma

Daniel McGillicuddy, MD*, Peter Rosen, MD

Department of Emergency Medicine, Beth Israel Deaconess Medical Center, One Deaconess Road, W/CC-2, Boston, MA 02215, USA

Blunt chest injuries are common encounters in the emergency department. The injuries can range from the fairly benign to the acutely life threatening, often with no obvious physical signs or symptoms of the underlying pathology. It is helpful to understand the mechanism of injury, to calculate the potential life threats associated with such mechanisms, and to employ the correct diagnostic approach and prudent management of blunt chest trauma and its associated injuries.

The initial evaluation of blunt chest trauma has become relatively standardized in recent years. The general application of the Advanced Trauma Life Support principles has been widely disseminated and practiced for over 20 years. Instead of a comprehensive review of blunt chest trauma, this article addresses current concepts relating to the evaluation of potential blunt thoracic aortic injuries, blunt myocardial injury, and blunt diaphragmatic injury. Topics also include the controversy surrounding the use of prophylactic antibiotics during chest tube thoracostomy insertion, the role of chest tube thoracostomy in occult pneumothorax, and the management of rib fractures in the elderly.

Blunt aortic injury

Blunt aortic injury is the second most common cause of death in blunt trauma patients [1]. Common mechanisms that induce blunt aortic injury are rapid deceleration injuries from motor vehicle or motorcycle crashes, falls, and crush injuries [2]. Blunt aortic injuries result in nearly 8000 deaths a year in the United States [3]. Classically, over 80% of patients who suffer

* Corresponding author.
E-mail address: dmcgilli@bidmc.harvard.edu (D. McGillicuddy).

0733-8627/07/$ - see front matter
doi:10.1016/j.emc.2007.06.004

emed.theclinics.com

blunt aortic injuries die on scene, whereas 13% to 15% of patients who survive the initial injury make it to the hospital alive [1].

Evaluation

Blunt thoracic aortic injuries usually occur at the aortic isthmus just distal to the origin of the left subclavian artery. There are several theories regarding the cause of blunt aortic injury. The sheering force theory postulates that the injury occurs at the isthmus due to the tethering of the ligamentum arteriosum. The osseous pinch theory suggests that the aorta is compressed between the sternum and thoracic spine in severe chest injury leading to disruption of the aorta. The water-hammer theory states that increased intra-abdominal pressure from rapid deceleration injuries increases the intraluminal pressure in the aorta causing aortic injury [2].

Patients with blunt aortic injury often complain of chest pain. The physical examination of a patient with a blunt aortic injury may reveal pseudocoarctation defined as elevated blood pressure in the upper extremities and lower blood pressure in the lower extremities. Furthermore, patients may have chest wall bruising, rib or sternal fractures, or an aortic insufficiency murmur on cardiac auscultation [2].

Patients who survive the initial accident often have no physical evidence of such a severe injury. There appears to be no clinical correlation between thoracic skeletal injury and blunt aortic injury. The lack of skeletal injury does not preclude the possibility of a blunt aortic injury [4]. Furthermore, Horton and colleagues [5] report that patients in motor vehicle crashes are not afforded protection from blunt aortic injury by the use of a restraint device. The mechanism of injury should make one think of potential aortic injuries. Rapid deceleration injuries from high-speed motor vehicle crashes, falls from heights of 4.5 m, ejection from a vehicle or motorcycle, and crushing between two objects such as a wall and the side of a truck or train are a few of the suggestive high-energy mechanisms [3]. Falls from heights as low as 5 ft and motor vehicle crashes with speeds of 10 miles per hour have also been linked to blunt aortic injury [6]. The classification of a serious predictive mechanism is subject to debate and often varies between institutions [7].

The initial imaging study in the evaluation of blunt aortic injury is the standard anteroposterior trauma chest radiograph. It would be preferable to use an upright posteroanterior view, but this is often precluded by the patient's instability or other injuries. Multiple findings on the chest radiographic study will suggest a blunt aortic injury (Box 1) [3].

The most common finding on chest radiography used to screen for potential blunt aortic injury is a widened mediastinum. Although many widths are reported, it is hard to pick any one width because there is no consensus on the level at which to measure the width of the mediastinum, and the technique of the radiographic study will also vary the width (eg, portable

Box 1. Findings on chest radiography suggestive of blunt aortic injury

Widened mediastinum
Deviated nasogastric tube
Apical capping
Depressed left main stem bronchus
Widened left paratracheal stripe
Loss of aortic knob contour

versus fixed tube.) The positive predictive value of a widened mediastinum is reported to be 5% to 20% [8]. False-positive findings of a widened mediastinum can be attributed to the technique of the portable anteroposterior chest radiograph, mediastinal fat pads, or unfolding of the aorta [8,9]. Studies evaluating the sensitivity and specificity of other radiographic chest findings in blunt aortic injury have had mixed results. No studies have shown that plain radiography of the chest is conclusive in diagnosing or ruling out blunt aortic injury [8,9]. One study attempted to use the mediastinal width, left mediastinal width, and the width ratio to increase the specificity of a chest radiograph in potential blunt aortic injury. A 100% negative predictive value was reported when using a mediastinal width less than 8 cm, a left mediastinal width of 6 cm, or a mediastinal width ratio of less than 0.6 in excluding blunt aortic injury. These measurements were used so as to not have any false negatives in the study because the outcomes were already known. An increase of specificity from 40% to 50% to 67.7% was reported when using the mediastinal width ratio and left mediastinal width to exclude blunt aortic injury. Because this small retrospective study was nonblinded and without confidence intervals, it would need to be prospectively validated before its widespread use in excluding aortic injury [8].

Many trauma centers will use the presence of a normal mediastinal width on chest radiography as being sufficient to rule out blunt aortic injury, even though there are many reports of blunt aortic injury detected on chest CT scan or aortic angiograms in patients with normal radiographic chest studies [6,8,10]. In one study of blunt chest trauma patients, 8% of patients with a normal radiographic chest study had a blunt aortic injury detected on chest CT scan [6]. In another study, Exadaktylos and colleagues [6] reported that approximately 50% of patients with blunt chest trauma and an appropriate mechanism for blunt aortic injury with a normal or negative radiographic chest study had an intrathoracic injury on chest CT scan. Patients with an appropriate mechanism for blunt aortic injury with a widened mediastinum on chest radiography require further evaluation of the aorta.

Although aortography is often described as the best imaging study to demonstrate a blunt aortic injury, the rapid development of multidetector CT scans and helical CT scans has altered the imaging evaluation of possible blunt aortic injury. The advantages of helical CT are its rapid availability, its ability to provide other intrathoracic injury information, and its lower dye load, lower stroke risk, and wider availability [11,12]. Older generation CT scanners and nonhelical CT scans have approximately a 3% false-negative rate [10]. Newer generation helical CT scanners have sensitivities and negative predictive values that approach 100% when compared with traditional angiograms [7,9,11,13]. The rapidity of the scan coupled with its high sensitivity and negative predictive value has led many centers to conclude that a negative chest CT essentially rules out a blunt aortic injury. Patients need a formal angiogram only with an equivocal chest CT or if clinical suggestion of the presence of the injury is very strong.

The presence of a mediastinal hematoma on a chest CT scan is a common finding in patients with blunt chest injury. In a recent study of 1104 patients, Mirvis and colleagues [10] found that over 10% (118 of 1104) of patients with blunt chest injury who underwent chest CT scan had a mediastinal hematoma detected. Twenty percent of the patients with mediastinal hematoma (24 of 118) had evidence of direct aortic injury. Of the patients with mediastinal hematoma without aortic injury detected on CT scan, 50% had hemorrhage related to thoracic spinal or sternal fracture.

A transesophageal echocardiogram has similar sensitivity to a helical CT scan for the accurate diagnosis of blunt aortic injury. A clear advantage of transesophageal echocardiography is that it can be performed at the bedside of patients too unstable for a CT scan. The disadvantages are its limited availability and the fact that the results are often operator dependent [9,14]. A negative spiral chest CT scan with an adequate intravenous contrast bolus may be used to exclude an aortic injury if the radiologist is experienced in reading chest CT angiograms [9,10,13,15,16]. The presence of a mediastinal hematoma not centered on a spinal fracture or the presence of a hematoma near a great vessel should prompt the clinician that the patient may require further evaluation. Conventional angiograms are still recommended when chest CT scans are equivocal in patients at high risk for aortic transaction [2,3].

Treatment

Once the diagnosis of blunt aortic injury has been made, the patient needs to be evaluated for surgical intervention. Before the mid-1990s, discussion of the operative repair of blunt aortic injury focused on the issue of cardiopulmonary bypass versus the cross-clamp and sew technique. There are advocates for both techniques, and major complications are involved in the use of either method. The most feared complication of the cross-clamp and sew technique is paraplegia from spinal cord ischemia; the major complication of bypass is the need for heparinization of a multiple trauma patient. Hunt and colleagues [17] demonstrated a significant reduction of the incidence of spinal cord injury in the bypass group compared with the clamp and sew group when the cross-clamp time exceeded 35 minutes.

Contemporary therapy shows an increase in the use of endovascular stent grafts in patients with blunt aortic injury. Several studies show promising results of endovascular repair in appropriate patients with low rates of morbidity and mortality when compared with traditional repair [18,19]. In a recent study, Ott and colleagues [18] reported a trend toward a decrease in mortality and paraplegia when using endovascular stents in comparison with traditional open repair. Cook and colleagues [20] demonstrated that selective use of medical therapy, endovascular and open repair, and delayed repair decreased the mortality rate from 65% to 26% in a comparison with historical controls. The current trend in operative repair of blunt aortic injury seems to be the increased use of endovascular repair when possible, although open operative repair is still common and necessary.

While the patient is awaiting definitive operative repair, blood pressure control may be necessary. Similar to the management of spontaneous aortic dissection, it may be advantageous to use both sodium nitroprusside and esmolol to reduce the transmural effect of hypertension on the aortic injury; however, many, if not all, patients with blunt aortic injury will also have sustained other traumatic injuries, and the use of vasoactive antihypertensive medications may be contraindicated (ie, intracranial hemorrhage or hemoperitoneum) [20]. The use of vasoactive agents in blunt trauma patients who have sustained blunt aortic injury has not been studied heavily to date, although their use is common in the surgical intensive care unit when delayed repair is being considered [17–19]. The use of vasoactive agents in blunt trauma patients should be left up to the consulting surgical service.

Blunt cardiac injury

Blunt cardiac injury is usually sustained in rapid deceleration injuries with direct blows to the chest. There is no standard definition of blunt cardiac injury and no straightforward or accurate way to establish the diagnosis. The exact incidence of blunt cardiac injury is unknown but is estimated to range from 8% to 71% of all blunt chest injured patients. This large variation in incidence and the lack of agreement between researchers as to the definition of blunt cardiac injury make standardized research and recommendations more difficult [21].

Evaluation

Patients with blunt cardiac injury may complain of chest pain or shortness of breath. The physical examination will often be nonspecific. Patients may have chest wall tenderness, a flail chest, or crepitus. They may also have sinus tachycardia and, occasionally, dysrhythmias or ectopy on the cardiac monitor or electrocardiogram [2].

Blunt cardiac injury has been associated with myocardial dysfunction leading to pump failure, electrical conduction disturbances leading to dysrhythmias, valvular dysfunction leading to heart failure, and, rarely, coronary artery injury leading to acute myocardial infarction.

All patients who sustain significant blunt chest injuries should undergo a screening electrocardiogram [2,21]. An otherwise uninjured patient with a normal EKG upon admission to the emergency department is at a low risk for complications of a blunt cardiac injury such as dysrhythmia or pump failure; therefore, these patients are safe to be discharged [22]. Some centers will hold these patients for 4 to 6 hours for serial EKGs. Patients with blunt chest trauma who are admitted for other reasons and who have a normal EKG are also at low risk for significant blunt cardiac injury and its complications, and further work-up for blunt cardiac injury is not indicated [23–25]. Patients with significant chest trauma (eg, multiple rib fractures, pulmonary contusions, hemothorax, major intrathoracic vascular injury) have a 13% incidence of significant blunt myocardial injury. In a small proportion of these patients who have an initial normal EKG, it is safe to rule out blunt cardiac injury by prior studies [26].

Predicting who will develop complications from blunt cardiac injury has proven as illusive as the diagnosis itself. There are multiple conflicting studies showing the benefit and lack of benefit of cardiac biomarkers, echocardiography, and radionuclide scans in predicting who will experience complications from blunt chest trauma. Previous studies have shown that cardiac biomarkers do not have clinical value in patients with blunt cardiac injuries [27,28]. Biffl and colleagues [27] studied cardiac biomarkers in blunt myocardial injury and found that in no patient were elevated biomarkers the sole predictor of cardiac complications. Furthermore in the study of Fabian and colleagues [28] of blunt myocardial injury, an elevated creatine kinase MB fraction correlated with dysrhythmias, but it was neither sensitive nor specific. More recent data evaluating the use of cardiac-specific troponin T and I have shown some predictive ability in patients with blunt chest trauma. Rajan and colleagues [29] reported that asymptomatic patients with blunt chest injuries with negative cardiac troponin I at 6 hours were at low risk for blunt cardiac injuries. They also showed that elevated troponin I levels were correlated with an increased risk of dysrhythmia and a decreased ejection fraction. A rise of troponin I by 1 μg/L was associated with an increased risk of dysrhythmia of 1.9% and a 0.4% decrease in ejection fraction. A second study by Lindstaedt and colleagues [30] reported the long-term outcomes of patients with the diagnosis of blunt cardiac injury. In that study, 93% of the patients diagnosed with blunt cardiac injury were in the ICU for other injuries. The incidence of blunt cardiac injury in this study was 19.4%. No patients diagnosed with blunt cardiac injury needed treatment for this injury during hospitalization, and at follow-up 3 and 12 months later, they still did not need treatment.

Patients who appear to have pump failure related to blunt cardiac injury may have valvular failure, acute pump failure, or an acute myocardial infarction. An EKG may help to identify those with cardiac ischemia as the etiology of pump failure but is often nonspecific and nondiagnostic. There are many reasons explaining why patients with blunt chest injury may be hypotensive, hypoxic, tachycardiac, or in heart failure, including pulmonary contusion, pneumothorax, hemorrhagic shock, and cardiac tamponade. A thorough investigation to rule out these potentially reversible causes of pump failure is mandated before focusing on blunt cardiac injury as the etiology. If it is determined that pump failure from blunt cardiac injury is the likely etiology of shock, the patient should undergo an immediate bedside echocardiogram to evaluate the function of the heart valves and ejection fraction. A ruptured valve is an indication for cardiothoracic surgery. A poor ejection fraction from injured myocardium may necessitate the addition of dopamine or an aortic balloon pump to increase cardiac output [21,31,32].

A small subset of patients with blunt cardiac injury present with symptoms consistent with acute myocardial infarction. Most of these patients do not have true coronary artery disease and develop signs and symptoms of ST elevation 5 to 7 days post trauma. They require angiography, but usually have developed the changes from local areas of contused myocardium, and the coronary arteries will be clear. A small number of patients experience thrombosis of the coronary artery and may have underlying clotting abnormalities. The left anterior descending artery, tricuspid valve, and right ventricle are the most commonly injured structures due to their anatomic position [33]. The exact mechanism of acute myocardial infarction with blunt cardiac injury is unknown. Acute thrombosis can occur in the setting of known atherosclerosis, and another mechanism for acute myocardial infarction is coronary artery dissection [34]. Cardiac catheterization and potential treatment of the lesion with angioplasty and stenting is only possible when other injuries do not prevent the use of anticoagulation associated with coronary artery bypass [35,36].

Blunt cardiac injury can be a difficult diagnosis for the emergency physician because the diagnosis is nebulous, and the outcomes are varied depending on the definition. One should use an initial EKG for help in decision making about this entity. If the patient is young, without significant comorbidities, and has a normal EKG, the probability for blunt cardiac injury is low enough that the patient is safe for discharge assuming he or she has no other injuries or reasons for admission. Older patients, patients with multiple cardiovascular comorbidities, those with multiple chest injuries, or those with an abnormal EKG require admission and monitoring. Cardiac enzymes and imaging studies may be of benefit in select patients with blunt myocardial injury. Cardiac-specific troponins may be used to evaluate for possible complications associated with blunt cardiac injury; however, no definitive studies have proven the utility of cardiac biomarkers in stable patients to date. Patients who are in cardiogenic shock should have an echocardiogram to evaluate valvular patency and the myocardial ejection fraction.

Blunt diaphragmatic rupture

Blunt diaphragmatic rupture most often occurs as a result of severe blunt chest and abdominal trauma resulting from motor vehicle crashes or vehicles striking pedestrians, as well as falls from a height of 10 ft or more. The reported incidence of blunt diaphragmatic rupture ranges from 0.5% to 8% of patients admitted to the emergency department as a result of automobile crashes or undergoing exploratory laparotomy for trauma [37–39]. Fifty percent to 80% of blunt diaphragmatic ruptures occur on the left side [40–42]. One percent to 2% of blunt diaphragmatic rupture is bilateral. Bilateral rupture has a much higher mortality than unilateral diaphragmatic rupture [37]. Right-sided diaphragmatic rupture is associated with a 50% rate of concomitant liver injury [43].

Evaluation

Common symptoms of blunt diaphragmatic rupture include coughing, shortness of breath, and chest pain. Common signs are a dullness to percussion on the side of diaphragmatic rupture, auscultating bowel sounds in the chest cavity, and decreased breath sounds on the side of diaphragmatic rupture [2,44].

Making the diagnosis of blunt diaphragmatic rupture is difficult [43]. If a rupture of the diaphragm is suggested clinically, a radiographic chest study should be performed. One should evaluate for elevated hemidiaphragms, an obscured diaphragmatic shadow, a displaced nasogastric tube position, and a boxlike appearance of the right hemidiaphragm when the right diaphragm is injured. With left hemidiaphragm rupture, it is more common to see bowel in the chest. With right side rupture, the box appearance is more often seen as the liver herniates into the thorax [38,41,45]. Unfortunately, chest radiography has poor sensitivity and specificity for the diagnosis of blunt diaphragmatic rupture [38,39]. In part, this is because the patient is usually too unstable to obtain an upright posteroanterior view, and the pathology is harder to demonstrate on a supine anteroposterior view (Fig. 1).

Studies evaluating the use of CT in the diagnosis of blunt diaphragmatic rupture report a wide range of sensitivities ranging from 50% to 73% [41,43,46]. More recent studies with helical CT scans have reported higher sensitivity in detecting blunt diaphragmatic rupture. The presence of a "hump sign," dependent viscera sign, or collar sign on a reformatted helical CT scan improves the sensitivity of the CT scan in the diagnosis of blunt diaphragmatic rupture [38]; however, even with a helical CT scan,

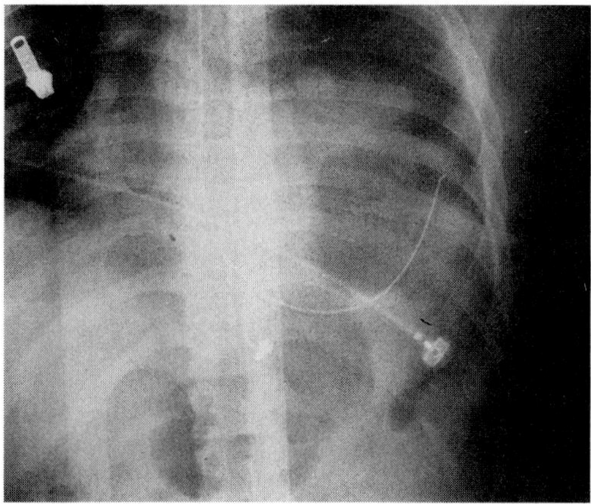

Fig. 1. X-ray of blunt diaphragmatic rupture. Displacement of the nasogastric tube in the left chest.

blunt diaphragmatic rupture injures are still missed. Other modalities including MRI and nuclear medicine tracer studies are effective but are unlikely to be used in the acute setting owing to logistical obstacles [41]. A CT scan showing a diaphragmatic injury is helpful in making the diagnosis; however, a negative CT scan for diaphragmatic injury is not sensitive enough to exclude the injury, and if there is concern for blunt diaphragmatic injury, further imaging or surgical evaluation is necessary.

Ultrasound has been used to diagnose blunt diaphragmatic rupture in patients with an equivocal CT scan [41,45]. All of the data on ultrasound use in diagnosing blunt diaphragmatic rupture are based on case reports. Blaivas and colleagues [45] recently published a case series of blunt diaphragmatic rupture diagnosed by bedside ultrasound. The diagnosis was suggested in the presence of abnormal movement or lack of movement of the diaphragm during the focused abdominal sonogram in trauma (FAST). Although no studies of FAST ultrasound in diagnosing blunt diaphragmatic rupture have been performed, the presence of abnormal diaphragmatic movement or the lack of movement may suggest an occult blunt diaphragmatic rupture.

Typically, there is minimal bleeding from the diaphragm itself, which leads to the low sensitivity of diagnostic peritoneal lavage in blunt diaphragmatic rupture [37,41,45]. If other intra-abdominal injuries are not sustained, it is difficult to demonstrate diaphragmatic injury. There are no documented cases of spontaneously healing blunt diaphragmatic ruptures, and it may be many years after the injury until the diagnosis is established. Owing to the negative intrathoracic pressure, visceral herniation into the thoracic cavity nearly always occurs. Patients may present with signs of bowel obstruction or abdominal sepsis from herniated viscera. They may also present in respiratory distress from a tension visceral thorax.

Thoracoscopy and laparoscopy have been proposed as possible screening mechanisms for blunt diaphragmatic rupture. Most studies that demonstrate the utility of laparoscopy for the evaluation of diaphragmatic injury have been performed in patients with penetrating trauma [41].

Missed blunt diaphragmatic rupture carries a high morbidity and mortality rate. Ten percent to 66% of blunt diaphragmatic injuries are missed on initial trauma evaluation [41,43]. Delayed presentations of missed blunt diaphragmatic rupture have been reported in most studies. Patients with missed or delayed diagnosis of blunt diaphragmatic rupture often present with nausea and vomiting secondary to a bowel obstruction from incarcerated bowel in the chest. Bowel sounds may be auscultated in the chest. Patients may also present with symptoms consistent with a tension pneumothorax when, in fact, they are sustaining tension viscerothorax. One study reported that only 72% of blunt diaphragmatic ruptures were noted preoperatively [37]. Shah and colleagues [40] report that 43.5% of injuries are noted preoperatively and 14.6% are delayed in their diagnosis.

Several researchers have noted a theoretical risk of increased missed blunt diaphragmatic rupture due to the emergence of nonoperative management of blunt hepatic and splenic injuries. Previously, many blunt diaphragmatic ruptures were discovered solely on laparotomy [41,43]. These missed injuries may be a cost of the decreased incidence of exploratory laparotomy.

Blunt diaphragmatic injuries are widely recognized as a marker of injury severity. Nevertheless, they are not cited as the immediate proximate cause of mortality, because the associated injuries are typically more severe [39].

Treatment

When the diagnosis of a blunt diaphragmatic rupture is established, a search for other injuries is required because the average Injury Severity Score of a patient with blunt diaphragmatic rupture is 25 [47]. Treatment for a blunt diaphragmatic rupture is always surgical. Either a transthoracic or transabdominal approach is acceptable, and the choice depends on the likelihood of other operative injuries. In the emergency department, rapid decompression of the intestines should be attempted with an oral or nasogastric tube, and an emergent surgical consult should be obtained. All patients with blunt diaphragmatic rupture should be admitted to a trauma or surgical service rather than orthopedic or neurosurgical unit despite concomitant injuries.

Current areas of controversy in the management of blunt chest trauma

The role of antibiotics in chest tube thoracostomy

Chest tube placement in blunt chest trauma is a common procedure. More than 100,000 chest tubes are placed annually in trauma patients

[48]. Large-bore chest tubes (36-F or higher) are often placed to drain traumatic hemothorax, traumatic pneumothorax, or in traumatic arrest. Complications with chest tube insertion are well known, and they include intra-abdominal tube placement, intrathoracic misplacement, lung parenchyma injury, intercostal artery or nerve injury, or post-procedural infectious complications [49].

Many of the complications of thoracostomy for chest tube insertion can be avoided by the use of careful technique. The chest tube insertion incision should never be placed lower than the fourth intercostal space, because the diaphragm can rise as high as the fifth interspace with expiration. With proper positioning, the chest tube cannot be inserted through the diaphragm into the liver or spleen. The operator must be careful to ensure the right direction of the tube and confirm that the last portal hole of the tube is inside the pleural cavity. This positioning can be achieved by making an adequate thoracostomy incision that will admit two fingers and by sweeping the pleural cavity before insertion of any tube. These steps will avoid penetration of any herniated abdominal viscera or penetration of the lung if it is adherent to the chest wall. Two fingers should also be placed in the pleural cavity as the tube is advanced posteriorly and superiorly. This action will avert interlobe placement of the tube or allowing the tube to bend upon itself or aim inferiorly. If the last portal hole is palpated within the pleural cavity, a large clamp should be placed on the chest tube at its junction with the chest wall. Before suturing the tube in place, the tube can be pushed back into this depth, ensuring that it has not inadvertently slipped out. This step prevents sewing the tube into a position where the last portal hole is in the subcutaneous tissue rather than the pleural cavity [50].

The use of prophylactic antibiotics to prevent post chest tube infections and empyema is a controversial subject. The potential etiologies of infection after chest tube insertion include iatrogenic infection of the pleural space, secondary infection from diaphragmatic or intra-abdominal disruption, inadequate drainage of hemothorax, and parapneumonic infection or bacteria introduced following penetrating trauma. The most common infectious organisms described are *Staphylococcus aureus* or *Streptococcus* sp, although more recent studies show the emergence of nosocomial organisms as infectious agents [51,52].

The incidence of post chest tube infections ranges from 2% to 25% [53]. Empyema is a less common post chest tube infection, with a reported incidence of 0% to 18% in the civilian population [49,52,54]. Empyemas often require more aggressive management including further chest tube insertion, surgical excision and drainage, and prolonged antibiotics [49,51,54].

Prophylactic antibiotics have been shown to reduce the incidence of infection in some types of surgery, but the efficacy of prophylactic antibiotics in preventing post chest tube thoracostomy infections is not well delineated.

The Eastern Association for the Surgery of Trauma guidelines do not support the use of prophylactic antibiotics in chest tube insertion owing to the lack of good randomized controlled studies powered to detect a difference in outcome [49]. Although multiple studies have evaluated the use of prophylactic antibiotics, methodologic flaws have included suboptimal antibiotics, prolonged dosing, or the types of injury involved. A large prospective double-blinded study by Maxwell and colleagues [51] attempted to answer the question of prophylactic antibiotics in preventing infections complications from chest tube insertion. This study ran for 39 months and was multi-institutional, but even with this large potential series, the study was able to obtain only 20% of the cases for a sufficient power analysis. The conclusion was that the incidence of empyema is small, and that prophylactic antibiotics do not seem to reduce the risk, but the study was underpowered to draw any definitive conclusions. Sanabria and colleagues [54] performed a meta-analysis of known randomized controlled trials of prophylactic antibiotics in chest tube thoracostomy. They concluded that the frequency of empyema was 1.1% in the antibiotic group and 7.6% in the placebo group. Furthermore, the pneumonia rate in the antibiotic group was 6.6% versus the placebo rate of 16%. Although these numbers may seem significant, in the study by Mandal and colleagues [55] of over 5000 patients, adequate drainage of hemothorax demonstrated an empyema rate of only 1.6%. Gonzales and Holevar [56] also performed a study that suggested that antibiotics reduced the risk of infection in chest tube insertion. In this study of 142 patients, 71 patients received placebo while 71 patients received cefazolin, 1 g every 8 hours, until chest tube removal. There were no infectious complications in the antibiotic group compared with four in the placebo group. Although the complication rate was low, it was statistically significant.

Although the question is still not settled, it appears that adequate drainage of any hemothorax and the use of appropriate sterile technique carries only a small risk of infection, and it does not appear that prophylactic antibiotics will further lower this risk. They also do not serve as a substitute for adequate drainage and effective technique [57].

Chest tube thoracostomy in occult pneumothorax

The detection of a pneumothorax on CT scan not seen on plain anteroposterior chest radiography in asymptomatic patients has revealed that the incidence of occult pneumothorax is greater than was experienced or recognized before the wider availability and use of a chest CT scan imaging study. With the increasing frequency of CT scans in trauma, as many as 72% of all pneumothoraces are now thought to be occult [58]. The management of occult pneumothorax has generated much debate. There appears to be a growing recognition and acceptance that occult pneumothorax can be safely treated without thoracostomy in non-ventilated patients [59–61]. Alternatively, some trauma physicians use small catheter drainage and avoid the use of a large chest tube.

There are conflicting data regarding the management of occult pneumothorax in patients who require positive pressure ventilation. Only two small prospective randomized controlled trials have been done, and these two studies provide conflicting results and recommendations. The studies are based on a total of 39 ventilated patients with occult pneumothorax. In the study by Enderson and colleagues, 8 of 21 patients managed without initial tube thoracostomy progressed in the size of their pneumothorax, became symptomatic, and required insertion of a chest tube. Three of these patients developed a tension pneumothorax. Enderson and colleagues [62] recommend that all patients with occult pneumothorax on positive pressure ventilation should have a chest tube placed. Conversely, Brasel and colleagues in a similar study of 18 patients on positive pressure ventilation with occult pneumothorax (9 managed with a chest tube and 9 without) found no difference in the overall complication rate, and only 2 of the 9 patients progressed and needed chest tube insertion. They concluded that patients with an occult pneumothorax who require ventilation can be managed safely without chest tube insertion if they are closely monitored for signs of respiratory distress in an ICU setting [62].

Currently, there are not enough data to suggest that an occult pneumothorax in a patient who requires ventilation should routinely be managed without a chest tube. Until more conclusive evidence appears, it is probably prudent to place a chest tube in these patients. A compromise may be to use a small catheter rather than a large chest tube.

If the patient is asymptomatic and does not require ventilation, it is safe to observe him or her without thoracostomy. If the patient has other injuries, is going to surgery for the management of other injuries (eg, for open reduction of extremity fractures), has any symptoms, or if there are insufficient personnel for effective close monitoring, the prudent management would be to insert a chest tube and not await the development of a larger or tension pneumothorax.

Management of rib fractures in the elderly

Rib fractures are commonly found in blunt chest injuries, with upwards of 10% of blunt trauma patients having evidence of rib fractures upon admission [63,64]. Rib fractures are associated with severe pain and delayed morbidity and mortality, often owing to pneumonia [65]. Rib fractures are often not sustained in isolation and may be associated with other significant injuries, including pulmonary contusion, hemothorax, aortic injury, intra-abdominal injury, or head injury. Flagel and colleagues [66] demonstrated that the presence of six or more rib fractures was associated with increased mortality from other injuries. The incidence of pneumonia nearly doubled, as did the incidence of acute respiratory distress syndrome in patients with six or more rib fractures. Flagel and colleagues also demonstrated that the number of fractured ribs was associated with an increased incidence of pneumothorax, aspiration pneumonia, and empyema.

Recently, it has been recognized that an increasing number of fractured ribs is associated with increasing morbidity and mortality in the elderly patient even when controlling for injury severity [63,65]. Bulger and colleagues [63] studied rib fractures in patients aged more than 65 years and found that, for each additional rib fracture, the mortality rate increased by 19% and the risk of pneumonia by 27%. Furthermore, Holcomb and colleagues [65] found that patients aged more than 45 years with more than four rib fractures remained intubated longer, with longer ICU stays and total hospital stays. Barnea and colleagues [67] also studied rib fractures in the elderly and were unable to find any other multivariate predictors of morbidity and mortality other than the number of rib fractures. The presence of other comorbidities was not predictive of outcome. This finding led the authors to conclude that elderly patients with rib fractures should be admitted.

Treatment

The treatment of rib fractures is supportive and consists of analgesia and pulmonary toilet (incentive spirometery, chest physiotherapy). The type of analgesia that is most effective is an open question, but it appears that epidural analgesia or intercostal blocks may be underutilized as compared with intravenous or oral analgesia [66,68]. In the study by Flagel and colleagues [66], patients were 50% more likely to receive epidural anesthesia if they had six or more rib fractures. The type of anesthesia that is most efficacious in pain control and in reducing morbidity and mortality has not yet been established [68]. Nevertheless, it is universally recognized that pain control is imperative in improving pulmonary toilet in patients with rib fractures.

The clinician must recognize that, although rib fractures may appear minor in an otherwise uninjured patient, they portend significant morbidity and mortality, particularly in the elderly. It is also reasonable to admit older patients with multiple rib fractures to achieve adequate pain control and teach proper pulmonary toilet techniques to decrease the incidence of pneumonia.

Summary

The management and evaluation of blunt chest trauma is an ever changing field. The use of helical CT scans has allowed for rapid diagnosis and exclusion of blunt aortic injury. The evaluation of blunt myocardial injury is difficult; however, a normal EKG in a patient with blunt chest trauma essentially rules out a significant risk of blunt myocardial injury. Blunt diaphragmatic injury is a relativity rare occurrence but carries a high morbidity and mortality if diagnosis is significantly delayed. The role of antibiotics in chest tube thoracostomy has not yet been fully defined but carries little risk but also little possible benefit. The management of occult pneumothorax is an area of active study, particularly in intubated patients. Currently, a chest tube should still be placed in patient with a pneumothorax who requires positive pressure ventilation; however, this paradigm may be shifting. The elderly patient with multiple rib fractures sustains substantial morbidity and mortality, and should be admitted for chest physiotherapy and analgesia to prevent the complications associated with rib fractures.

References

[1] Fabian TC, et al. Prospective study of blunt aortic injury: multicenter trial of the American Association for the Surgery of Trauma. J Trauma 1997;42(3):374–80 [discussion: 380–3].

[2] Markovchick VJ. Clinical practice of emergency medicine. In: Wolfson A, et al, editors. Harwood-Nuss. Philadelphia: Lippincott Williams & Wilkins; 2005. p. 681–90.

[3] Nagy K, et al. Guidelines for the diagnosis and management of blunt aortic injury: an EAST Practice Management Guidelines Work Group. J Trauma 2000;48(6):1128–43.

[4] Lee J, et al. Noncorrelation between thoracic skeletal injuries and acute traumatic aortic tear. J Trauma 1997;43(3):400–4.

[5] Horton TG, et al. Identification of trauma patients at risk of thoracic aortic tear by mechanism of injury. J Trauma 2000;48(6):1008–13 [discussion: 1013–4].

[6] Exadaktylos AK, et al. Do we really need routine computed tomographic scanning in the primary evaluation of blunt chest trauma in patients with "normal" chest radiograph? J Trauma 2001;51(6):1173–6.

[7] Dyer DS, et al. Thoracic aortic injury: how predictive is mechanism and is chest computed tomography a reliable screening tool? A prospective study of 1561 patients. J Trauma 2000;48(4):673–82 [discussion: 682–3].

[8] Wong YC, et al. Left mediastinal width and mediastinal width ratio are better radiographic criteria than general mediastinal width for predicting blunt aortic injury. J Trauma 2004; 57(1):88–94.

[9] Wintermark M, Wicky S, Schnyder P. Imaging of acute traumatic injuries of the thoracic aorta. Eur Radiol 2002;12(2):431–42.

[10] Mirvis SE, et al. Use of spiral computed tomography for the assessment of blunt trauma patients with potential aortic injury. J Trauma 1998;45(5):922–30.

[11] Parker MS, et al. Making the transition: the role of helical CT in the evaluation of potentially acute thoracic aortic injuries. AJR Am J Roentgenol 2001;176(5):1267–72.

[12] Collier B, et al. Is helical computed tomography effective for diagnosis of blunt aortic injury? Am J Emerg Med 2002;20(6):558–61.

[13] Demetriades D, et al. Routine helical computed tomographic evaluation of the mediastinum in high-risk blunt trauma patients. Arch Surg 1998;133(10):1084–8.

[14] Vignon P, et al. Transesophageal echocardiography and therapeutic management of patients sustaining blunt aortic injuries. J Trauma 2005;58(6):1150–8.

[15] Bruckner BA, et al. Critical evaluation of chest computed tomography scans for blunt descending thoracic aortic injury. Ann Thorac Surg 2006;81(4):1339–46.

[16] Chen MY, et al. The trend of using computed tomography in the detection of acute thoracic aortic and branch vessel injury after blunt thoracic trauma: single-center experience over 13 years. J Trauma 2004;56(4):783–5.

[17] Hunt JP, et al. Thoracic aorta injuries: management and outcome of 144 patients. J Trauma 1996;40(4):547–55 [discussion: 555–6].

[18] Ott MC, et al. Management of blunt thoracic aortic injuries: endovascular stents versus open repair. J Trauma 2004;56(3):565–70.

[19] Peterson BG, et al. Percutaneous endovascular repair of blunt thoracic aortic transection. J Trauma 2005;59(5):1062–5.

[20] Cook J, et al. The effect of changing presentation and management on the outcome of blunt rupture of the thoracic aorta. J Thorac Cardiovasc Surg 2006;131(3):594–600.
[21] Pasquale M, Nagy K, Clarke J. Practice management guidelines for screening of blunt cardiac injury. Available at: www.east.org. Accessed 1998.
[22] Dowd MD, Krug S. Pediatric blunt cardiac injury: epidemiology, clinical features, and diagnosis. Pediatric Emergency Medicine Collaborative Research Committee: Working Group on Blunt Cardiac Injury. J Trauma 1996;40(1):61–7.
[23] Helling TS, et al. A prospective evaluation of 68 patients suffering blunt chest trauma for evidence of cardiac injury. J Trauma 1989;29(7):961–5 [discussion: 965–6].
[24] Foil MB, et al. The asymptomatic patient with suspected myocardial contusion. Am J Surg 1990;160(6):638–42 [discussion: 642–3].
[25] Illig KA, et al. A rational screening and treatment strategy based on the electrocardiogram alone for suspected cardiac contusion. Am J Surg 1991;162(6):537–43 [discussion: 544].
[26] Velmahos GC, et al. Normal electrocardiography and serum troponin I levels preclude the presence of clinically significant blunt cardiac injury. J Trauma 2003;54(1):45–50 [discussion: 50–1].
[27] Biffl WL, et al. Cardiac enzymes are irrelevant in the patient with suspected myocardial contusion. Am J Surg 1994;168(6):523–7 [discussion: 527–8].
[28] Fabian TC, et al. A prospective evaluation of myocardial contusion: correlation of significant arrhythmias and cardiac output with CPK-MB measurements. J Trauma 1991;31(5): 653–9 [discussion: 659–60].
[29] Rajan GP, Zellweger R. Cardiac troponin I as a predictor of arrhythmia and ventricular dysfunction in trauma patients with myocardial contusion. J Trauma 2004;57(4):801–8 [discussion: 808].
[30] Lindstaedt M, et al. Acute and long-term clinical significance of myocardial contusion following blunt thoracic trauma: results of a prospective study. J Trauma 2002;52(3): 479–85.
[31] Ismailov RM, et al. Trauma associated with acute myocardial infarction in a multi-state hospitalized population. Int J Cardiol 2005;105(2):141–6.
[32] Ismailov RM, et al. Blunt cardiac injury associated with cardiac valve insufficiency: trauma links to chronic disease? Injury 2005;36(9):1022–8.
[33] Tsoukas A, et al. Myocardial contusion presented as acute myocardial infarction after chest trauma. Echocardiography 2001;18(2):167–70.
[34] Kohli S, et al. Coronary artery dissection secondary to blunt chest trauma. Cathet Cardiovasc Diagn 1988;15(3):179–83.
[35] Naseer N, et al. Circumflex coronary artery occlusion after blunt chest trauma. Heart Dis 2003;5(3):184–6.
[36] Goktekin O, et al. Traumatic total occlusion of left main coronary artery caused by blunt chest trauma. J Invasive Cardiol 2002;14(8):463–5.
[37] Athanassiadi K, et al. Blunt diaphragmatic rupture. Eur J Cardiothorac Surg 1999;15(4): 469–74.
[38] Rees O, Mirvis SE, Shanmuganathan K. Multidetector-row CT of right hemidiaphragmatic rupture caused by blunt trauma: a review of 12 cases. Clin Radiol 2005;60(12): 1280–9.
[39] Barsness KA, et al. Blunt diaphragmatic rupture in children. J Trauma 2004;56(1):80–2.
[40] Shah R, et al. Traumatic rupture of diaphragm. Ann Thorac Surg 1995;60(5):1444–9.
[41] Guth AA, Pachter HL, Kim U. Pitfalls in the diagnosis of blunt diaphragmatic injury. Am J Surg 1995;170(1):5–9.
[42] Eren S, Kantarci M, Okur A. Imaging of diaphragmatic rupture after trauma. Clin Radiol 2006;61(6):467–77.
[43] Reber PU, et al. Missed diaphragmatic injuries and their long-term sequelae. J Trauma 1998; 44(1):183–8.

[44] Blaivas M, Lyon M, Duggal S. A prospective comparison of supine chest radiography and bedside ultrasound for the diagnosis of traumatic pneumothorax. Acad Emerg Med 2005; 12(9):844–9.
[45] Blaivas M, et al. Bedside emergency ultrasonographic diagnosis of diaphragmatic rupture in blunt abdominal trauma. Am J Emerg Med 2004;22(7):601–4.
[46] Demos TC, et al. Computed tomography in traumatic defects of the diaphragm. Clin Imaging 1989;13(1):62–7.
[47] Bergeron E, et al. Impact of deferred treatment of blunt diaphragmatic rupture: a 15-year experience in six trauma centers in Quebec. J Trauma 2002;52(4):633–40.
[48] LoCicero J 3rd, Mattox KL. Epidemiology of chest trauma. Surg Clin North Am 1989;69(1): 15–9.
[49] Luchette F, Barie P, Oswanski M, et al. Practice management guidelines for prophylactic antibiotic use in tube thoracostomy for traumatic hemopneumothorax: EAST Practice Management Guidelines Work Group. J Trauma 2000;48(4):753–7.
[50] Rosen P, Chan T, Vilke G, et al. Atlas of emergency procedures. St Louis (MO): Mosby; 2001. p. 40–5.
[51] Maxwell RA, et al. Use of presumptive antibiotics following tube thoracostomy for traumatic hemopneumothorax in the prevention of empyema and pneumonia–a multi-center trial. J Trauma 2004;57(4):742–8 [discussion: 748–9].
[52] Cant PJ, Smyth S, Smart DO. Antibiotic prophylaxis is indicated for chest stab wounds requiring closed tube thoracostomy. Br J Surg 1993;80(4):464–6.
[53] Eddy AC, Luna GK, Copass M. Empyema thoracic in patients undergoing emergent closed tube thoracostomy for thoracic trauma. Am J Surg 1989;157(5):494–7.
[54] Sanabria A, et al. Prophylactic antibiotics in chest trauma: a meta-analysis of high-quality studies. World J Surg 2006;30(10):1843–7.
[55] Mandal AK, Thadepalli H, Chettipalli U. Posttraumatic empyema thoracis: a 24-year experience at a major trauma center. J Trauma 1997;43(5):764–71.
[56] Gonzalez RP, Holevar MR. Role of prophylactic antibiotics for tube thoracostomy in chest trauma. Am Surg 1998;64(7):617–20 [discussion: 620–1].
[57] Adrales G, et al. A thoracostomy tube guideline improves management efficiency in trauma patients. J Trauma 2002;52(2):210–4 [discussion: 214–6].
[58] Ball CG, et al. Are occult pneumothoraces truly occult or simply missed? J Trauma 2006; 60(2):294–8 [discussion: 298–9].
[59] Ball CG, et al. Factors related to the failure of radiographic recognition of occult posttraumatic pneumothoraces. Am J Surg 2005;189(5):541–6 [discussion: 546].
[60] Ball CG, et al. Occult pneumothorax in the mechanically ventilated trauma patient. Can J Surg 2003;46(5):373–9.
[61] Ball CG, et al. Incidence, risk factors, and outcomes for occult pneumothoraces in victims of major trauma. J Trauma 2005;59(4):917–24 [discussion: 924–5].
[62] Enderson BL, et al. Tube thoracostomy for occult pneumothorax: a prospective randomized study of its use. J Trauma 1993;35(5):726–9 [discussion: 729–30].
[63] Bulger EM, et al. Rib fractures in the elderly. J Trauma 2000;48(6):1040–6 [discussion: 1046–7].
[64] Martinez R, Sharieff G, Hooper J. Three-point restraints as a risk factor for chest injury in the elderly. J Trauma 1994;37(6):980–4.
[65] Holcomb JB, et al. Morbidity from rib fractures increases after age 45. J Am Coll Surg 2003; 196(4):549–55.
[66] Flagel BT, et al. Half-a-dozen ribs: the breakpoint for mortality. Surgery 2005;138(4):717–23 [discussion: 723–5].
[67] Barnea Y, et al. Isolated rib fractures in elderly patients: mortality and morbidity. Can J Surg 2002;45(1):43–6.
[68] Karmakar MK, Ho AM. Acute pain management of patients with multiple fractured ribs. J Trauma 2003;54(3):615–25.

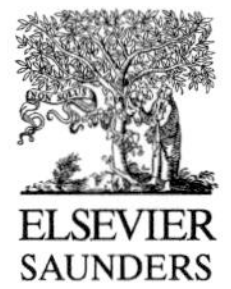

ELSEVIER
SAUNDERS

EMERGENCY
MEDICINE
CLINICS OF
NORTH AMERICA

Emerg Med Clin N Am 25 (2007) 713–733

Advances in Abdominal Trauma

Jennifer L. Isenhour, MD[a,b,*], John Marx, MD[a,b]

[a]*Department of Emergency Medicine, Carolinas Medical Center, 1000 Blythe Boulevard, Charlotte, NC 28203, USA*

[b]*Department of Emergency Medicine, University of North Carolina, P.O. Box 32861, Charlotte, NC 28232-2861, USA*

Emergency practitioners routinely encounter patients who suffer from abdominal trauma, be it blunt or penetrating. These injuries are often confounded by altered mental status, distracting injuries, or lack of historical information, and may present challenges in management. However, in the last several years new approaches to the diagnosis and management of abdominal trauma, including bedside ultrasound, newer generation computed tomography scans, laparoscopy, and the ability for selected nonoperative management expedite identification of life threatening injury and offer new options in treatment.

Blunt abdominal trauma

Background

Historically, blunt abdominal trauma (BAT) is more frequently encountered in the emergency department (ED) than penetrating abdominal trauma, and usually results from a motor vehicle collision (MVC). When combined with pedestrian versus auto accidents, these types of abdominal traumas account for up to 75% of cases seen, while direct abdominal blows and falls comprise the remainder [1,2]. The spleen is the most often injured organ and may be the only intra-abdominal injury in over 60% of cases. Liver and hollow viscus injuries follow in decreasing incidence [1]. Blunt abdominal trauma may herald occult domestic violence or child abuse.

* Corresponding author. Department of Emergency Medicine, Carolinas Medical Center, 1000 Blythe Boulevard, Charlotte, NC 28203.

E-mail address: jennifer.isenhour@carolinashealthcare.org (J.L. Isenhour).

doi:10.1016/j.emc.2007.06.002

emed.theclinics.com

Initial assessment

Historical data, while often lacking, may provide invaluable information to the emergency practitioner when evaluating a patient with abdominal trauma. If the patient was involved in a MVC, information regarding fatalities at the scene, vehicle type and velocity, roll over, intrusion, steering wheel deformity, use of seatbelts and air bags, and the patient's location within the vehicle offer guidance in management [3–5].

Physical examination

While some studies cite physical examination as only 55% to 65% sensitive for diagnosing injury in those sustaining BAT, it is still the cornerstone for primary assessment [6]. Patients with BAT may present to the ED anywhere on the spectrum from normotensive and alert to obtunded and in shock. Careful attention to physical findings helps drive decision making and proper sequencing of diagnostic tests.

Hypotension after BAT typically results from visceral organ injury and hemorrhage, usually of the spleen [1]. These patients need emergent evaluation of the peritoneal cavity, and coincident appraisal of any extra-abdominal injury creating hemorrhage or hemodynamic instability, such as long bone fracture, scalp laceration, hemothorax, pneumothorax, or, in infants, severe head injury [7].

In awake, hemodynamically stable patients with isolated BAT, abdominal pain, tenderness, and peritoneal signs are the most reliable findings for intra-abdominal injury and can be found in up to 90% of those with injury. However, several studies demonstrate that even in these patients, significant injury may be missed with physical exam alone. Therefore, absence of physical findings does not preclude injury and the need for further observation and diagnostic testing [8,9].

Salim and colleagues' study [9], published in 2006, evaluated 592 subjects with significant blunt multisystem trauma, who had no visible chest or abdomen injury, were hemodynamically stable, and had a normal abdominal physical examination. Of these, 19.6% had clinically significant findings on chest computed tomography (CT) and 7.1% on abdominal CT, leading to a change in clinical management in almost 19% of the subjects.

When extra-abdominal injuries are present, suspicion for concomitant intra-abdominal injury is paramount. Up to 10 % of those with closed head injury, and 7% of those with a distracting extremity injury, will have an abdominal injury even with no signs or symptoms of abdominal trauma [10,11]. Pleuritic left costal margin pain may indicate underlying splenic injury [12]. Ecchymosis across the lower abdomen, a "seatbelt sign," portends intra-abdominal injury in up to one third of patients [13].

Some recent small studies suggest that in awake, hemodynamically stable adult patients who are going to the operating room for extra-abdominal injuries, physical exam will exclude most intra-abdominal injuries requiring immediate operative intervention [14–16]. In 2004, Gonzalez and colleagues [15] evaluated 162 hemodynamically stable patients after BAT and with extra-abdominal injuries requiring operative repair. These patients had a Glasgow Coma Score (GCS) greater than or equal to 14, no findings on physical examination of the lower ribs, abdomen, and pelvis, and no neurologic deficits. Two injuries (a grade one splenic laceration and a small bowel mesenteric hematoma) were missed by physical examination but detected on CT. Neither of these patients required surgical intervention or transfusion. Thus, the investigators conclude that physical examination alone may be sufficient for evaluating for surgically significant injury in patients with extra-abdominal injury. However, they suggest that larger prospective studies are still needed.

Laboratory testing

Most hematologic and blood chemistries serve only as adjuvants in the management of patients with abdominal trauma. A baseline hematocrit may be useful, but rarely will alter emergent management. Blood typing should routinely be sent for any patient with abdominal trauma and signs of hemorrhage or potential need for transfusion. Base deficit is often used as a marker for hemorrhagic shock, but as with all laboratory values, it must be interpreted in context of the clinical scenario and what resuscitation has occurred, as correction of the metabolic acidosis will lag behind physiologic correction [17,18]. White blood cell count, pancreatic enzymes, and liver function tests have all been used as markers of intra-abdominal injury in the past; however, most studies now show these are nonspecific and may not provide much guidance in the acute decision-making for patients with abdominal trauma [19,20]. Urinalysis with detection of hematuria (both microscopic and gross) indicates renal injury, and coupled with abdominal tenderness predicts intra-abdominal injury following BAT with 65% sensitivity and 94% specificity [21,22]. Toxicologic studies have little value in the acute management of abdominal trauma, unless there is unexplained altered mental status [23].

Emergency management

Unstable patients

Determining need for emergent operative care is the top priority in the evaluation of patients sustaining BAT. In those patients who are hemodynamically unstable, the presence of intra-abdominal hemorrhage must be expeditiously established. Risk of death from isolated intra-abdominal injury increases with time spent in the emergency department and severity of hypotension (Fig. 1) [24].

Clarke and colleagues' review [24] of the Pennsylvania Trauma Systems Foundation trauma registry, from October 1986 until July 1999, identified 243 hypotensive patients with intra-abdominal injury who were initially evaluated in a trauma center. Using logistic regression, the probability of

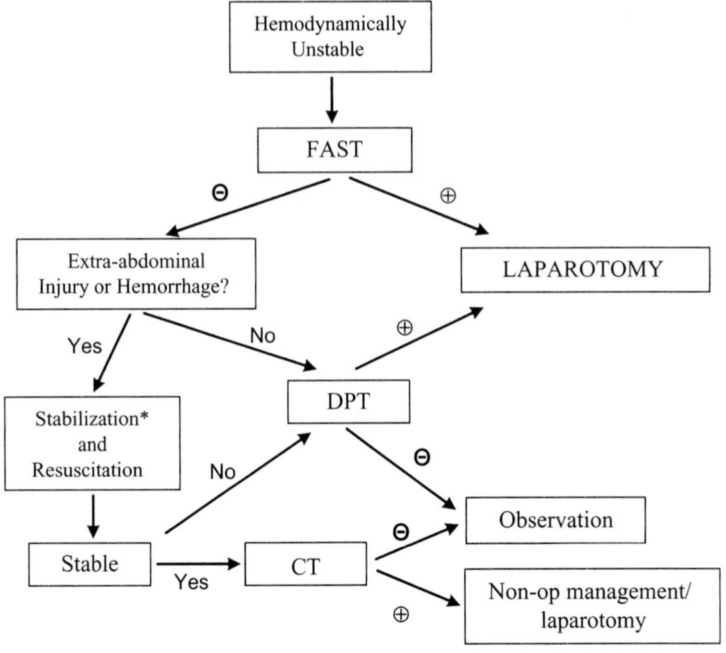

*Pelvic wrap, chest tube placement, whip stitch
FAST – Focused Abdominal Sonography for Trauma
DPT – Diagnostic Peritoneal Tap; ⊕ if ≥10 cc gross blood aspirated
CT – Computed Tomagraphy

Fig. 1. Unstable patients with blunt abdominal trauma. ⊕, ≥10 cc blood aspirated; DPT ⊖, <10 cc blood aspirated

death increased as time spent in the ED increased up to 90 minutes. Also, those patients with initial systolic blood pressures of less than 60 mm Hg had a significantly higher risk of death, while those with a systolic blood pressure of greater than 80 mm Hg had a significantly lower risk of death. Traditionally, bedside diagnostic peritoneal lavage or tap (DPL or DPT) quickly triages unstable patients with multisystem trauma. If 10 cc of gross blood is aspirated then intra-abdominal hemorrhage is present and the patient requires urgent laparotomy. This knowledge is especially useful when multisystem trauma is present and the physician must decide which therapeutic path to tread, be it exploratory laparotomy or angiography with embolization. However, with the advent of bedside ultrasonography (US), DPL is being employed less and is no longer the standard diagnostic procedure in these unstable patients.

Recent literature shows mixed opinion on the use of US in the unstable patient. While some studies cite near 100% sensitivity for hemoperitoneum requiring surgical intervention in the hypotensive patient [25], others show a wide range of sensitivity and caution against its sole use in this patient population, especially when no intraperitoneal free fluid is detected [26].

Farahmand and colleagues' [25] retrospective review of 128 hypotensive BAT patients demonstrated an assessment of focused abdominal sonography for trauma (FAST) sensitivity of 85% for detection of any intra-abdominal injury. When only those injuries requiring surgical intervention were included, sensitivity rose to 97%, and it was 100% sensitive for all fatal injuries. The only missed surgical injury was a mesenteric injury. Of the other missed injuries, 63% were extraperitoneal. Thus, the investigators concluded that FAST in the hypotensive patient is an effective screening tool and, when coupled with risk assessment, can effectively rule out intra-abdominal injury requiring surgical intervention.

A recent study of 7047 patients demonstrated lower accuracy in those subjects with additional closed head injury and low GCS [27]. However, in most centers, hemodynamically unstable patients with a positive FAST exam proceed to exploratory laparotomy.

Because intra-abdominal injury can not be entirely ruled out in those unstable patients with a negative FAST, further diagnostic testing, bedside DPL or DPT, or—once more stable—CT, must be performed to completely evaluate for intra-abdominal injury, while concurrently pursuing possible extra-abdominal injury as a cause of instability (Fig. 2).

Chest and pelvic radiographs determine the presence of extra-abdominal causes of hypotension or hemorrhage, namely pneumothorax or hemothorax and pelvic ring fracture, respectively (Fig. 3). Needle decompression, chest tube placement, or pelvic wrapping and subsequent angiography

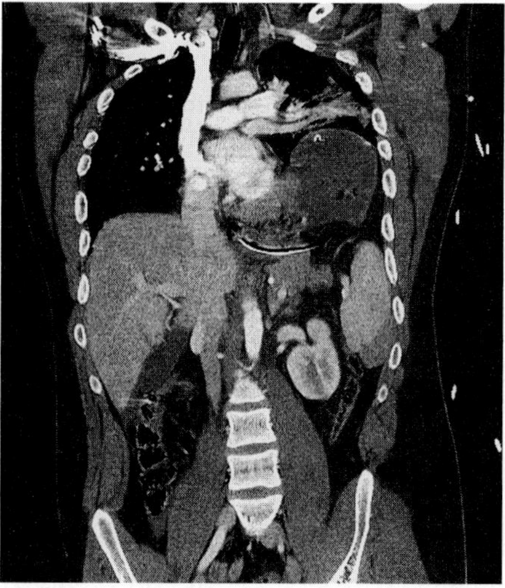

Fig. 2. Ruptured left diaphragm and grade 3 splenic laceration.

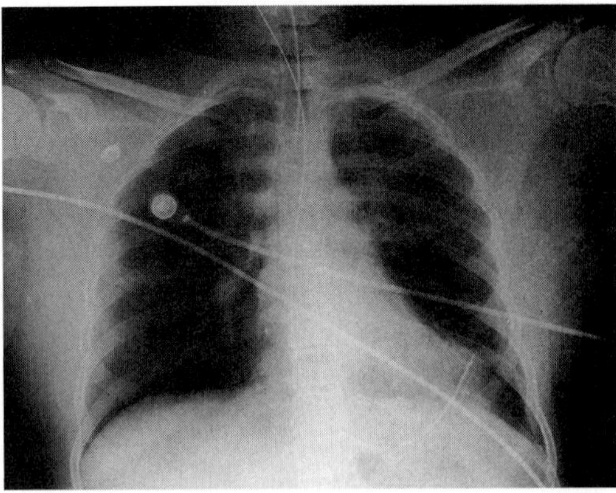

Fig. 3. Nasogastric tube in left chest with diaphragmatic rupture.

control further blood loss and aid in resuscitation. Large scalp lacerations may also prove a source of hemorrhage and should be whip-stitched (or Rainey clipped) closed.

Stable patients

New advances in computed tomography and ultrasound continue to alter the management of stable patients with BAT (Fig. 4). Hemodynamically stable patients allow for a more time intensive evaluation and alternative testing to diagnose intra-abdominal injury. While physical exam in the stable, alert, nonintoxicated patient is reasonably accurate, it is not infallible and clinical observation with serial examinations is warranted [8]. Furthermore, one recent study advocates for CT evaluation in all patients sustaining BAT. The authors cite missed significant injury, one requiring alteration of treatment, at a rate of 7% in a patient population with no signs of external trauma and normal abdominal examination [9].

Most centers employ US as part of their initial survey in trauma resuscitation. Studies demonstrate a range in sensitivity for hemoperitoneum from 65% to 95%, although most recent studies cite ranges of 86% to 89% [28–30]. If the FAST is noted to be positive, these stable patients then proceed to CT for delineation of intraperitoneal injury and quantification of the hemoperitoneum (Fig. 5).

If the FAST is negative, concern for intra-abdominal injury is still present, as US is notoriously poor at identifying solid organ subcapsular injury, bowel injury, or injury to the retroperitoneum or diaphragm [26,31,32]. However, some report that a negative FAST coupled with a negative physical exam, followed by an observation period of 12 to 24 hours in an alert, stable patient virtually excludes intra-abdominal injury [33]. Others recommend serial abdominal US to increase the sensitivity of the FAST exam [34,35].

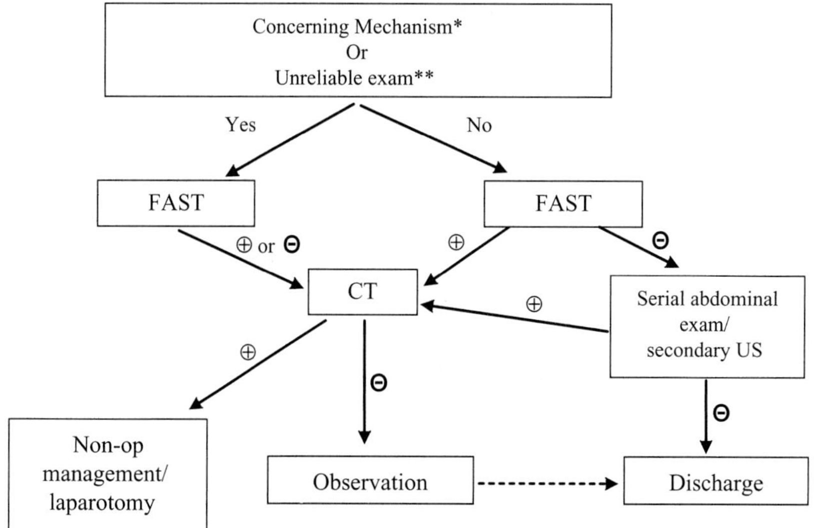

* Concerning mechanism: fatality at scene, rollover, intrusion, prolonged extrication
** Unreliable exam: altered mental status, intoxication, distracting injury

FAST – Focused Abdominal Sonography for Trauma
CT – Computed Tomagraphy

Fig. 4. Stable patients with blunt abdominal trauma. DPT ⊕, ≥10 cc blood aspirated; DPT ⊖, <10 cc blood aspirated.

A recently published study prospectively illustrates that US use in patients with abdominal trauma changed management decisions in 32.8% of cases and decreased the need for CT and DPL or DPT. This prospective study compared 419 patients who required trauma team activation. A convenience sample of 194 subjects received an initial bedside FAST after the trauma team leader specified the patient management plan. After the FAST, the plan was reviewed and a revised plan was documented. The remaining 225 subjects did not undergo FAST examination and proceeded with the trauma leader's original plan. Of those with a FAST examination, the subsequent use of CT decreased from 47% to 34% and DPL from 9% to 1% [36]. Other studies cite decreased time to laparotomy and improved use of hospital resources when US was part of the initial trauma evaluation in those with abdominal trauma.

Branney and colleagues [37] prospectively evaluated 486 BAT patients who followed an ultrasound-based key clinical pathway during a 3-month period. He compared these with a similar cohort for 3 months and found that those using the US pathway had significant reductions in the use of CT (56% to 26%) and DPL (17% to 4%).

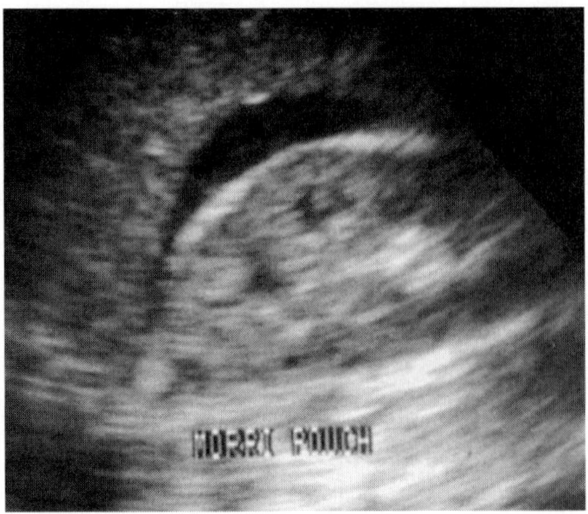

Fig. 5. Free fluid in Morrison's Pouch.

Most recently Melniker and colleagues' [38] point-of-care limited ultrasonography (PLUS) for trauma study prospectively evaluated the amount of time from ED arrival to transfer to operative care. The 29 subjects in the PLUS group who went to the operating room had a decrease of 64% in time to operative care when compared with the 34 controls. Secondary measures noted a coincident decrease in use of CT, length of stay, and complications for the 111 subjects in the PLUS cohort when compared with the 106 control subjects.

The advent of 64-slice helical CT scanners has improved diagnosis of both solid and hollow viscus injury post-BAT (see Fig. 3). Recent studies advocate the use of CT, even in patients with no signs of injury, be it intra- or extra-abdominal [9]. Most admit to its low yield in those patients who are alert with no signs of trauma; however, missed injury in these studies was at times significant and, therefore, routine use of CT can not be abandoned in certain patient populations, namely those with extra-abdominal injuries, ethanol ingestion, and otherwise unreliable abdominal examination [8,14,39].

The 2004 American College of Emergency Physicians Clinical Policy statement, based on review of the literature, touts CT as reliably excluding liver and spleen injury after BAT. This clinical policy also states that CT alone could not reliably rule out hollow viscus, diaphragmatic, or pancreatic injury [40].

Hollow viscus injury (HVI) remains difficult to detect despite advances in diagnostic modalities. Coincident solid organ injury often masks CT findings of HVI, increasing morbidity and mortality because of delay in diagnosis [41]. Recent studies suggest physical examination for signs of peritonitis, coupled with CT with intravascular (IV) contrast only, may be adequate for diagnosing bowel injury [42–45]. However, the low incidence of HVI makes large prospective studies for noncontrast CT identification difficult.

Stuhlfaut and colleagues [43], restrospectively evaluated 1082 patients with BAT who had a noncontrast CT of the abdomen and pelvis. Eleven patients were diagnosed with HVI requiring operative repair. Noncontrast CT had a sensitivity of 82% and specificity of 99% for detecting these injuries.

In 2004 Allen and colleagues [54] prospectively evaluated 500 patients after blunt abdominal trauma with noncontrast CT of the abdomen and pelvis. A CT was considered positive for HVI if there was presence of bowel wall thickening, bowel perforation, free intraperitoneal air, free fluid without solid organ injury, and mesenteric laceration or hematoma. Of these 500, 19 of 20 subjects with HVI were detected on initial CT read (a duodenal perforation was missed). There were two false-positive studies that were read as suspicious for bowel injury but at laparotomy had only splenic injury, and another misinterpreted as a gastric hematoma on the initial CT read, but correctly refuted on immediate follow up CT with oral contrast. In this study, noncontrast CT had a sensitivity of 95% and specificity of 99.6% for HVI.

In 2003 the Eastern Association for the Surgery of Trauma (EAST) multi-institutional hollow viscus injury study reviewed trauma registries from 95 trauma centers over 2 years. They concluded that no test or combination of findings could reliably exclude colonic injury. They noted that, though only used in 22 % of cases, DPL was the only diagnostic test with a sensitivity of 97% and negative predictive value of 80% for HVI [42].

If liver or splenic injury is detected by CT in a hemodynamically stable patient, nonoperative management with close observation, serial examinations, and hematocrits is now standard [46–48]. This is in part due to improved resolution on CT, which allows better definition of the injury and quantification of hemorrhage [47]. Even high-grade liver lacerations can be initially managed nonoperatively; however, complications and the possible need for therapeutic laparotomy should be expected [48].

In 2005, Kozar and colleagues [48] evaluated 230 patients with grade 3 or higher blunt hepatic injury initially managed nonoperatively. Of these, 25 had complications (11%) including bleeding, biliary tract related complications, abdominal compartment syndrome, liver abscesses, and liver necrosis. Grade 5 injuries had a 63% complication rate, whereas only one of the grade 3 patients had a complication (a peripheral bile duct leak). Operative intervention was required in 5.2% of all study subjects initially managed nonoperatively.

Special considerations

Pelvic fracture is routinely managed nonoperatively with angiography. Therefore determination of concurrent hemoperitoneum in unstable patients is paramount, as need for laparotomy in these patients may require external fixator placement in the operating room for fracture stabilization.

Ultrasound and DPT have both proven efficacious in the management of this patient population [49].

Closed head injury renders physical exam less useful in the triage of patients with BAT. Furthermore, the ability perform more time intensive diagnostic testing, such as CT, may be limited. When no lateralizing signs are present, the need for urgent craniotomy is less and a quick head CT follow by abdominal CT may be possible. However, those with lateralizing signs and hemodynamic instability may need a burr hole with concurrent laparotomy. Others that respond to resuscitative measures may have time for a "quick" head CT just before abdominal CT [50,51].

There is evidence that patients with serious abdominal trauma, especially those requiring surgical intervention, do better at regional trauma centers. Consultation and transfer should occur early in the evaluation of patients. However, a subset of patients with hemodynamic instability and known hemoperitoneum will benefit from laparotomy with hemorrhage control before transfer [52].

Penetrating abdominal trauma

Background

Penetrating trauma is increasing because of the growth of violence in our society. Stab wounds are encountered three times more often than gunshot wounds, but have a lower mortality because of their lower velocity and less invasive tract. As a result of their greater force and extensive missile tract, gunshot wounds account for up to 90% of the mortality associated with penetrating abdominal trauma. Injury to the bowel (small, then large) is most often found, followed by hepatic injury, regardless of type of penetrating injury [53].

Initial assessment

For those with penetrating abdominal trauma, it is important to note in stab wounds the implement used, its trajectory, and length, and in gunshot wounds, the type of gun, number of shots heard, the position of the patient during the assault, and the distance of the patient from the gun. Shotgun wounds create a special scenario, as their velocity and trajectories differ from gunshot wounds. As distance is gained, shotgun pellets disperse and thus mortality is decreased; however, debris carried into these resulting multiple wounds increases morbidity [54].

Physical examination

It is vital that patients sustaining penetrating trauma be completely undressed and thoroughly examined for injury. Often these patients will present with an obvious wound to the anterior abdomen, only to have a secondary wound in an axilla, perineum, scalp, or skin fold that may be unnoticed and perhaps lethal.

The tenet of evaluating penetrating abdominal trauma is to determine peritoneal violation and then peritoneal injury. Physical exam may reveal peritonitis, evisceration, or other indications of peritoneal violation, and thus the need for operative management [55]. Those patients with unstable vital signs may have an intra-abdominal injury with hemorrhage; however, tension pneumothorax, hemothorax, and pericardial tamponade must be considered and evaluated.

Emergency management

With the advent of anesthesia, sterilization, and surgical training, post World War I treatment of penetrating injury to the abdomen was mandatory laparotomy. This dogmatic approach was predicated by battlefield experience with trauma laparotomies and translated to civilian populations in the post-war era. However, as nontheraputic laparotomy rates approached 30%, surgeons found that the injuries and morbidity associated with noncombat penetrating wounds differed from those produced by military weapons. In 1960 Shaftan [56] published a paper advocating nonoperative management in select patient populations sustaining stab wounds, and the tenet of mandatory laparotomy was lost. Today, nonoperative treatment of abdominal gunshot wounds is also gaining favor [57–60].

Indication for mandatory laparotomy

The mainstay of evaluation of those with penetrating abdominal trauma is identification of the need for immediate surgical intervention. Physicians agree that immediate laparotomy is indicated if there is hemodynamic instability or the presence of peritoneal signs on physical examination [9,57,61–69].

When evisceration is present, surgical intervention is generally accepted as the next step in management. Nagy and colleagues' [63] prospective study in 1999 included 81 patients with abdominal stab wounds and evisceration: either omentum (75%), small intestine (22%), colon (1%), or both small bowel and colon (1%). Peritoneal signs or hemodynamic instability were absent in 76% and evisceration was therefore the sole indication for surgical exploration. A necessary laparotomy was performed in 76% of this subgroup, and of those with only omental evisceration, the necessary laparotomy rate was 73%. This high incidence of intra-abdominal injury following stab wounds with evisceration has made exploratory laparotomy in these patients standard [9,61–63].

Newer studies are challenging this standard in those with anterior stab wounds. Arikan [64] published a small study in 2005, evaluating nonoperative management for abdominal stab wounds with evisceration. Thirty-one patients were managed non-operatively, despite evisceration of omentum (28) or organ (3). Of these, 24 were discharged home without exploratory laparotomy, including two with organ evisceration. Seven patients were explored because of development of concerning physical exam findings during the observation period. There were two negative, five therapeutic, and no nontheraputic laparotomies. Those patients with nonoperative management had decreased hospital length of stay and complication rates when compared with a group of 21 patients managed with mandatory laparotomy. Patients with refractory hypotension, peritonitis, blood from a nasogastric tube, or obviously perforated bowel were excluded. Evisceration after gunshot wounds mandates immediate laparotomy because of increase injury and contamination associated with these injuries [57].

Identification of peritoneal injury

Stab wounds

Stab wounds produce peritoneal violation in up to 70% of instances, but of these only one fourth to one third will require operative intervention (Fig. 6) [65,70]. For those patients without evisceration, peritonitis, or hemodynamic instability, studies show that judicious use of local wound exploration, CT, DPL, laparoscopy, and US, coupled with physical examination, can safely select patients appropriate for nonoperative management [66,69,71].

Local wound exploration is easily and safely performed at the bedside in those patients with abdominal stab wounds. If the stab wound tract ends before violation of the abdominal fascia, studies show these patients are safe for discharge. However, if the tract is not completely visualized because of body habitus, other injuries, or technical inability then further testing is necessary.

Most centers employ CT as the next step in evaluation of these stable patients as it is noninvasive, offers information about the extent of injury to visceral organs, and can help plan both operative and nonoperative management [9,72,73]. While triple contrast CT is still routinely used for its 97% sensitivity and 98% specificity [72], one recent study evaluated the use of CT with only IV contrast and found a similar sensitivity and specificity. This protocol reserves use of oral and rectal contrast for specific patient populations, thus decreasing the amount of time needed to perform the diagnostic test in most patients [59]. Injuries to the bowel, diaphragm, and pancreas are poorly visualized on CT (even with triple contrast), and in those patients with high suspicion for injury (such as those with hepatic injury and right-sided hemothorax), further diagnostic testing with laparascopy or DPL may be warranted despite negative CT [60,72].

The role of ultrasound in penetrating abdominal trauma is still evolving. A positive FAST may indicate intraperitoneal hemorrhage and injury, but in this group of stable patients, more definitive testing must follow as there is potential for nonoperative management. A negative FAST does not exclude injury and requires further evaluation [74]. A small study of 35

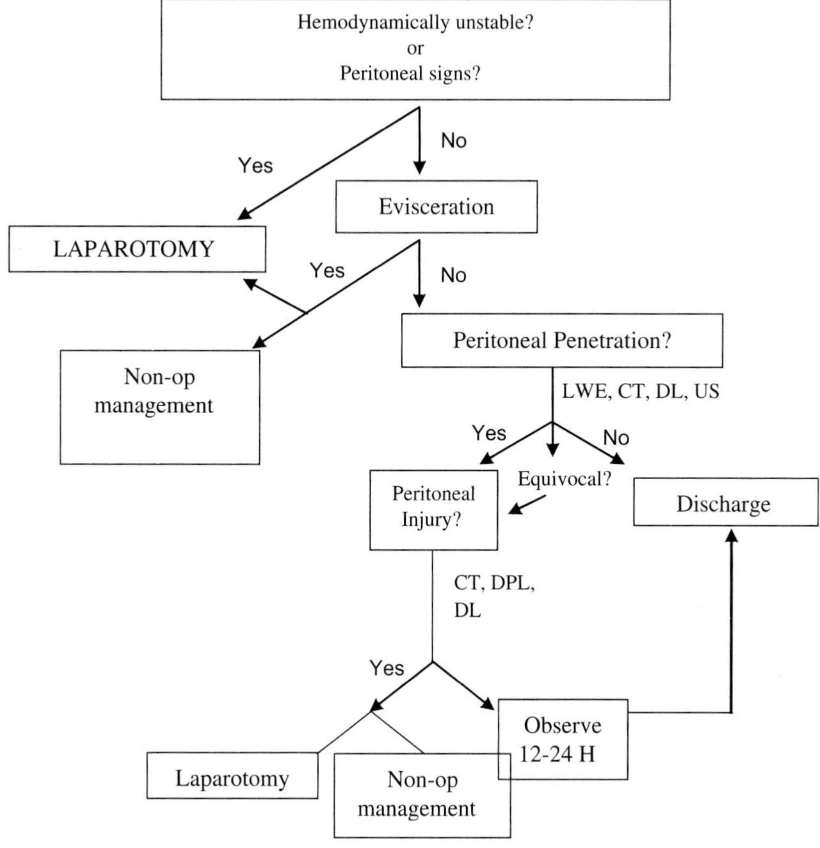

LWE Local Wound Exploration
CT Computed Tomagraphy
DL Diagnostic Laparoscopy
DPL Diagnostic Peritoneal Lavage

Fig. 6. Abdominal stab wounds. US, ultrasonography.

hemodynamically stable patients with anterior abdominal stab wounds used US to determine fascial violation. After anesthetizing the wound, the 8.0 MHz probe was used to assess abdominal fascial integrity directly beneath the wound and in a 10-cm by 10-cm area surrounding the injury. All stab wounds were then evaluated with standard local wound exploration. While overall sensitivity was only 59%, this increased as the operator's years of training increased (specificity was 100%) [75]. As emergency practitioners become more facile with alternative applications of US, this less invasive test for peritoneal violation may play a larger role.

At some centers, diagnostic laparoscopy (DL) is used as a screening tool for those with abdominal stab wounds. It is useful for inspecting the diaphragm and evaluating the depth of wound tracts [67,76,77]. Its routine use for penetrating trauma, however, is controversial.

A small prospective study of 232 subjects demonstrated that in patients with clear peritoneal violation (43 subjects), diagnostic laparoscopy (N = 20) performed no better than exploratory laparotomy (N = 23). In this study, no therapeutic laparoscopies were performed and nine subjects were converted from DL to laparotomy. However, in those 63 subjects with local wound exploration showing equivocal penetration, those randomized to laparoscopy (N = 28) had more minor and occult organ injury detected than those in the selected nonoperative management group (N = 31). But, this was at the expense of increased length of stay, hospital cost, and time to recovery in the DL group, leading the investigators to recommend against routine use of DL in penetrating abdominal trauma [78].

Other advocates of DL point to decreased cost and length of stay when laparoscopy is employed rather than exploratory laparotomy; albeit, this is at centers adept at DL [67,79]. Simon and colleague's [79] 5-year review of over 9,000 trauma patients at Jacobi Medical Center in New York found 344 explorations for penetrating abdominal trauma (300 laparotomies and 44 laparoscopies). During the last 4 years of the study period, he noted a rise in the use of DL for stab wound evaluation from 19.4% to 27%, which correlated to a decrease in the negative laparotomy rate during that time period. Of the 44 laparoscopies, 22 were positive for peritoneal violation and 15 of those required conversion to laparotomy for repair (there was 1 nontheraputic laparotomy). The remaining seven were three non-bleeding liver lacerations managed nonoperatively and four left diaphragmatic injuries repaired laparoscopically. There were 238 positive, 31 nontheraputic, and 31 negative laparotomies in those patients managed with initial laparotomy.

Length of stay for those patients with no other injuries and a negative laparotomy (N = 21; length of hospital stay 4.0 plus or minus 1.7 days) and those with no other injuries and a negative DL (N = 5; length of hospital stay 2.2 plus or minus 1.1 days) were compared and noted to be significantly less in the DL group ($P = .0349$). Neither of these groups had any significant complications. The investigators concluded that in a trauma center with an aggressive DL program, patients with anterior stab wound can benefit from this approach [79].

A small prospective study of 52 subjects with penetrating abdominal trauma, by Ahmed and colleagues [67], demonstrated that 77% of stable patients could avoid laparotomy when DL was employed. Of the 38% with visceral injury, almost half were managed nonoperatively. In this small series, only 12 subjects required open therapeutic laparotomy. When compared with National Trauma Data Bank matched patients, the use of DL was estimated to reduce hospitalization by over 55% in this series.

Diagnostic peritoneal lavage performed at the bedside determines both peritoneal violation and peritoneal injury. This rapid, yet invasive, test provides information about solid viscus, bowel, and diaphragmatic injury. While there has been debate over what red blood cell counts to use for detecting injury, most agree that the presence of greater than 10,000 red blood cells per high-power field (RBCs/hpf) indicates visceral injury in penetrating abdominal wounds [55,80]. A reduced range of 5 to 10,000 RBCs/hpf should be used for thoracoabdominal wounds [54]. When coupled with physical examination, DPL helps identify those patients who are candidates for nonoperative management [66,68,71]. However, as other less invasive diagnostic modalities are gaining favor, routine use of DPL is decreasing [57].

Gunshot wounds

Determining trajectory of gunshot wounds helps to determine the presence of intraperitoneal injury (Fig. 7). Once a thorough physical exam is completed and the number of wounds counted, plain film radiographs elucidate the missile path. Radio-opaque markers on any wounds, coupled with anteroposterior and lateral films, create a three dimensional estimation of trajectory path. Caution should prevail, as even wounds suggesting a superficial path may have intraperitoneal injury. If an odd number of wounds are present, careful attention to radiographs should reveal the missile location [57].

Computed tomography scanning is frequently employed after abdominal gunshot wounds, as it allows for determination of trajectory path, identifies organ injury and, therefore, optimal patients for nonoperative management [57,59,72]. As discussed previously, sensitivity and specificity remain high for this modality, even when IV contrast is solely used [59]. Many studies use CT as an adjuvant to nonoperative management [57,60,69,73]. It is especially helpful for defining hepatic injury that may be ideal for conservative treatment with observation only.

While more invasive, DPL has known high sensitivity for intra-abdominal injury after gunshot wounds [55,57,80]. It is an excellent means of determining peritoneal violation: using 10,000 RBCs/hpf as the threshold, it has a sensitivity of 96% [55]. Brakenridge and colleagues [80] also demonstrated its utility in shotgun wounds, citing a sensitivity of 87.5% in these patients. But, while DPL is sensitive for hemoperitoneum, it does not give specific information regarding organ injury and is therefore less useful in determining nonoperative management in stable patients, and its use as a screening exam in these patients is declining [57].

Conversely, laparoscopy is slowly gaining favor in the management of abdominal gunshot wounds. Laparoscopy serves primarily to determine the presence of peritoneal violation and to inspect the diaphragm. Drawbacks include the need for anesthesia, inability to repair certain injuries (requiring conversion to laparotomy), and difficulty in visualizing the posterior

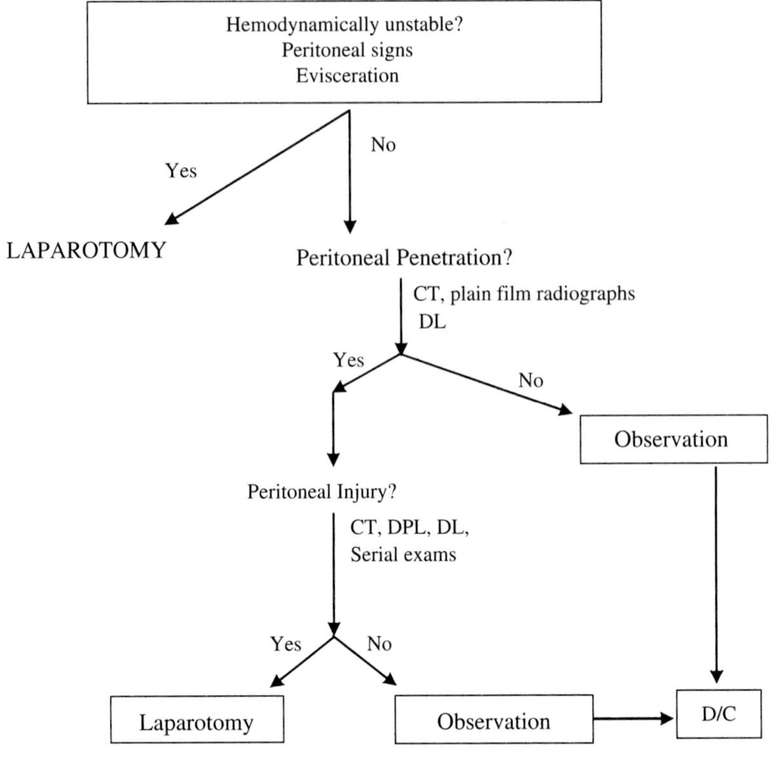

CT Computed Tomagraphy
DL Diagnostic Laparoscopy
DPL Diagnostic Peritoneal Lavage

Fig. 7. Abdominal gunshot wounds.

diaphragm, subtle bowel injuries, and the retroperitoneum [57,67,76]. As for stab wounds, as trauma centers become more adept at this procedure laparoscopy may be used more frequently, especially in those patients with left sided thoracoabdominal injuries in which diaphragmatic injury must be ruled out [57].

Selective nonoperative management

Once the need for mandatory laparatomy is ruled out, patients may be triaged to nonoperative management. These patients must be serially observed with frequent physical examination. If peritoneal signs develop, conversion to laparotomy follows. Some centers use additional diagnostic testing (as described above) to further stratify patients for nonoperative management. Numerous studies have touted this approach for management of abdominal stab wounds, showing it safely reduces rates of nontheraputic and negative laparotomies, as well as decreasing the length of hospital stay and cost [60,69,71].

Now studies confirm that similar algorithms for abdominal gunshot wounds are also safe practice in centers able to perform frequent re-examination of patients and transition to laparotomy when indicated [57–60,72]. Velmahos and colleagues' study [59] of 100 subjects with nontangential abdominal gunshot wounds selected for nonoperative management showed CT had a sensitivity of 90.5% and specificity of 96% for identifying injury. In this study, 26 subjects went on to laparotomy, of which 5 were nontheraputic. In another study of nonoperative management of penetrating abdominal trauma, 41 patients with gunshot wounds were evaluated. Of these, 17 had a positive CT and 24 had a negative CT. There were no false-negative CTs in this select group. Thirteen went on to laparotomy, of which 11 were therapeutic, 1 was nontheraputic and 1 was negative (this patient had a negative CT but clinical indications for laparotomy). There were five nonoperative hepatic injuries, three hepatic injuries that had angioembolization, and one video-assisted thorascopic diaphragm repair [72].

Special considerations

Flank and back penetrating injury present a difficult situation, as visualization of those areas via local wound exploration, US, DPL, and laparoscopy is challenging, if not impossible. Computed tomographic scan with triple contrast has become the test of choice in hemodynamically stable patients, and may safely allow triage to nonoperative management [58,81]. There is growing evidence for nonoperative management, but these studies remain small and are only applicable at trauma centers. As most patients with these injuries have indication for mandatory laparotomy, larger more translatable studies are probably not forthcoming [57].

Thoracoabdominal wounds are especially difficult, as the trajectory of penetration cannot be reliably determined because of movement of the diaphragm. As noted above, if DPL is used in this group, then a lowered RBC/hpf threshold of 5000 must be used [54]. While exploratory lapartomy has been mandatory for these types of injuries in the past, use of laparoscopy continues to gain favor. This approach reduces negative and nontheraputic laparotomy rates previously documented [57].

Summary

Several advances in diagnostic modalities challenge the traditional dogmatic approach to abdominal trauma. Ultrasonography is now routinely used in the initial assessment of those with blunt abdominal trauma, and its role in penetrating trauma is being defined. Improved CT resolution with multislice and helical CT scanners allows for better identification of injuries with improved ability to grade their severity. This in turn, offers a nonoperative approach for certain patients with penetrating or blunt abdominal trauma. As competence with laparoscopy continues to evolve, this more invasive screening tool shows promise for evaluation of certain types of patients with penetrating injury, and may lead to less morbity and more cost-effective use of hospital resources. Finally, selective nonoperative management for both BAT and abdominal stab wounds and gunshot wounds is no longer a novelty, finally accumulating the literature necessary to make its practice standard in most trauma centers.

References

[1] Davis JJ, Cohn I Jr, Nance FC, et al. Diagnosis and management of blunt abdominal trauma. Ann Surg 1976;183:672–8.

[2] Demetriades D, Murray JA, Brown C, et al. High-level falls: type and severity of injuries and survival outcome according to age. J Trauma 2005;58:342–5.

[3] Rivara FP, Koepsell TD, Grossman DC, et al. Effectiveness of automatic shoulder belt systems in motor vehicle crashes. JAMA 2000;283:2826–8.

[4] Brasel KJ, Nirula R. What mechanism justifies abdominal evaluation in motor vehicle crashes. J Trauma 2005;59:1057–61.

[5] Newgard CD, Lewis RJ, Kraus JF. Steering wheel deformity and serious thoracic or abdominal injury among drivers and passengers involved in motor vehicle crashes. Ann Emerg Med 2005;45:43–50.

[6] Brown CK, Dunn KA, Wilson K, et al. Diagnostic evaluation of patients with blunt abdominal trauma: a decision analysis [see comment]. Acad Emerg Med 2000;7:385–96.

[7] Mahoney EJ, Biffl WL, Harrington DT, et al. Isolated brain injury as a cause of hypotension in the blunt trauma patient. J Trauma 2003;55:1065–9.

[8] Poletti PA, Mirvis SE, Shanmuganathan K, et al. Blunt abdominal trauma patients: can organ injury be excluded without performing computed tomography? J Trauma 2004;57: 1072–81.

[9] Salim A, Sangthong B, Martin M, et al. Whole body imaging in blunt multisystem trauma patients without obvious signs of injury: results of a prospective study. Arch Surg 2006; 141:468–73.

[10] Schurink GW, Bode PJ, van Luijt PA, et al. The value of physical examination in the diagnosis of patients with blunt abdominal trauma: a retrospective study. Injury 1997;28:261–5.

[11] Ferrera PC, Verdile VP, Bartfield JM, et al. Injuries distracting from intraabdominal injuries after blunt trauma. Am J Emerg Med 1998;16:145–9.

[12] Holmes JF, Ngyuen H, Jacoby RC, et al. Do all patients with left costal margin injuries require radiographic evaluation for intraabdominal injury. Ann Emerg Med 2005;46: 232–6.

[13] Velmahos GC, Tatevossian R, Demetriades D, et al. The "seat belt mark" sign: a call for increased vigilance among physicians treating victims of motor vehicle accidents. Am Surg 1999;65:181–5.

[14] Schauer BA, Nguyen H, Wisner DH, et al. Is definitive abdominal evaluation required in blunt trauma victims undergoing urgent extra abdominal surgery. Acad Emerg Med 2005; 12:707–11.

[15] Gonzalez RP, Han M, Turk B, et al. Screening for abdominal injury prior to emergent extra-abdominal trauma surgery: A prospective study. J Trauma 2004;57:739–41.

[16] Gonzalez RP, Dziurzynski K, Maunu M. Emergent extra-abdominal trauma surgery: is abdominal screening necessary. J Trauma 2000;49:195–9.
[17] Davis JW, Mackersie RC, Holbrook TL, et al. Base deficit as an indicator of significant abdominal injury [see comment]. Ann Emerg Med 1991;20:842–4.
[18] Davis JW, Kaups KL, Parks SN, et al. Base deficit is superior to pH in evaluating clearance of acidosis after traumatic shock. J Trauma 1998;44:114–8.
[19] Asimos AW, Gibbs MA, Marx JA, et al. Value of point-of-care blood testing in emergent trauma management. J Trauma 2000;48:1101–8.
[20] Takishima T, Sugimoto K, Hirata M, et al. Serum amylase level on admission in the diagnosis of blunt injury to the pancreas Its significance and limitations. Ann Emerg Med 1997;226:70–6.
[21] Knudson MM, McAninch JW, Gomez R, et al. Hematuria as a predictor of abdominal injury after blunt trauma. Am J Surg 1992;164:482–5.
[22] Richards JR, Derlet RW, Richards JR, et al. Computed tomography for blunt abdominal trauma in the ED: a prospective study. Am J Emerg Med 1998;16:338–42.
[23] Sloan EP, Zalenski RJ, Smith RF, et al. Toxicology screening in urban trauma patients: drug prevalence and its relationship to trauma severity and management. J Trauma 1989;29:1647–53.
[24] Clarke JR, Trooskin SZ, Doshi PJ, et al. Time to laparotomy for intra-abdominal bleeding from trauma does affect survival for delays up to 90 minutes. J Trauma 2002;52:420–5.
[25] Farahmand N, Sirlin CB, Brown MA, et al. Hypotensive patients with blunt abdominal trauma: performance of screening US. Radiology 2005;235:436–43.
[26] Holmes JF, Harris D, Battistella FD, et al. Performance of abdominal ultrasonography in blunt trauma patients with out-of-hospital or emergency department hypotension. Ann Emerg Med 2004;43:354–61.
[27] Soffer D, Schulman CI, Mckenney MG, et al. What does ultrasonography miss in blunt trauma patients with a low glasgow coma score (GCS). J Trauma 2006;60:1184–8.
[28] Chiu WC, Cushing BM, Rodriguez A, et al. Abdominal injuries without hemoperitoneum: a potential limitation of focused abdominal sonography for trauma (FAST). J Trauma 1997;42:617–25.
[29] Dolich MO, McKenney MG, Varela JE, et al. 2,576 ultrasounds for blunt abdominal trauma. J Trauma 2001;50:108–12.
[30] Bode PJ, Edwards MJ, Kruit MC, et al. Sonography in clinical algorithm for early evaluation of 1671 patients with blunt abdominal trauma. AJR Am J Roentgenol 1999;172:905–11.
[31] Fakhry SM, Watts DD, Luchette FA, et al. Current diagnostic approaches lack sensitivity in the diagnosis of perforated blunt small bowel injury: analysis from 275,557 trauma admissions from the EAST multi-institutional HVI trial. J Trauma 2003;54:295–306.
[32] Lorente-Ramos RM, Santiago-Hernando A, Del Valle-Sanz Y, et al. Sonographic diagnosis of intramural duodenal hematomas. J Clin Ultrasound 1999;27:213–6.
[33] Sirlin CB, Brown MA, Andrade-Barreto OA, et al. Blunt abdominal trauma: clinical value of negative screening US scans. Radiology 2004;230:661–8.
[34] Henderson SO, Sung J, Mandavia D, et al. Serial abdominal ultrasound in the setting of trauma. J Emerg Med 2000;18:79–81.
[35] Blackbourne LH, Soffer D, Mckenney MG, et al. Secondary ultrasound examination increases the sensitivity of the FAST exam in blunt trauma. J Trauma 2004;57:934–8.
[36] Ollerton JE, Sugrue M, Balogh Z, et al. Prospective study to evaluate the influence of FAST on trauma patient management [see comment]. J Trauma 2006;60:785–91.
[37] Branney SW, Moore EE, Cantrill SV, et al. Ultrasound based key clinical pathway reduces the use of hospital resources for the evaluation of blunt abdominal trauma [see comment]. J Trauma 1997;42:1086–90.
[38] Melniker LA, Leibner E, McKenney MG, et al. Randomized controlled clinical trial of point-of-care, limited ultrasonography for trauma in the emergency department: the first

sonography outcomes assessment program trial [see comment]. Ann Emerg Med 2006;48: 227–35.
[39] Beck D, Marley R, Salvator A, et al. Prospective study of the clinical predictors of a positive abdominal computed tomography in blunt trauma patients. J Trauma 2004;57:296–300.
[40] ACEP Clinical Policies Committee, Clinical Policies Subcommittee on Acute Blunt Abdominal Trauma. Clinical policy: critical issues in the evaluation of adult patients presenting to the emergency department with acute blunt abdominal trauma. Ann Emerg Med 2004;43: 278–90.
[41] Hackam DJ, Ali J, Jastaniah SS. Effects of other intra-abdominal injuries on the diagnosis, management, and outcome of small bowel trauma. J Trauma 2006;49:606–10.
[42] Williams MD, Watts D, Fakhry S. Colon injury after blunt abdominal trauma: Results of the EAST multi-institutional hollow viscus injury study. J Trauma 2003;55:906–12.
[43] Stuhlfaut JW, Soto JA, Lucey BC, et al. Blunt abdominal trauma: performance of CT without oral contrast material. Radiology 2004;233:689–94.
[44] Mitsuhide K, Junichi S, Atsushi N, et al. Computed tomographic scanning and selective laparoscopy in the diagnosis of blunt bowel injury: a prospective study. J Trauma 2005;58: 696–701.
[45] Allen TL. Computed tomographic scanning without oral contrast solution for blunt bowel and mesenteric injuries in abdominal trauma. J Trauma 2004;56:314–22.
[46] Clancy TV, Ramshaw DG, Maxwell JG, et al. Management outcomes in splenic injury: a statewide trauma center review. Ann Surg 1997;226:17–24.
[47] Malhotra AK, Fabian TC, Croce MA, et al. Blunt hepatic injury: a paradigm shift from operative to nonoperative management in the 1990s. Ann Emerg Med 2000;231:804–13.
[48] Kozar RA, Moore JB, Niles SE, et al. Complications of nonoperative management of high-grade blunt hepatic injuries. J Trauma 2005;59:1066–71.
[49] Mendez C, Gubler KD, Maier RV, et al. Diagnostic accuracy of peritoneal lavage in patients with pelvic fractures. Ann Surg 1994;129:477–81.
[50] Thomason M, Messick J, Rutledge R, et al. Head CT scanning versus urgent exploration in the hypotensive blunt trauma patient [see comment]. J Trauma 1993;34:40–4.
[51] Winchell RJ, Hoyt DB, Simons RK, et al. Use of computed tomography of the head in the hypotensive blunt-trauma patient. Ann Emerg Med 1995;25:737–42.
[52] Weinberg JA, McKinley K, Petersen SR, et al. Trauma laparotomy in a rural setting before transfer to a regional center: Does it save lives. J Trauma 2003;54:823–8.
[53] Nicholas JM, Rix EP, Easley KA, et al. Changing patterns in the management of penetrating abdominal trauma: the more things change, the more they stay the same. J Trauma 2003;55: 1095–110.
[54] Marx JA, Isenhour JL. Abdominal trauma. In: Marx JA, editor. Rosen's emergency medicine: concepts and clinical practice. 6th edition. Philadelphia: Mosby; 2006.
[55] Nagy KK, Krosner SM, Joseph KT, et al. A method of determining peritoneal penetration in gunshot wounds to the abdomen. J Trauma 1997;43:242–6.
[56] Shaftan GW. Indications for operation in abdominal trauma. Am J Surg 1960;99:657–64.
[57] Pryor JP, Reilly PM, Dabrowski GP, et al. Nonoperative management of abdominal gunshot wounds. Ann Emerg Med 2004;43:344–53.
[58] Ginzburg E, Carrillo EH, Kopelman T, et al. The role of computed tomography in selective management of gunshot wounds to the abdomen and flank. J Trauma 1998;45:1005–9.
[59] Velmahos GC, Constantinou C, Tillou A, et al. Abdominal computed tomographic scan for patients with gunshot wounds to the abdomen selected for nonoperative management. J Trauma 2005;59:1155–61.
[60] Velmahos GC, Demetriades D, Toutouzas KG, et al. Selective nonoperative management in 1,856 patients with abdominal gunshot wounds: Should routine laparotomy still be the standard of care. Ann Emerg Med 2001;234:395–403.

[61] Leppaniemi AK, Haapiainen RK, Leppaniemi AK, et al. Selective nonoperative management of abdominal stab wounds: prospective, randomized study. World J Surg 1996;20: 1101–5.
[62] Leppaniemi AK, Voutilainen PE, Haapiainen RK, et al. Indications for early mandatory laparotomy in abdominal stab wounds. Br J Surg 1999;86:76–80.
[63] Nagy KK, Roberts RR, Joseph KT, et al. Evisceration after abdominal stab wounds: Is laparotomy required. J Trauma 1999;47:622–30.
[64] Arikan S, Kocakusak A, Yucel AF, et al. A prospective comparison of the selective observation and routine exploration methods for penetrating abdominal stab wounds with organ or omentum evisceration. J Trauma 2005;58:526–32.
[65] Nance FC, Wennar MH, Johnson LW, et al. Surgical judgment in the management of penetrating wounds of the abdomen: experience with 2212 patients. Ann Surg 1974;179: 639–46.
[66] Ertekin C, Yanar H, Taviloglu K, et al. Unnecessary laparotomy by using physical examination and different diagnostic modalities for penetrating abdominal stab wounds. Emerg Med J 2005;22:790–4.
[67] Ahmed N, Whelan J, Brownlee J, et al. The contribution of laparoscopy in evaluation of penetrating abdominal wounds. J Am Coll Surg 2005;201:213–6.
[68] Alzamel HA, Cohn SM, Alzamel HA, et al. When is it safe to discharge asymptomatic patients with abdominal stab wounds? J Trauma 2005;58:523–5.
[69] Conrad MF, Patton JH Jr, Parikshak M, et al. Selective management of penetrating truncal injuries: is emergency department discharge a reasonable goal? Am Surg 2003;69:266–72.
[70] Demetriades D, Rabinowitz B, Demetriades D, et al. Indications for operation in abdominal stab wounds. A prospective study of 651 patients. Ann Surg 1987;205:129–32.
[71] Tsikitis V, Biffl WL, Majercik S, et al. Selective clinical management of anterior abdominal stab wounds. Am J Surg 2004;188:807–12.
[72] Chiu WC, Shanmuganathan K, Mirvis SE, et al. Determining the need for laparotomy in penetrating torso trauma: a prospective study using triple contrast enhanced abdominopelvic computed tomography. J Trauma 2001;51:860–9.
[73] Shanmuganathan K, Mirvis SE, Chiu WC, et al. Penetrating torso trauma: triple-contrast helical CT in peritoneal violation and organ injury—a prospective study in 200 patients. Radiology 2004;231:775–84.
[74] Udobi KF, Rodriguez A, Chiu WC, et al. Role of ultrasonography in penetrating abdominal trauma: a prospective clinical study. J Trauma 2001;50:475–9.
[75] Murphy JT, Hall J, Provost D. Fascial ultrasound for evaluation of anterior abdominal stab wound injury. J Trauma 2005;59:843–6.
[76] Friese RS, Coln E, Gentilello LM. Laparoscopy is sufficient to exclude occult diaphragm injury after penetrating abdominal wounds. J Trauma 2005;58:789–92.
[77] Leppäniemi A, Haapiainen R. Occult diaphragmatic injuries caused by stab wounds. J Trauma 2003;55:646–50.
[78] Leppäniemi A, Haapiainen R. Diagnostic laparoscopy in abdominal stab wounds: a prospective, randomized study. J Trauma 2003;55:636–45.
[79] Simon RJ, Rabin J, Kuhls D. Impact of increased use of laparoscopy on negative laparotomy rates after penetrating trauma. J Trauma 2002;53:297–302.
[80] Brakenridge SC, Nagy KK, Joseph KT, et al. Detection of intra-abdominal injury using diagnostic peritoneal lavage after shotgun wound to abdomen. J Trauma 2003;54:329–31.
[81] Albrecht RM, Vigil A, Schermer CR, et al. Stab wounds to the back/flank in hemodynamically stable patients: evaluation using triple-contrast computed tomography. Am Surg 1999; 65:683–7.

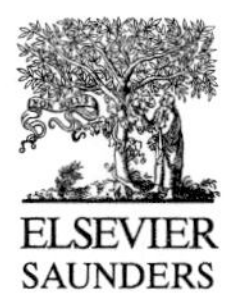

ELSEVIER
SAUNDERS

Emerg Med Clin N Am 25 (2007) 735–750

EMERGENCY
MEDICINE
CLINICS OF
NORTH AMERICA

Imaging of Spinal Cord Injuries

Amy Kaji, MD*, Robert Hockberger, MD

Department of Emergency Medicine, Harbor-UCLA Medical Center, 1000 West Carson Street, #21, Torrance, CA 90509, USA

Worldwide, spinal cord injury (SCI) occurs with an annual incidence of 15 to 40 cases per million [1]. In the United States, approximately 11,000 incident cases of SCI occur each year [2], and the annual prevalence is estimated to be 253,000 persons. According to the National Spinal Cord Injury Database, the average age of injury has increased as the median age of the general population of the United States has increased. As of 2000, the average age of injury was 38 years, and the percentage of persons over 60 years of age increased from 4.7% before 1980 to 11.5% among injuries occurring since 2000. Among incident cases, 77.8% of SCIs occur among males. Blunt mechanisms of injury, such as motor vehicle crashes, account for 46.9% of SCIs, followed by falls, acts of human violence (eg, gunshot wounds and assaults), and sports-related injuries [3]. Penetrating trauma accounts for approximately 10% to 20% of spinal injuries [4]. Although lifetime costs attributable to SCI depend on the age, level, and severity of injury, estimates range from $472,000 to $2,924,000 [3]. According to a systematic review performed by Sekhon and Fehlings [1], 55% of all spine injuries involve the cervical spine, with a lesser but approximately equal percentage involving the lumbosacral (15%), throracolumbar (15%), and thoracic (15%) regions, respectively.

Spinal cord injury without radiographic abnormality (SCIWORA) is defined as the presence of neurologic deficits in the absence of an apparent injury on a complete, technically adequate plain radiographic series. The injury pattern has been attributed to various causes, including ligamentous injuries, disc prolapse, and cervical spondylosis. SCIWORA is reported more commonly among the pediatric population, and it accounts for up to two thirds of severe cervical injuries in children under 8 years of age [5]. However, SCIWORA is not uncommon among middle-aged and elderly patients,

* Corresponding author.
E-mail address: akaji@emedharbor.edu (A. Kaji).

doi:10.1016/j.emc.2007.06.012

accounting for up to 12% of cases of adult SCI [6]. In fact, in a subanalysis performed on the large database of the National Emergency X-radiography Utilization Study (NEXUS), only 27 of the 818 total patients with cervical spine injury were diagnosed with SCIWORA, none of whom were children despite the inclusion of over 3000 pediatric patients [7].

According to the National Spinal Cord Injury Resource Association Center, 45% of all injuries are classified as *complete* injuries, which result in total loss of sensation and function below the injury level. Overall, a little more than 50% of the injuries result in quadriplegia [8]. Although all SCI patients can improve from the initial classification of having a *complete* or *incomplete* injury, no more than 0.9% of patients fully recover. In fact, many SCI patients suffer progressive neurologic deterioration due to myelomalacia, syrinx formation, progressive cord compression, or cord tethering due to adhesions [4].

Early diagnosis and management of SCI is critical in minimizing complications and the severity of injury. This article reviews the test characteristics and evidence-based indications for imaging modalities of SCI.

Routine radiographs

Cervical spine injuries

Three-view radiographic series

Indicative of the relatively high mortality associated with cervical spine injuries, the incidence of cervical spine injuries is greater than its prevalence (52% versus 40%). Reviewing the data from NEXUS, of 818 cervical spine injuries among the cohort of 34,069 patients, fractures of C2 accounted for the majority (24%) of fractures, whereas injuries involving the sixth and seventh vertebrae accounted for over one third of cervical fractures (39%) [9]. In 2000, there was an estimated 800,000 plain cervical radiographs ordered [10], and large studies have been conducted to develop decision rules to decrease the number of radiographs that are obtained. According to the National Hospital Ambulatory Care Survey, only 4% of all cervical spine radiographs demonstrate a fracture [11]; furthermore, the cost of imaging is tremendous, especially when one considers the space and time used to continue immobilizing patients on a backboard for many hours in a busy emergency department. Moreover, there is great practice variation among emergency physicians, with a sixfold range in radiography ordering rates [12].

In an effort to standardize clinical practice and guide physicians to be more selective in their use of radiography without jeopardizing patient care, two clinical decision rules have been developed. The first rule to be developed was the NEXUS Low-risk Criteria (NLC), which was based on a multicenter prospective observational study that tested a five-part decision rule to predict patients with a spinal injury (Box 1) [10]. All patients with

Box 1. National Emergency X-Radiography Utilization Study Criteria

All low risk criteria met?
1. No posterior midline cervical spine tenderness
2. No evidence of intoxication
3. Normal level of alertness
4. No focal neurologic deficit
5. No painful distracting injuries

If yes, no radiography. If no, then radiography is indicated.

blunt trauma who underwent radiography of the cervical spine at one of the 21 participating emergency departments were included in the study. The NLC decision instrument stipulates that radiography is unnecessary if patients satisfy all five of the following low- risk criteria: absence of midline tenderness, normal level of alertness, no evidence of intoxication, no abnormal neurologic findings, and no painful distracting injuries [10]. Insignificant injuries were defined as those that would not lead to any consequences, if left undiagnosed. The NEXUS investigators evaluated 34,069 patients who underwent radiography of the cervical spine, comprised of either a three-view cervical spine radiograph or a cervical spine CT scan after blunt trauma. The sensitivity, specificity, and negative predictive value of the NLC were calculated and were found to be 99.6%, 12.9%, and 99.8%, respectively [10].

Due to the low specificity of 12.9%, Stiell and colleagues [13] expressed concern that the use of the NLC would actually increase the use of radiography in some regions of the United States and in the majority of countries outside of the United States. Thus, Stiell subsequently developed the Canadian C-spine rule (CCR) (Box 2), based upon three clinical questions that were derived from 25 positive and negative clinical predictor variables associated with spine injury [13]. First, patients who are judged to be at high risk due to age, dangerous mechanism of injury, or the presence of paresthesias must undergo radiography. Second, patients with any one of five low- risk characteristics may undergo assessment of active range of motion. Third, patients who are able to actively rotate their neck 45 degrees to the left and right, regardless of pain, do not require radiography [13]. In the derivation study, the CCR demonstrated a sensitivity of 100% and a specificity of 42.5% for identifying clinically important cervical spine injuries [13]. In 2003, the CCR was prospectively studied and compared with the NLC in the emergency departments of nine Canadian tertiary care hospitals. Of 8283 patients, 162 were found to have clinically significant injuries, and the sensitivity, specificity, and negative predictive values were 99.4%, 45.1%, and 100%, respectively [14]. The investigators reported that the

Box 2. Canadian C-spine Rules

A. *Any* high-risk factor that mandates radiography? If yes, then radiograph; if no, then proceed to questions in section B.
   1. Age >65 years
   2. Dangerous mechanism (fall from ≥3 feet or 5 stairs; axial load to the head; motor vehicle accident at a high speed [>100 km/h]), rollover, or ejection; collision involving a motorized recreational vehicle; bicycle collision
   3. Paresthesias in extremities

B. Any low-risk factor that allows safe range of motion assessment? If no, then radiograph; if yes, then proceed to question in section C.
   1. Simple rear-end motor vehicle accident
   2. Sitting position in the emergency department
   3. Ambulatory at any time
   4. Delayed neck pain onset
   5. No midline cervical tenderness

C. Able to rotate neck actively (45 degrees left and right)? If no, radiograph; if yes, then no radiography is indicated.

CCR would have missed one patient with a clinically important cervical spine injury, while the NLC would have missed 16 patients.

There is some controversy as to which of the two rules to implement. In contrast to the NEXUS study, in which the NLC was demonstrated to have a sensitivity of 99.6% and a specificity of 12.9%, Stiell and colleagues [14] reported different results, with a lower NLC sensitivity of 90.7% and a higher specificity of 36.8%. The discrepancy may be due to methodologic differences in the respective study designs. For example, the inclusion criteria were different for the two studies. Although the Canadian group excluded those under the age of 16 years and subjects with a Glasgow Coma Score of less than 15, these subjects were included among the NEXUS cohort. Additionally, whereas NEXUS investigators excluded all those in whom x-rays were deemed unnecessary, the Canadian investigators included individuals in whom x-rays were not obtained with a clinical follow-up protocol. Thus, due to selection bias, it is possible that there were a lower number of false negatives and true negatives reported in the Canadian study sample, potentially inflating both the sensitivity and specificity of the CCR [15]. Finally, the prospective validation phase of the CCR was performed in the same institutions in which the criteria were derived, raising concerns about improved performance of the CCR due to local and regional familiarity with the rule. Before the widespread application of any prediction rule, outside validation is necessary to assess its generalizability, since degradation in the performance of decision rules is often seen when implemented in a new setting [16].

Flexion–extension radiographic series

Flexion–extension (F/E) radiographs of the cervical spine are often used in patients with blunt trauma when the physician is unable to assess an unconscious or obtunded trauma patient or when the physician is concerned about ligamentous injuries despite negative standard radiographs. Instability of the cervical spine is suggested by any of the following: more than 3.5 mm of horizontal displacement between the disks, displaced apophyseal joints, widened disk spaces, loss of $>30\%$ of the disk height, or the presence of a prevertebral hematoma [4].

Unfortunately, F/E radiographs in the acute setting have unacceptably high false negative and false positive rates [17]. In a retrospective chart review of 123 blunt trauma victims with normal three-view plain radiographs who could not be assessed clinically due to altered mental status, 4 of 7 patients with documented cervical spine injuries were not detected on F/E views [18]. In a subgroup analysis of the NEXUS study, of the 818 patients ultimately found to have a cervical spine injury, 86 (10.5%) underwent F/E imaging. Two patients sustained bony injuries, and 4 patients sustained subluxation injuries detected only on F/E views, but all others had injuries apparent on routine plain radiographs of the cervical spine [19]. Similarly, in a retrospective review of 276 traumatic brain-injured patients who underwent cervical spine plain radiographs, CT with three-dimensional reconstructions, and F/E views as part of a routine protocol, dynamic F/E with fluoroscopy identified no new fractures or instability. In fact, F/E was inadequate in 9 patients, truly negative in 260 of 276 (94%) patients, falsely positive in 6 (2.2%) patients, and falsely negative in 1 (0.4%) patient [20]. Thus, F/E appears to have a limited role in the cervical spine clearance protocol for blunt spinal injury patients, as it adds little new information to plain radiographs and CT with three-dimensional reconstructions.

Spinal cord evaluation in the unevaluable blunt trauma patient

The mechanism for clearing the cervical spine in patients with a persistently altered sensorium or those with a distracting injury remains controversial. The potential for ligamentous injury may mandate prolonged neck immobilization with a hard collar, even after CT and plain radiographs demonstrate no fracture. The Eastern Association for the Surgery of Trauma (EAST) practice management guidelines recommend clearance of the cervical spine after performance of a CT of C1-C2 and three views of the cervical spine in the unreliable patient. In a 3-year retrospective analysis of over 14,000 patients, it was demonstrated that ligamentous injuries without fractures of the cervical spine were extremely rare (0.5%) when applying the EAST guidelines; the authors thus concluded that application of the EAST guidelines would facilitate early removal of the cervical collar in the obtunded or unreliable trauma patient [21]. In contrast, the Joint Recommendation of the American Association of Neurological Surgeons and the Congress of Neurological Surgeons Joint Section on Trauma recommends MRI or fluoroscopy with F/E in the obtunded patient, with the implication that normal MRI and/or normal F/E would allow removal of the cervical collar [22]. For the emergency physician, the trauma patient with distracting injuries or a persistently altered sensorium will, in all likelihood, be admitted, and it would be reasonable to keep the cervical collar in place for the duration of the patients' emergency department course.

Thoracic and lumbar spine injuries

Among blunt trauma patients admitted to the hospital, the rate of thoracic and lumbar spine injuries is 2% to 5% [23–25]. Although this is a small percentage of blunt trauma patients, thoracic and lumbar spine injuries are associated with a relatively high mortality and morbidity rate. In fact, up to 50% of these injuries may be associated with a neurologic deficit [4]. In a prospective study of a consecutive sample of blunt trauma patients presenting to a level I trauma center, Holmes and colleagues [26] reported the prevalence of thoracolumar (TL) spine injury patients who underwent TL spine imaging to be 6.3%. Of 260 injuries, the most common anatomic levels of injury were L1, L2, L3, and T12, with 42 (16.2%) occurring at L1, 38 (14.6%) at L2, 29 (11.1%) at L3, and 27 (10.4%) at T12. Whereas vertebral body compression fractures were the most common injury seen in the thoracic spine, transverse process fractures were the most common injury type in the lumbar spine [26].

Unlike the many studies performed to develop guidelines for imaging cervical spine trauma, there are far fewer studies assessing the validity of decision rules for TL imaging. There are retrospective reviews identifying potential predictors of thoracic and lumbar spine injuries [24,25,27,28], which include the following: altered mental status; pain or tenderness over the spine; local sign of injury (step-off, bruising, or hematoma) along the spine; neurologic deficit; high-force mechanism (fall greater than 3 m or 10 feet, ejection from a vehicle, moderate velocity motor vehicle or motorcycle crash, or automobile versus pedestrian); distracting injury; and the presence of another identified spine injury. To develop a decision rule from predictors identified in the literature, Hsu and colleagues [29] performed a chart review in which 100 subjects with TL spine fractures were compared with 100 randomly selected controls who were multiple trauma patients. If a subject had blunt multi-trauma (necessitating trauma team activation) or a high energy mechanism of injury (fall greater than 3 m, moderate velocity motor vehicle crash or motorcycle crash, or automobile versus pedestrian), and there were any high-risk criteria (Glasgow Coma Score <15, neurologic deficit, distracting injury, local signs of injury [eg, step-off, bruising, or hematoma]), alcohol or drug intoxication, pain or tenderness over the spine, or the presence of another identified spine fracture (eg, in the cervical spine), then the patient was to undergo radiography. The presence of any of the high-risk criteria predicted a TL injury with a sensitivity of 100%, specificity of 11.3%, and a negative predictive value of 100%. The most sensitive criteria was the presence of back pain or midline tenderness with a sensitivity of 62.1%, while the criterion with the highest specificity (100%) was the presence of a palpable step-off over the spine [29].

In a prospective cohort of 2404 patients undergoing TL spine radiographs after blunt trauma, Holmes and colleagues [30] assessed six clinical predictors: (1) complaints of TL spine pain; (2) TL spine tenderness; (3) decreased level of consciousness; (4) intoxication with alcohol or drugs; (5) neurologic deficits; and (6) a painful, distracting injury. The presence of any of the high-risk criteria identified all 152 patients with TL fractures, demonstrating a sensitivity and positive predictive value of 100%. However, the criteria had a very low specificity of 3.9% and a positive predictive value of only 6.6%.

CT and MRI

CT and MRI play an increasing role in the clinical evaluation of spine injuries [4,31–33], potentially obviating the role of plain radiographs. Investigators have assessed whether CT data obtained for the evaluation of chest and abdominal injuries provides sufficient data to screen for spinal fractures, thereby decreasing the time and cost of spine injury evaluation. In a retrospective review of 3,537 blunt trauma patients of whom 236 (7%) sustained a cervical, thoracic, or lumbar fracture, Brown and colleagues [34] reported that CT identified 99.3% of all fractures. The one cervical and one thoracic fracture missed by CT required minimal treatment with a rigid cervical collar or no treatment, respectively [34]. In a registry-based retrospective analysis of 573 trauma patients comparing plain radiography with CT, of whom 54 sustained SCI, Antevil and colleagues [35] demonstrated a sensitivity of 70% for plain radiography and 100% for CT.

MRI is widely accepted as the imaging modality that best delineates the integrity of the spinal cord itself, intervertebral discs, surrounding soft tissue, ligamentous structures, the vertebral arteries, and SCIWORA [36]. The most common MRI findings among SCIWORA patients include central disc herniation, spinal stenosis, cord edema, and contusion (Fig. 1) [7,37]. MRI has also been shown to have prognostic value in SCIWORA, because patients with minimal cord changes have the best outcome, followed by those with cord edema, hemorrhage, and finally, contusion [6].

In addition to aiding in the determination of acuity of bony injuries, MRI is helpful in diagnosing the causes of delayed and progressive neurologic deterioration in spinal injury patients. There are characteristic findings indicative of myelomalacia, syrinx formation, cord tethering, and progressive cord compression [4]. Thus, with both diagnostic and prognostic capability

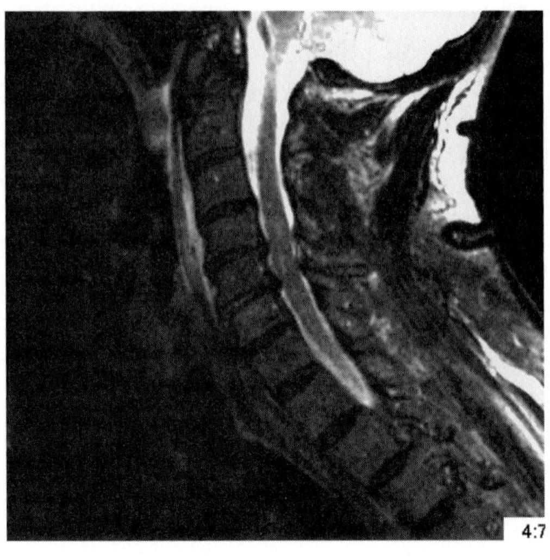

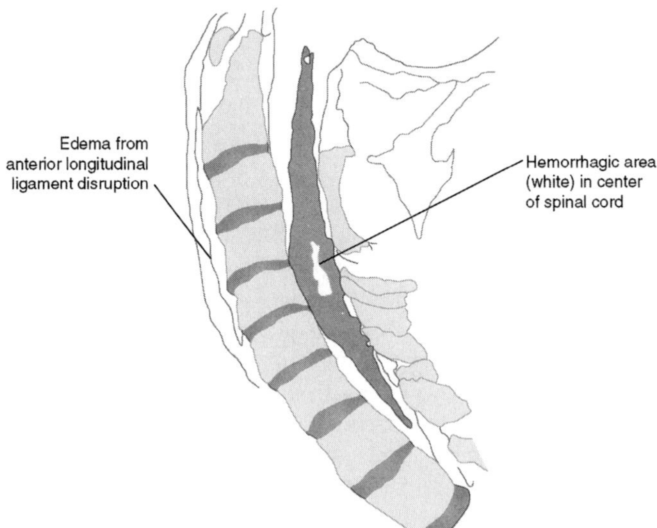

Fig. 1. MRI scan showing a small area of central cord hemorrhage and both anterior and posterior ligamentous disruption. (*From* Hockberger RS, Kaji AK, Newton E. Spinal injuries. In: Marx JA, Hockberger RS, Walls RM, et al, editors. Rosen's emergency medicine. Philadelphia: Mosby, Inc.; 2006. p. 434; with permission.)

in the acute and subacute setting, MRI can help discriminate between neurologic deficits caused by hemorrhage or edema, as well as injury to the cord itself from those caused by extrinsic compression [38].

CT and MRI in the evaluation of cervical spine injuries

Controversy persists regarding the most efficient and effective method of cervical spine imaging after blunt trauma, and no standard has been explicitly defined. Plain radiographs may be inadequate to visualize the complete cervical spine in up to 72% of cases, and the sensitivity and specificity of plain films to detect fractures may be as low as 31.6% and 99.2%, respectively [39]. A single lateral radiograph detects only 60% to 80% of cervical spine fractures [17]. Plain radiographs, even when swimmer's views and/or oblique views are performed, are often inadequate and miss 12% to 16% of cervical spine fractures [40]. In a study of 2690 admissions for blunt trauma, the test characteristics of plain radiographs were compared with those of CT scans. The investigators found that whereas CT identified 67 of 70 patients, plain films identified only 38 of 70 patients with injuries to the cervical spine [41]. Similarly, in a retrospective review of 1199 patients who underwent both plain radiography and CT, plain radiographs missed 41 of 116 (35.3%) injuries, resulting in a sensitivity of 64.5% (95% CI 55.5–77.6). Notably, all 41 patients required treatment, and 13 of these were unstable fractures requiring surgical stabilization [42]. CT also appears to be more time-efficient than plain radiography [43,44]. One retrospective review demonstrated that blunt trauma patients with a normal motor examination and a normal cervical spine CT do not require further radiologic examination before clearing the cervical spine [45].

After penetrating neck trauma, although conventional angiography is still considered the gold standard for the diagnosis of pseudoaneurysms and fistulas, CT and CT angiography may be superior to delineate the trajectory after penetrating neck trauma [46,47].

MRI is much less sensitive than CT for the detection of fractures of the posterior elements of the spine and injuries to the craniocervical junction [17]. However, it is superior to CT in detecting injuries to ligamentous structures, the disc interspace, and the spinal cord itself. High-resolution T2-weighted sequences may be useful to diagnose nerve root avulsions, hematomas, and the formation of pseudomeningoceles [4]. However, MRI is associated with delays in time to complete cervical clearance, and it increases the risks associated with complex transports [40]. Ventilators, monitors, and other devices must be compatible with the MRI machine.

Another indication for MRI or magnetic resonance arteriography (MRA) in cervical spine injury may be to screen for vascular injury. The incidence of vertebral artery injury after blunt neck trauma is estimated to be as high as 24% to 46%, although most of these lesions are asymptomatic [48]. Physicians should be suspicious for vascular injury if patients have experienced severe blunt force to the neck or significant hyperextension and hyperflexion injuries to the neck or demonstrate unexplained neurologic deficits. Additional indications for screening for vascular injury include skull base fractures, cervical vertebral fractures adjacent to or involving vascular foramina and penetrating injuries adjacent to vascular structures [49]. MRI and MRA may be useful to detect pseudoaneurysms, arteriovenous fistulas, dissections of vital vessels, and mural hematomas.

The disadvantages of CT imaging of the cervical spine include the delivery of a higher dose of radiation, with a 50% increase in mean radiation dose to the cervical spine in pediatric patients for helical CT compared with conventional radiography [50]. Rybicki and colleagues [51] demonstrated a 10-fold increase in radiation dose to the skin (28 versus 2.89 mGy) and a 14-fold increase in dose to the thyroid (26 versus 1.8 mGy) when comparing cervical CT scanning to a five-view radiographic series. Children, especially those under the age of 5, are more prone to radiation-induced malignancies due to increased radiosensitivity of certain organs and a longer time during which to develop cancer [52]. Estimated lifetime cancer mortality risks attributable to the radiation exposure from CT for a 1-year-old child is approximately 0.07% to 0.18%, which is a risk that is an order of magnitude higher than that for adults who are exposed to a CT of the cervical spine [53]. CT is also limited in patients with severe degenerative disease. Moreover, although CT detects 97% to 100% of all fractures, its accuracy in the detection of purely ligamentous injuries has not been well studied [17].

CT and MRI in the evaluation of thoracic and lumbar spine injuries

In a retrospective chart review of all trauma patients undergoing abdominal and pelvic CT, Berry and colleagues [54] compared plain radiographs to CT in evaluating the TL spine. Seven (27%) of the thoracolumbar spine fractures were missed on plain radiographs, while all 26 patients diagnosed with fractures were diagnosed by CT, Thus, CT demonstrated a sensitivity of 100%, specificity of 97%, and a negative predictive value of 100%, while plain radiographs were 73% sensitive, 100% specific, and had a negative predictive value of 92%. In this study, CT also appeared to improve time efficiency, because it was routinely performed shortly after presentation to evaluate all patients with suspected thoracic or abdominal trauma, whereas the average additional time to completion of plain films was 8 hours (range, 44 minutes to 38 hours, and median time of 2 hours and 48 minutes) [54].

A prospective evaluation of 222 consecutive trauma patients requiring TL spine screening because of clinical findings or altered mental status similarly demonstrated the superior accuracy of helical CT. Whereas the accuracy for plain radiographs was only 87% (95% CI 82–92), the accuracy of CT for TL fractures was 99% (95% CI 96–100) (Figs. 2A–D) [55]. A systematic review performed by Inaba and colleagues [56] corroborated the superior sensitivity and interobserver reliability for a reformatted CT, compared with plain radiographic screening of the lumbar and thoracic spine. Furthermore, CT did not require further patient transportation, radiation exposure, cost, or time. In contrast to the higher radiation exposure with cervical CT compared with plain radiography, CT of the TL spine involves lower levels of radiation exposure compared with plain films (4 milliSieverts [mSv] versus 26 mSv) [35].

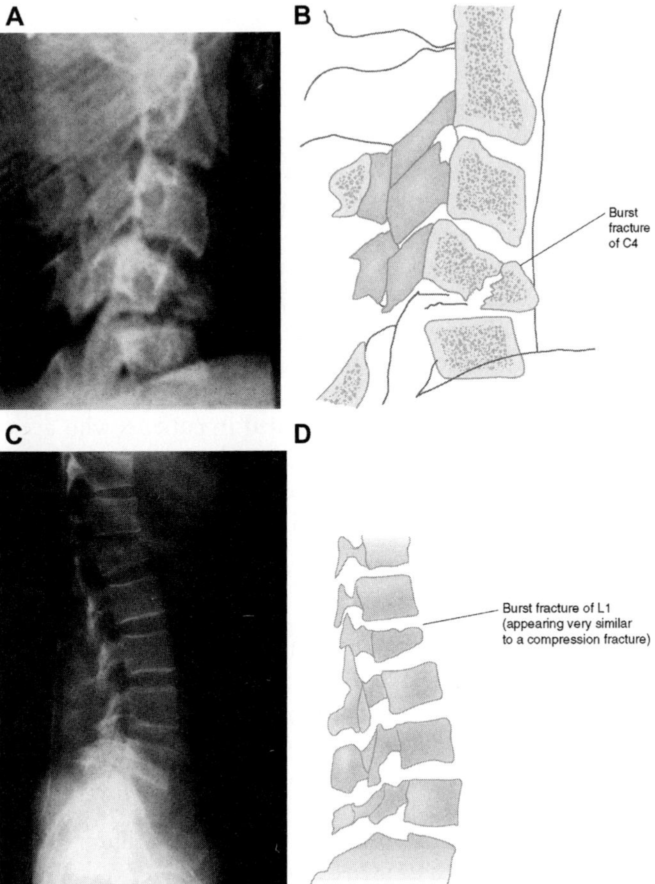

Fig. 2. Burst fracture of a vertebral body. (*A, B*) Lateral plain radiograph showing a burst fracture of L1. (*C, D*) Computed tomographic scan of L1 in the same patient, showing comminution of the fracture and retropulsion of fragments into the spinal canal. (*From* Hockberger RS, Kaji AK, Newton E. Spinal injuries. In: Marx JA, Hockberger RS, Walls M, et al, editors. Rosen's emergency medicine. Philadelphia: Mosby, Inc.; 2006. p. 434; with permission.)

Cost-effective analyses comparing CT with TL plain radiography have demonstrated that although CT has a higher initial fixed cost, it is offset by a decreased need for the number of repeat radiographic examinations needed due to inadequate films, lower medico-legal costs (including costs of prolonged hospitalizations, rehabilitation, lost productivity, and malpractice suits from missed injuries), and fixed personnel costs [57,58].

Pediatric spinal injuries

Pediatric injuries comprise only 2% to 5% of all spine injuries [59]. Similar to adults, motor vehicle crashes account for the majority of spine injuries, but rather than falls, sports injuries account for the second most common cause [60]. When retrospective epidemiologic analyses of subgroups are performed, spine injuries are found to be more common in children over 8 years of age [61].

In contrast, SCIWORA is reported to account for up to two thirds of severe cervical injuries in children under 8 years of age [5]. Children are thought to be at greater risk for SCIWORA due to pediatric spinal anatomy and their associated ligamentous flexibility [62,63]. As with other SCIs, SCIWORA is caused by motor vehicle accidents, serious falls, sporting injuries, and child abuse. Often delayed for several days, the symptoms of SCIWORA may present as complete or incomplete cord lesions, with a better prognosis for incomplete lesions. Because MRI is considered the imaging modality of choice to diagnose SCIWORA and has also been shown to have prognostic value, MRI is recommended in patients who are suspected of having SCIWORA after nondiagnostic or negative plain radiographs [6,36]. Recurrent SCIWORA has also been reported; a recent meta-analysis demonstrated that immobilization for 12 weeks may help prevent recurrences among patients who are moderately injured [64].

To evaluate indications for imaging the pediatric cervical spine after blunt trauma, Viccellio and colleagues [65] performed a subanalysis of the the NLC (midline cervical tenderness, altered level of alertness, evidence of intoxication, neurologic abnormality, and presence of painful distracting injury) in patients under 18 years of age. This subgroup accounted for 3065 patients (9% of all NEXUS patients), 30 (0.98%) of whom sustained a cervical spine injury. Fractures at C5-C7 accounted for 45.9% of the cervical spine injury, all of whom were over 2 years of age, and the majority (26/30) were over 9 years of age. The NLC identified all pediatric cervical spine injury subjects with a sensitivity of 100% (95% CI 87.8–100), a specificity of 19.9% (95% CI 18.5–21.3), and a negative predictive value of 100% (95% CI 99.2–100) [65].

Geriatric spinal injuries

The elderly account for a disproportionate majority of total spine injuries. In the NEXUS observational study, age greater than 65 years was associated with a relative risk of 2.09 (95% CI 1.77–2.59) [10], while the Canadian C-spine derivation study demonstrated that age greater than 65 years was associated with an odds ratio of 3.7 (95% CI 2.4–5.6) [13]. Moreover, a cross-sectional study using the National Spinal Cord Injury Statistical Center database demonstrated that older age is consistently associated with greater morbidity, with decreased self-reported favorable outcomes in functional independence, overall life satisfaction, physical independence, mobility, occupational functioning, and social integration [66].

One of the CCR's high-risk criteria includes age greater than 65 years, and such patients therefore automatically undergo radiologic studies. In contrast, age is not one of the criteria of the NLC. To evaluate the performance of the NLC in the elderly, a subgroup analysis of 2943 subjects (8.6%) over 65 years of age was performed [67]. The instruments' test characteristics were as follows: sensitivity of 100% (95% CI 97.1–100), specificity of 14.7% (95% CI 14.6–14.7), and negative predictive value of 100% (95% CI 99.1–100) [67].

Summary

Spinal injuries can cause significant morbidity and mortality, underscoring the importance of early diagnosis. Clinical trials have resulted in improved guidelines and predictions rules, such as the NLC and CCR, to help clinicians to judiciously screen and use plain radiographs. Other studies demonstrate that F/E views add little information to the evaluation in spinal trauma. With superior diagnostic accuracy, as well as improved cost and time efficiency, CT is playing an increasingly important role in the diagnosis and management of spinal trauma, although clinicians must be cognizant of the associated increased radiation exposure. MRI is indicated when the clinician needs more detailed imaging of the spinal ligaments, discs, and the spinal cord itself. In addition to having prognostic capability, MRI is also useful in diagnosing the etiology of delayed and progressive neurologic deterioration in patients with SCI. Both CT angiography and MRA, as well as conventional angiography, have roles in the detection and management of vascular injuries associated with SCIs.

References

[1] Sekhon LH, Fehlings MG. Epidemiology, demographics, and pathophysiology of acute spinal cord injury. Spine 2001;26(Suppl 24):S2–12.
[2] Available at: www.spinalcord.uab.edu. Accessed July 1, 2006.
[3] NSCISC. Spinal cord injury facts and figures at a glance. Birmingham (AL): National Spinal Cord Injury Statistical Center; 2006.
[4] Bagley LJ. Imaging of spinal trauma. Radiol Clin North Am 2006;44(1):1–14.
[5] Available at: http://www.wheelessonline.com/ortho/sciwora_syndrome_spinal_cord_injury_w_o_radiologic_abnormality. Accessed August 26, 2006.
[6] Tewari MK, Gifti DS, Singh P, et al. Diagnosis and prognostication of adult spinal cord injury without radiographic abnormality using magnetic resonance imaging: analysis of 40 patients. Surg Neurol 2005;63(3):204–9.
[7] Hendey GW, Wolfson AB, Mower WR, et al. National Emergency X-Radiography Utilization Study in blunt cervical trauma. Spinal cord injury without radiographic abnormality: results of the NEXUS in blunt cervical trauma. J Trauma 2002;53(1):1–4.
[8] Available at: http://www.makoa.org/nscia/fact02.html. Accessed August 26, 2006.
[9] Goldberg W, Mueller C, Panacek E, et al. Distribution and patterns of blunt traumatic cervical spine injury. Ann Emerg Med 2001;38(1):17–21.
[10] Hoffman JR, Mower WR, Wolfson AB, et al. Validity of a set of clinical criteria to rule out injury to the cervical spine in patients with blunt trauma. National Emergency X-radiography Utilization Study Group. N Engl J Med 2000;343(2):94–9.
[11] McCaig LF, Burt CW. National hospital ambulatory medical care survey: 2003 emergency department summary. Adv Data 2005;358:1–38.

[12] Stiell IG, Wells GA, Vandemheen K, et al. Variation in emergency department use of cervical spine radiography for alert, stable trauma patients. CMAJ 1997;156:1537–44.
[13] Stiell IG, Wells GA, Vandemheen KL, et al. The Canadian C-spine rule for radiography in alert and stable trauma patients. JAMA 2001;286(15):1841–8.
[14] Stiell IG, Clement CM, McKnight RD, et al. The Canadian C-spine rule versus the NEXUS low-risk criteria in patients with trauma. N Engl J Med 2003;349:2510–8.
[15] Mower WR, Hoffman J. Comparison of the Canadian C-spine rule and NEXUS decision instrument in evaluating blunt trauma patients for cervical spine injury. Ann Emerg Med 2004;43(4):515–7.
[16] Yealy DM, Auble TE. Choosing between clinical prediction rules. N Engl J Med 2003; 349(26):2553–5.
[17] Crim JR, Moore K, Brodke D. Clearance of the cervical spine in multitrauma patients: the role of advanced imaging. Semin Ultrasound CT MR 2001;22(4):283–305.
[18] Freedman I, van Gelderen D, Cooper DJ, et al. Cervical spine assessment in the unconscious trauma patient: a major trauma service's experience with passive flexion-extension radiography. J Trauma 2005;58(6):1183–8.
[19] Pollack CV Jr, Hendey GW, Martin DR, et al. NEXUS group. Use of flexion-extension radiographs of the cervical spine in blunt trauma. Ann Emerg Med 2001;38(1):8–11.
[20] Padayachee L, Cooper DJ, Irons S, et al. Cervical spine clearance in unconscious traumatic brain injury patients:dynamic flexion-extension fluoroscopy versus computed tomography with three dimensional reconstruction. J Trauma 2006;60(2):341–5.
[21] Chiu WC, Haan JM, Cushing BM, et al. Ligamentous injuries of the cervical spine in unreliable blunt trauma patients: incidence, evaluation, and outcome. J Trauma 2001;50(3): 457–64.
[22] Available at: http://www.spineuniverse.com/pdf/traumaguide. Accessed April 15, 2007.
[23] Samuels LE, Kerstein MD. "Routine" radiologic evaluation of the thoracolumbar spine in blunt trauma patients; a reappraisal. J Trauma 1993;34:85–9.
[24] Cooper C, Dunham CM, Rodriguez A. Falls and major injuries are risk factors for thoracolumbar injuries: cognitive impairment and multiple injuries impede the detection of back pain and tenderness. J Trauma 1995;38:692–5.
[25] Frankel HL, Rozycki GS, Ochsner GM, et al. Indications for obtaining surveillance thoracic and lumbar spine radiographs. J Trauma 1994;37:673–6.
[26] Holmes JF, Miller PQ, Panacek EA, et al. Epidemiology of thoracolumbar spine injury in blunt trauma. Acad Emerg Med 2001;8(9):866–72.
[27] Durham RM, Luchtefeld WB, Wibbenmeyer L, et al. Evaluation of the thoracic and lumbar spine after blunt trauma. Am J Surg 1995;170(6):681–4.
[28] Meldon SW, Moettus LN. Thoracolumbar spine fractures: clinical presentation and the effect of altered sensorium and major injury. J Trauma 1995;39(6):1110–4.
[29] Hsu JM, Joseph T, Ellis AM. Thoracolumbar fracture in blunt trauma patients: guidelines for diagnosis and imaging. Injury 2003;34(6):426–33.
[30] Holmes JF, Panacek EA, Miller PQ, et al. Prospective evaluation of criteria for obtaining thoracolumbar radiographs in trauma patients. J Emerg Med 2003;24(1):1–7.
[31] Brandt MM, Wahl WL, Yeom K, et al. Computed tomographic scanning reduces cost and time of complete spine evaluation. J Trauma 2004;56(5):1022–6.
[32] Rhee PM, Bridgeman A, Acosta JA, et al. Lumbar fractures in adult blunt trauma: axial and single slice helical abdominal and pelvic computed tomographic scans versus portable plain films. J Trauma 2002;53(4):663–7.
[33] Gestring ML, Gracias VH, Felicaino MA, et al. Evaluation of the lower spine after blunt trauma using abdominal computed tomographic scanning supplemented with lateral scanograms. J Trauma 2002;53(1):9–14.
[34] Brown CV, Antevil JL, Sise MJ, et al. Spiral computed tomography for the diagnosis of cervical, thoracic, and lumbar spine fractures: its time has come. J Trauma 2005;58(5):890–5.

[35] Antevil JL, Sise MJ, Sack DI, et al. Spiral computed tomography for the initial evaluation of spine trauma: a new standard of care? J Trauma 2006;61(2):382–7.
[36] Cohen WA, Giauque AP, Hallam DK, et al. Evidence-based approach to use of MR imaging in acute spinal trauma. Eur J Radiol 2003;48(1):49–60.
[37] Dare AO, Dias MS, Li V. Magnetic resonance imaging correlation in pediatric spinal cord injury without radiographic abnormality. J Neurosurg 2002;97(Suppl 1):33–9.
[38] el-Khoury GY, Kathol MH, Daniel WW. Imaging of acute injuries of the cervical spine: value of plain radiography, CT, and MR imaging. AJR Am J Roentgenol 1995;164(1): 43–50.
[39] Gale SC, Gracias VH, Reilly PM, et al. The inefficiency of plain radiography to evaluate the cervical spine after blunt trauma. J Trauma 2005;59(5):1121–5.
[40] Cooper DJ, Ackland HM. Clearing the cervical spine in unconscious head injured patients—the evidence. Crit Care Resusc 2005;7(3):181–4.
[41] Schenarts PJ, Diaz J, Kaiser C, et al. Prospective comparison of admission computed tomographic scan and plain films of the upper cervical spine in trauma patients with altered mental status. J Trauma 2001;51(4):663–8.
[42] Griffen MM, Frykberg ER, Kerwin AJ, et al. Radiographic clearance of blunt cervical spine injury: plain radiograph or computed tomography scan? J Trauma 2003;55(2):222–6.
[43] Daffner RH. Cervical radiography for trauma patients: a time-effective technique? AJR Am J Roentgenol 2000;175:1309–11.
[44] Daffner RH. Helical CT of the cervical spine for trauma patients: a time study. AJR Am J Roentgenol 2001;177:677–9.
[45] Schuster R, Waxman K, Sanchez B, et al. Magnetic resonance imaging is not needed to clear cervical spines in blunt trauma patients with normal computed tomographic results and no motor deficits. Arch Surg 2005;140(8):762–6.
[46] Ofer A, Nitecki SS, Braun J, et al. CT angiography of the carotid arteries in trauma to the neck. Eur J Vasc Endovasc Surg 2001;21:401–7.
[47] Munera F, Soto JA, Nunez D. Penetrating injuries of the neck and the increasing role of CTA. Emerg Radiol 2004;10(6):303–9.
[48] Cothren CC, Moore EE, Biffl WL, et al. Cervical spine fracture patterns predictive of vertebral artery injury. J Trauma 2003;55:811–3.
[49] Biffl WL, Moore EE, Offner PJ, et al. Blunt carotid and vertebral artery injuries. World J Surg 2001;25:1036–43.
[50] Adelgias KM, Grossman DC, Langer SG, et al. Use of helical computed tomography for imaging the pediatric cervical spine. Acad Emerg Med 2004;11(3):228–36.
[51] Rybicki F, Nawfel RD, Judy PF, et al. Skin and thyroid dosimetry in cervical spine screening: two methods for evaluation and a comparison between a helical CT and radiographic trauma series. AJR Am J Roentgenol 2002;179:933–7.
[52] Frush DP, Donnelly LF, Rosen NS. Computed tomography and radiation risks: what pediatric healthcare providers should know. Pediatrics 2003;112:951–7.
[53] Brenner D, Elliston C, Hall E, et al. Estimated risks of radiation-induced fatal cancer from pediatric CT. Am J Roentgenol 2001;176(2):289–96.
[54] Berry GE, Adams S, Harris MB, et al. Are plain radiographs of the spine necessary during evaluation after blunt trauma? Accuracy of screening torso computed tomography in thoracic/lumbar spine fracture diagnosis. J Trauma 2005;59(6):1410–3.
[55] Hauser CJ, Visvikis G, Hinrichs C, et al. Prospective validation of computed tomographic screening of the thoracolumbar spine in trauma. J Trauma 2003;55(2):228–34.
[56] Inaba K, Munera M, Schulman C, et al. Visceral torso computed tomography for clearance of the thoracolumbar spine in trauma: a review of the literature. J Trauma 2006;60(4): 915–20.
[57] Blackmore CC, Ramsey SD, Mann FA, et al. Cervical spine screening with CT in trauma patients: a cost effectiveness analysis. Radiology 1999;212:117–25.

[58] Grogan EL, Morris JA, Dittus RS, et al. Cervical spine evaluation in urban trauma centers: lowering institutional costs and complications through helical CT scan. J Am Coll Surg 2005; 200:160–5.

[59] Lowery DW, Wald MM, Browne BJ, et al. Epidemiology of cervical spine injury victims. Ann Emerg Med 2001;38(1):12–6.

[60] Brown RL, Brunn MA, Garcia VF. Cervical spine injuries in children: a review of 103 patients treated consecutively at a level 1 pediatric trauma center. J Pediatr Surg 2001;36(8): 1107–14.

[61] d'Amato C. Pediatric spinal trauma: injuries in very young children. Clin Orthop Relat Res 2005;432:34–40.

[62] Pang D, Pollack IF. Spinal cord injury without radiographic abnormality in children—the SCIWORA syndrome. J Trauma 1989;29(5):654–64.

[63] Pang D, Wilberger JE Jr. Spinal cord injury without radiographic abnormalities in children. J Neurosurg 1982;57(1):114–29.

[64] Launay F, Leet AI, Sponseller PD. Pediatric spinal cord injury without radiographic abnormality: a meta-analysis. Clin Orthop Relat Res 2005;433:166–70.

[65] Viccellio P, Simon H, Pressman BD, et al. NEXUS group. A prospective multicenter study of cervical spine injury in children. Pediatrics 2001;108(2):E20.

[66] Putzke JD, Barrett JJ, Richards JS, et al. Age and spinal cord injury: an emphasis on outcomes among the elderly. J Spinal Cord Med 2003;26(1):37–44.

[67] Touger M, Gennis P, Nathanson N, et al. Validity of a decision rule to reduce cervical spine radiography in elderly patients with blunt trauma. Ann Emerg Med 2002;40(3):287–93.

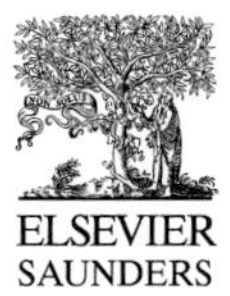

ELSEVIER
SAUNDERS

EMERGENCY
MEDICINE
CLINICS OF
NORTH AMERICA

Emerg Med Clin N Am 25 (2007) 751–761

Acute Complications of Extremity Trauma

Edward J. Newton, MD

Department of Emergency Medicine, Keck School of Medicine, LAC+USC Medical Center, Building GNH 1011, 1200 North State Street, Los Angeles, CA 90033, USA

In addition to the large number of patients with isolated limb injuries, many patients with major blunt or penetrating trauma harbor extremity injuries as a component of their overall clinical picture. In these cases, diagnosis and treatment of extremity injuries takes a lower priority, as resuscitation focuses on life-threatening injuries. Extremity injuries range from gross deformities and amputations to more subtle injuries, potentially difficult to diagnose. Injuries may also escape detection in unconscious or intoxicated patients. However, many soft tissue and vascular injuries require time sensitive interventions to ensure salvage of the limb and the best outcome for the patient. This article reviews the acute management of vascular and soft tissue injuries in the emergency department (ED).

Crush injury

Crush injury of an extremity occurs when a limb is compressed between two hard surfaces, to the point where vascular supply is impaired and vulnerable tissues undergo necrosis. Most commonly, limbs are crushed during auto versus pedestrian accidents, motor vehicle crashes, and industrial accidents. However, during natural disasters such as earthquakes, building collapses, landslides, mine cave-ins, and acts of war with mass civilian casualties, epidemics of limb crush injuries can occur. The large number of casualties requiring specialized medical care can easily overwhelm medical systems, particularly if medical facilities are simultaneously affected by the disaster.

E-mail address: ednewton@usc.edu

0733-8627/07/$ - see front matter. Published by Elsevier Inc.
doi:10.1016/j.emc.2007.06.003

emed.theclinics.com

Pathophysiology

The severity of the crush injury depends on both the degree of compression as well as its duration. Changes that occur in the trapped extremity are analogous to those seen in compartment syndrome, in which internal pressure precludes effective perfusion. In crush injury the pressure is applied externally but the effects on limb perfusion are similar. A crushed extremity can contain multiple injured structures, but most importantly the blood vessels supplying the limb may be disrupted or occluded for sufficient time to cause ischemic injury to nerves and muscles. The term "crush syndrome" refers to the consequences of crushed limbs that sustain prolonged ischemia, muscle necrosis, and release of cellular components into the circulation when the trapped limb is freed and reperfused. Third space fluid losses in the injured limb can cause severe hypovolemia and shock. Release of potassium, calcium, and myoglobin from damaged muscle can have life-threatening effects on cardiac conduction and renal function. Release of lactic acid and other organic acids leads to systemic acidosis, worsening the arrhythmogenic effects of hyperkalemia. Systemic release of myoglobin has several consequences, particularly on renal function. Myoglobin is a large molecule but is still easily filtered by the glomerulus. In an acidic environment myoglobin forms a gel that occludes the tubule, preventing function of the nephron and ultimately causing renal failure.

Clinical presentation

As with compartment syndrome, the key to making the diagnosis is a high clinical suspicion. Patients may present with obvious mangled extremities that suggest the possibility of crush syndrome. In other cases, such as a patient with coma or drug overdose who remains in the same position for a prolonged time, there may be few external signs of injury to the limb. Immediately on release of an entrapped limb, reestablishment of the circulation to the limb results in massive fluid sequestration and progressive swelling. Vital signs will usually reflect the resultant hypovolemia as tachycardia and hypotension. Hypovolemic shock is the most common cause of death in the first 48 hours of crush syndrome [1]. Myoglobinuria results in dark "smoky" colored urine, but urine output may be markedly decreased or absent so that this clue may be lacking. Increase in potassium can generate cardiac arrhythmias, especially in the presence of acute renal failure, and cardiac arrest can be the initial presentation of this syndrome.

Management

Diagnosis of crush syndrome relies on the clinical evidence described above, as well as laboratory confirmation. Myoglobinuria can be inferred when the urinalysis dips strongly positive for blood but few red blood cells (RBC) are seen on microscopic examination. Direct measurement of myoglobin is difficult, so serum creatine phosphokinase (CPK) is followed as a surrogate marker for rhabdomyolysis. Serum creatine phosphokinase reflects the extent of muscle damage and levels exceeding 30,000 to 100,000 units are routinely seen with crush syndrome involving large muscle groups. It is important to serially measure serum chemistry to determine renal function, serum bicarbonate, electrolytes, and especially potassium level. These measurements may become progressively abnormal over the first 24 hours after injury and should be followed frequently until an improving trend is noted. Crush syndrome and compartment syndrome may coexist or evolve into one another, so measurement of compartment pressure in the crushed limb may be indicated.

Ideally, treatment of crush injury should begin in the field simultaneous with extrication efforts. In anticipation of hypovolemia upon release of the entrapped extremity, fluid resuscitation should be initiated if venous access is available during extrication. Similarly, airway management can at times be instituted if access to the patient and positioning of the patient allows. The affected limb should be splinted and the patient transported as expeditiously as possible. Supplemental oxygen may be useful when an ischemic extremity injury is present, even if there is no respiratory compromise.

In the ED, treatment of crush syndrome is aimed at restoring effective circulating blood volume, correcting electrolyte and pH imbalance, and supporting renal function while attempting to reverse renal injury. Airway management is conducted as per protocols, except that it is prudent to avoid using succinylcholine as a paralytic agent in these cases because of the possibility of hyperkalemia. Volume resuscitation is guided by vital signs and urine output. Monitoring central venous pressure is helpful in guiding volume replacement in the elderly, patients with cardiac or pulmonary disease, and in those with anuric renal failure, to avoid overhydration. The use of sodium bicarbonate in this setting is controversial because it does not affect mortality but it may be effective in mobilizing precipitated myoglobin from the renal tubules [2,3]. Glucose, insulin, and sodium bicarbonate rely on shifting potassium intracellularly across intact cell membranes to reduce serum potassium. If sufficient muscle mass has been damaged, these traditional treatments for hyperkalemia may be less effective. Administration of calcium is indicated for arrhythmias related to hyperkalemia or for cardiac arrest. Dialysis if often needed to support renal function, at least as a bridging measure until renal function recovers. A recent study of patients with rhabdomyolysis determined that patients who develop acute renal failure have significantly higher mortality than those who do not (59% versus 22%) [4]. Most patients recover renal function over a period of weeks to months, although some patients remain dialysis dependent. The shortage of dialysis machines and technicians is almost always a second disaster in developing countries that are suddenly faced with mass casualties who develop renal failure, and this is a priority for relief organizations responding to this type of large-scale disaster [1,5].

Compartment syndrome

There are two types of compartment syndrome (CS), acute and chronic. Chronic CS occurs in distance runners, resulting in exercise-related symptoms, primarily in the anterolateral compartment of the leg. Acute CS is a surgical emergency in which pressure must be relieved in the compartment to avoid permanent damage to its contents. There are over 40 compartments in the body, including the abdomen, thorax, eye, and cranial vault, and CS has been reported in virtually all of them. However, almost 70% of CS occurrences are associated with fractures and half of those are caused by tibia fractures [6].

An extremity compartment is defined as an anatomic space confined by unyielding fascia and bone and containing compressible structures such as muscle, nerves, and blood vessels. Increasing the contents of the compartment, through edema formation or hemorrhage or excessive external compression, causes compartment pressure to rise precipitously. As the pressure reaches a critical threshold it compresses venules, ending venous outflow. As arterial perfusion continues, further edema develops and compartment pressure continues to increase. Once the pressure is sufficient to cause collapse of arterioles, effective perfusion of muscle and nerves ends and CS occurs. Inadequate perfusion is assumed to occur once compartment pressure is within 20 mm Hg of diastolic blood pressure, or within 30 mm Hg of mean arterial pressure [7]. It is important to interpret compartment pressure with this in mind, as a hypotensive patient may develop CS at pressures that are not usually considered dangerous. Patients with pre-existing vascular disease may develop irreversible necrosis more quickly and at lower compartment pressures. Muscles and nerves can tolerate 4 hours of warm (body temperature) ischemia without permanent injury; after 6 hours most muscle will recover complete function but some portion of the muscle often sustains irreversible necrosis; after 8 hours, most nerve and muscle tissue will have undergone necrosis [8]. Once nerves and muscle undergo necrosis, scarring and contractures eventually result in a deformed, insensate, nonfunctional limb.

Compartment syndrome can occur from a variety of causes, including intravenous and intraosseous fluid infiltration, snakebite, burns, nephrotic syndrome, diabetes, drug overdose or injection, and a variety of medications such as pressors, anticoagulants, and platelet inhibitors. However, by far the most common cause is fracture of a long bone. Fractures of the tibia and forearm are particularly prone to develop CS and account for a majority of cases. The syndrome can occur with open fractures as well. In one series, CS was more common in open than closed fractures of the tibia, reflecting the greater force of trauma and soft tissue injury associated with open fractures [9]. Compressive dressings and casts can also cause compartment syndrome and, in fact, caused the first case reported by Volkman [10]. Finally, arterial injury or occlusion can cause CS, although the occurrence of elevated compartment pressures distal to an arterial occlusion is unclear and certainly not inevitable.

The five "Ps" (pain, pallor, pulselessness, paresthesias, and paralysis) associated with arterial injury are often mistakenly applied to CS. Of these, the only reliable sign is pain. Patients with extremity fracture usually do not experience severe pain once the fracture has been reduced and the limb is immobilized and at rest. Patients with a burning quality of pain, delayed onset or increasing severity of pain, or pain on a passive stretch of the compartment, merit evaluation for CS. For example, dorsiflexing the foot and toes will cause pain in the posterior calf compartments if compartment pressure is elevated. Paresthesias and paralysis are late findings in this syndrome but also merit investigation, but arterial pulses may persist indefinitely because compartment pressure is almost always less than systolic blood pressure. The soft tissues are often visibly swollen and the compartment will usually have a tense "woody" feeling on palpation. The presence of fracture blisters suggests increased compartment pressure, but they are not reliably present.

Diagnosis of CS relies first on clinical suspicion of the condition. Use of pulse oximetry to measure tissue oxygenation is sometimes used for diagnosis, but it is not generally reliable, with a sensitivity of only 40% [11]. Pulse oximetry relies on superficial skin HbO_2/Hb measurement, whereas in CS this may be normal in spite of severe deeper tissue ischemia. Near-infra red spectroscopy (NIRS) can measure the oxygen saturation in tissues at depths up to 10 cm, and is increasingly being used to diagnose CS [12,13]. NIRS can penetrate skin, muscle, and bone with adjustable depths, and can provide continuous monitoring of compartment perfusion [14,15]. However, there are several limitations to this technology that may make it less reliable than direct measurement of compartment pressure. Patients with shock, severe anemia, and hypoxia may have false-positive results with NIRS because all tissue perfusion and oxygenation is reduced. Similarly, a large hematoma surrounding a fracture and containing desaturated blood may give a false-positive reading [14]. Despite these limitations, refined NIRS technology will likely become more accurate and more clinically applicable in the near future.

Currently, the most reliable means of diagnosing CS is to directly measure pressure in the compartment. Automated devices, such as the Stryker, are most commonly used but must be calibrated carefully before relying on the measurement. The device should be inserted within 5 cm from the fracture site to avoid falsely low readings, and sterile technique is used to prevent infection of the fracture hematoma (Fig. 1) [8].

Each compartment contiguous with the fracture should be assessed. For example, in tibia fractures, all four compartments of the leg, including the deep posterior compartment, should have the pressure measured. Pressures greater than 30 mm Hg are suspect but a more physiologic measure is the difference between diastolic blood pressure and compartment pressure (Δp). When Δp is less than 20 mm Hg, compartment syndrome is likely and

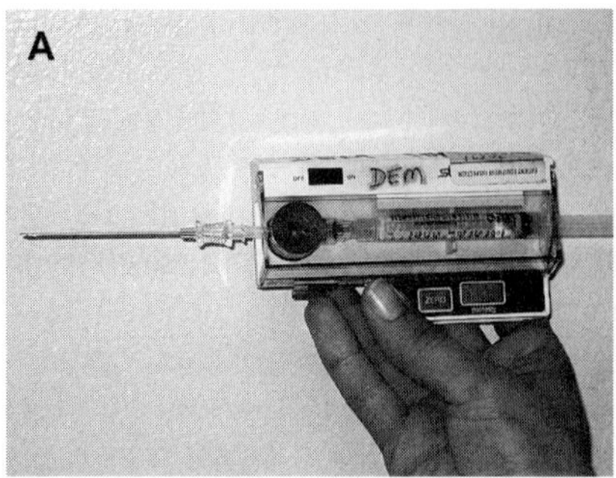

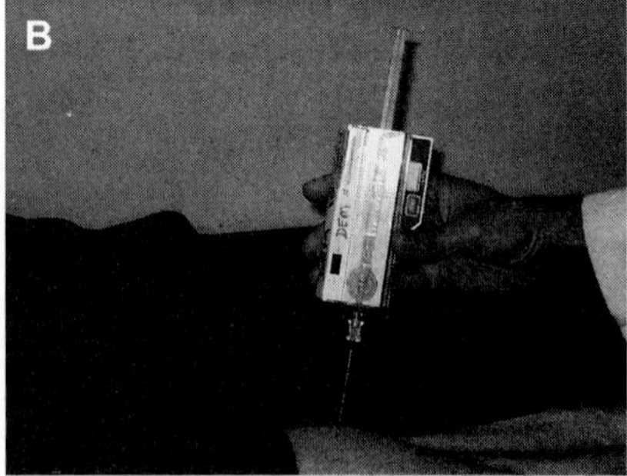

Fig. 1. (*A*) The Stryker device for measurement of intracompartmental pressure. (*B*) The Stryker device being inserted into the calf compartment under local anesthesia.

fasciotomy is indicated [8,16]. There are several limitations in using a single measurement of compartment pressure to detect CS. First, compartment pressures may increase progressively over 24 to 48 hours and second, the patient's hemodynamic status may change over time, with subsequent development of hypotension (eg, intraoperatively). Clearly, a single early measurement of compartment pressure is inadequate in detecting later deterioration. Repeated measurements or continuous monitoring of compartment pressure may be indicated. Additional diagnostic tests are indicated to look for rhabdomyolysis, myoglobinuria, renal failure, and hyperkalemia.

The treatment of CS should begin with removal of any constricting bandages or cast. The limb should be kept in neutral elevation because elevating the leg may aggravate the condition by decreasing perfusion pressure without decreasing compartment pressure [11]. Once the diagnosis of CS is established, fasciotomy should be completed, ideally within 6 hours of its onset. Fasciotomy needs to include wide incisions to completely release the constraining fascia. Repeat pressure measurement should verify that pressures have been reduced. The patient needs to be admitted for continuing debridement of necrotic tissue, prophylactic antibiotics, analgesia, and monitoring of renal function. Closure of the wounds may require skin flaps or grafts. Recently, use of mannitol, to decrease tissue edema, and hyperbaric oxygen, to increase tissue oxygenation, have been reported to improve the outcome in CS, and in some cases avoid the need for fasciotomy despite high compartment pressures [11,17]. Additional study of these modalities is indicated. Patients who present beyond the 6-hour window of warm ischemia with an insensate "dead" limb do not benefit from fasciotomy and experience increased complications, such as wound infection, if performed [16].

Penetrating arterial injuries

The evaluating practitioner's role in penetrating arterial injuries is to diagnose the injury, stabilize the patient, and mobilize the specialized resources needed to perform arterial repair within the 6-hour window of warm ischemia. Physical findings are divided into "hard" and "soft" signs of arterial injury. Hard findings include a pulsatile or rapidly enlarging hematoma, obvious pulsatile arterial bleeding from open wounds, a bruit or thrill on palpating the arterial pulse, and any of the five "Ps" indicating arterial insufficiency (pain, pallor, pulselessness, paresthesias and paralysis). However, absence of a peripheral pulse may be misleading in up to 27% of cases in which no arterial injury is found, and pulses can be maintained in the presence of arterial injury in up to 42% of cases [18]. Consequently, even with the hard finding of a pulse deficit, many centers proceed with further investigations if the patient is stable. Soft findings are presence of a diminished pulse compared with the uninjured side, delayed capillary refill, isolated peripheral nerve injury, and a nonpulsatile stable hematoma. Up to 35% of patients with soft findings have an arterial injury, although most of these injuries do not require surgical repair [19]. Patients with hard findings usually require surgical exploration and arterial repair. If ischemic time and the patient's clinical status allow, many surgeons prefer to have a preoperative arteriogram before operating, to locate and define the injury. Arteriography solely based on the location of the wounds is not indicated. "Proximity wounds" are variably defined as wounds within 1 cm, 5 cm, or 1 inch of a major vessel. The vast majority of these wounds have negative studies in the absence of hard or soft findings of arterial injury [20].

Patients with soft findings require further investigation. In the past this investigation invariably consisted of formal arteriography; however, in recent years alternative studies have often been used instead of arteriography. Comparison of the systolic arterial pressure in the injured limb compared with the uninjured limb (arterial pressure index or API) or comparison of the injured limb to the uninjured arm or leg (ankle brachial index or ABI) can reliably detect arterial injury [21]. An index of 0.9 or less is a sensitive and specific indicator of arterial injury. However, some arteries do not normally have palpable pulses (eg, peroneal artery), so that injury to these arteries and any venous injuries are not detectable by this method.

Duplex ultrasound is useful in evaluating possible arterial injuries, as absence of arterial and venous blood flow is usually readily apparent. The advantage of ultrasound is that it can be performed at the bedside while resuscitation is ongoing, and it can diagnose major venous injuries. Abnormal pressure indices, or Doppler flow studies, are an indication for surgical exploration and repair of the damaged artery. Indeterminate Doppler studies, or ABIs between 0.9 and 0.99, are managed by local wound care and observation. If all of these studies are normal, some patients can be safely discharged. In recent years, some centers have begun using computed tomography angiography (CTA) in the place of standard angiography. Preliminary data reports high sensitivity for the detection of arterial injury. Busquets and colleagues [22] compared 97 CT angiograms to either surgery or formal angiography, and found CTA detected 21 injuries and had no missed injuries. Inaba and colleagues [23] recently published a retrospective review of 63 CTA with 22 detected injuries. This study reported both a sensitivity and specificity of 100%. Early data on CTA for penetrating arterial injury is promising, but future prospective trials should be performed.

Open fractures

Open fractures occur frequently because of external penetration by gunshots, stab wounds, impalement with various objects that fracture the bone, or penetration from within by sharp fragments of bone fractured during blunt trauma. In the last case, the wound produced by fractured bone often causes innocuous-appearing small wounds that may be several centimeters removed from the site of the fracture. Any wound in the vicinity of a fracture should be considered an open fracture until proven otherwise by exploration of the wound or by radiography. The evaluating practitioner's role in these injuries is to diagnose the injury, stabilize the patient, and mobilize the specialized resources needed to perform arterial repair within the 6-hour window of warm ischemia. The Gustilo and Anderson classification is used to grade open fractures according to the degree of soft tissue damage and contamination and the presence of arterial injury [24].

Treatment of open fractures involves analgesia, debridement of the wound, reduction of the fracture, administration of appropriate antibiotics, and prophylactic treatment to prevent tetanus. Broad spectrum antibiotics, such as a first generation cephalosporin, are used with the addition of an aminoglycoside for more severely contaminated wounds. Alternatives, such as ertapenem, are also appropriate. Tetanus toxoid is given for previously immunized patients and tetanus immune globulin for particularly tetanus prone wounds or for patients who have not received a complete primary tetanus immunization series. The timing of surgical debridement and irrigation of open fractures is controversial. In the past it was thought that surgical debridement had to be done within 6 hours of injury to prevent subsequent osteomyelitis. Recently however, there are several large series that refute this principle, finding no increase in osteomyelitis if debridement is completed within the first 24 hours, providing appropriate antibiotics are begun in the ED [25,26]. Most of these series dealt with low energy tibial fractures, or fractures in children whose excellent vascular status may decrease the incidence of osteomyelitis, regardless of treatment. Fractures with high-energy mechanisms, severe soft tissue injury, or severe contamination should still be prioritized for early debridement [27].

Amputation

It is estimated that up to 50,000 traumatic amputations occur every year in the United States. Conn and colleagues [28] estimated that in 2001–2 there were 30,673 nonwork-related amputations alone. Of all amputations, less than one third are considered suitable for replantation or revascularization if there is an incomplete amputation. Most amputations occur in the workplace or are caused by home accidents involving power tools. The nature of the wound ranges from sharp incisions to wounds with severely crushed and devitalized parts, and this is one of the main criteria for deciding to replant the amputated part. Public expectations regarding replantation greatly exceed the reality, and failure to replant amputated parts is often a source of litigation or patient dissatisfaction. Replantation services are not uniformly available throughout the nation and the need to transfer patients to qualified centers is problematic because of the time involved in these transfers.

Replantation should be considered for amputations involving whole limbs, the thumb, and single or multiple digits amputated distal to the insertion of the flexor superficialis tendon. Pediatric amputations have a much better prognosis and should be considered regardless of the level [29]. Contraindications to replantation include amputations in which warm ischemic time is greater than 6 hours or cold ischemic time is greater than 12 hours, crushed or avulsed parts in which multiple tendons have ruptured, multiple levels of amputation, the presence of significant vascular disease or diabetes, self-inflicted amputations, and hemodynamically unstable patients.

ED care of patients with amputation consists of basic trauma management with priority focus on life-threatening injuries. An amputation is often visually striking and tends to distract attention from potentially more serious injuries. Hemorrhage from the limb can occur, but massive arterial bleeding is actually relatively uncommon, as the arteries retract and constrict when severed. Nevertheless, serious bleeding can occur and is best dealt with by direct compression of the bleeding vessel rather than clamping. Placement of a tourniquet is rarely necessary, but if used it should be kept on less than 3 hours.

The handling of the amputated part is important. In a complete amputation the severed part is wrapped in a sterile saline-soaked gauze and placed in a thin plastic bag that is then placed in a container of ice. The ideal temperature for cooling is 4°C and freezing should be avoided. Even if the part is unsuitable for replantation it should be preserved as a potential source of skin and bone for revision of the stump. In partial amputation, cooling the partially severed component is controversial. If there is evidence of perfusion to the part, cooling is avoided. If the part shows no evidence of perfusion, it should be cooled as if completely amputated [29]. Prophylactic antibiotics are indicated if replantation is considered likely. Replanted limbs and digits are psychologically desirable for the patient but often have limited function. Almost all replanted parts have sensory deficits with decreased two-point discrimination, and many have limited range of motion and strength. Rehabilitation after replantation is prolonged. With the advent of fairly functional prosthetic limbs, many patients would be better served by completion of the amputation, revision of the stump, and fitting with a prosthesis.

References

[1] Malinoski DJ, Slater MS, Mullins RJ. Crush injury and rhabdomyolysis. Crit Care Clin 2004;20:171–92.
[2] Brown CV, Rhee P, Chan L, et al. Preventing renal failure in patients with rhabdomyolysis: do bicarbonate and mannitol make a difference? J Trauma 2004;56:1191–6.
[3] Ozguc H, Kavechi N, Akkose S, et al. Effects of different resuscitation fluids on tissue blood flow and oxidant injury in experimental rhabdolyolysis. Crit Care Med 2005;33: 2579–86.
[4] de Meijer AR, Fikkers BG, de Keijzer MH, et al. Serum creatine kinase as predictor of clinical course in rhabdomyolysis: a 5-year intensive care study. Intensive Care Med 2003;29: 1121–5.
[5] Sever MS, Erek E, Vanholder R, et al. Lessons learned from the catastrophic Maramara earthquake: factors influencing the final outcome of renal victims. Clin Nephrol 2004;61: 413–21.
[6] McQueen MM, Gaston P, Court-Brown CM. Acute compartment syndrome. Who is at risk? J Bone Joint Surg (Br) 2000;82:200–3.
[7] Olson SA, Glasgow RR. Acute compartment syndrome in lower extremity musculoskeletal trauma. J Am Acad Orthop Surg 2005;13:436–44.
[8] Whitesides TE, Heckman MM. Acute compartment syndrome: update on diagnosis and treatment. J Am Acad Orthop 1996;4:209–18.
[9] Delee JL, Stiehl JB. Open tibia fracture with compartment syndrome. Clin Orthop 1981;160: 175–84.
[10] Seiler JG III, Casey PJ. Binford SA Compartment syndrome of the upper extremity. J South Orthop Assoc 2000;9:233–47.
[11] Wattel F, Mathieu D, Neviere R, et al. Acute peripheral ischemia and compartment syndrome: a role for hyperbaric oxygenation. Anaesthesia 1998;53(Suppl 2):63–5.
[12] Velmahos GC, Toutouzas K. Vascular trauma and compartment syndromes. Surg Clin North Am 2002;82:125–41.
[13] Tobias JD, Hoernschemeyer DG. Near-infrared spectroscopy identifies compartment syndrome in an infant. J Pediatr Orthop 2007;27:311–3.
[14] Gentilello LM, Sanzone A, Wang L, et al. Near-infrared spectroscopy versus compartment pressure for the diagnosis of lower extremity compartmental syndrome using electromyography-determined measurements of neuromuscular function. J Trauma 2001;51:1–8.
[15] Garr JL, Gentilello LM, Cole PA, et al. Monitoring for compartmental syndrome using near-infrared spectrospcopy: a noninvasive, continuous, transcutaneous monitoring technique. J Trauma 1999;46:613–6.
[16] Pearse FP, Harry L, Nanchahal J. Acute compartment syndrome of the leg. BMJ 2002;325: 557–8.
[17] Better OS, Zinman C, Reis DN, et al. Hypertonic mannitol ameliorates intracompartmental tamponade in model compartment syndrome in dogs. Nephron 1991;58:344–6.
[18] Fields CF, Latifi R, Ivatury RR. Brachial and forearm vessel injuries. Surg Clin North Am 2002;82:105–14.
[19] Espinosa GA, Chiu JC, Sammett EJ. Clinical assessment and arteriography for patients with penetrating extremity injuries: a review of 500 cases with the Veterans Affairs West Side Medical Center. Mil Med 1997;162:19–23.
[20] Gillespie DL, Woodson J, Kaufman J, et al. Role of arteriography for blunt or penetrating injuries in proximity to major vascular structures: an evolution in management. Ann Vasc Surg 1993;7:145–9.

[21] Hood DB, Weaver FA, Yellin AE. Changing perspectives in the diagnosis of peripheral vascular trauma. Semin Vasc Surg 1998;11:255–60.
[22] Busquets AR, Acosta J, Colon E, et al. Helical computed tomographic angiography for the diagnosis of traumatic arterial injuries of the extremities. J Trauma 2004;56:625–8.
[23] Inaba K, Munera F, McKenney M, et al. Multi-slice CT angiography for arterial evaluation in the injured lower extremity. J Trauma 2006;60:502–7.
[24] Gustilo RB, Anderson JT. Prevention of infection in the treatment of one thousand and twenty five open fractures of long bones: retrospective and prospective analyses. J Bone Joint Surg (Am) 1976;58:453–8.
[25] Yang EC, Eisler J. Treatment of isolated type I open fractures: is emergent operative debridement necessary? Clin Orthop Rel Res 2003;410:289–94.
[26] Skaggs DL, Friend L, Alman B, et al. The effect of surgical delay on acute infection following 554 open fractures in children. J Bone Joint Surg (Am) 2005;87:8–12.
[27] Khatod M, Botte MJ, Hoyt DB, et al. Outcomes in open tibia fractures: relationship between delay in treatment and infection. J Trauma 2003;55:949–54.
[28] Conn JM, Annest JL, Ryan GW, et al. Non-work-related finger amputations in the United States, 2001–2. Ann Emerg Med 2005;45:630–5.
[29] Langdorf M, Kazzi ZN. Replantation. E-Medicine on-line medical text. Boston: Boston Medical Publishing; 2007.

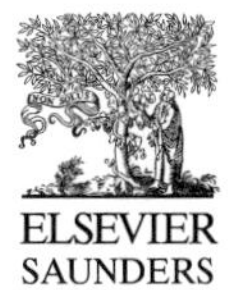
ELSEVIER
SAUNDERS

Emerg Med Clin N Am 25 (2007) 763–793

EMERGENCY
MEDICINE
CLINICS OF
NORTH AMERICA

Emergency Department Management of Selected Orthopedic Injuries

Edward J. Newton[a,*], John Love, MD[b]

[a]*Department of Emergency Medicine, Keck School of Medicine, LAC+USC Medical Center, Building GNH 1011, 1200 North State Street, Los Angeles, CA 90033, USA*

[b]*Keck School of Medicine and LAC+USC Medical Center, 1200 North State Street, Unit I, Room 1011, Los Angeles, CA 90033, USA*

Upper extremity

Scapulothoracic dissociation

Traumatic scapulothoracic dissociation (TSD) is an unusual, devastating shoulder girdle injury resulting from a sudden and severe traction to the upper extremity. Conceptually, TSD is characterized as a closed dislocation of the scapula from the thoracic wall. The injury frequently is missed on initial presentation, particularly in patients who present with multiple injuries. An important initial diagnostic clue is noting a laterally displaced scapula on chest radiograph.

Clinical presentation

The most common reported mechanisms of injury for TSD include a life-threatening fall, or a high-speed motorcycle or motor vehicle accident. However, isolated TSD injuries have occurred in industrial and farming accidents. An important clue is to recognize the potential for a severe lateral traction force applied to the shoulder girdle.

The patient typically presents with extensive soft tissue swelling and ecchymosis around the shoulder and upper extremity. Unfortunately, neurovascular deficits are common and often complete. The overlying skin is usually intact, and the extensive soft tissue swelling, tenderness, and neurovascular injury may be attributed inappropriately to commonly associated fractures of the shoulder girdle.

* Corresponding author.
E-mail address: ednewton@usc.edu (E.J. Newton).

0733-8627/07/$ - see front matter
doi:10.1016/j.emc.2007.07.003 **_emed.theclinics.com_**

The vascular injury is often proximal and most commonly involves the subclavian or axillary artery. Distal pulses are frequently nonpalpable. However, other signs of severe limb ischemia are uncommon because the shoulder has an extensive collateral vascular network. Vascular injury is reported in 90% of TSD cases. Unstable hemorrhage from the vascular injury occurs in approximately 10% of cases and requires urgent operative control [1]. Vascular repair in the stable patient with a flaccid arm and no signs of severe limb ischemia is controversial because it may not change the final neurovascular outcome [2].

Brachial plexus injury is the most devastating consequence of TSD. The reported incidence is 94% and often the avulsion is complete [3]. Overall, the final outcome is poor because of the severe neurovascular injury. The patient typically has a nonfunctional, flail upper extremity. Above the elbow amputation is typically recommended. If the brachial plexus injury is incomplete, then partial functional recovery is possible, but is not typical (Fig. 1).

Radiographic findings

The classic finding is a laterally displaced scapula noted on initial chest radiograph. The key is a bilateral comparison of the medial scapular border from the midline thoracic spine. Of particular concern is lateral scapular displacement greater than 1 cm [4]. Ideally, the arms are positioned

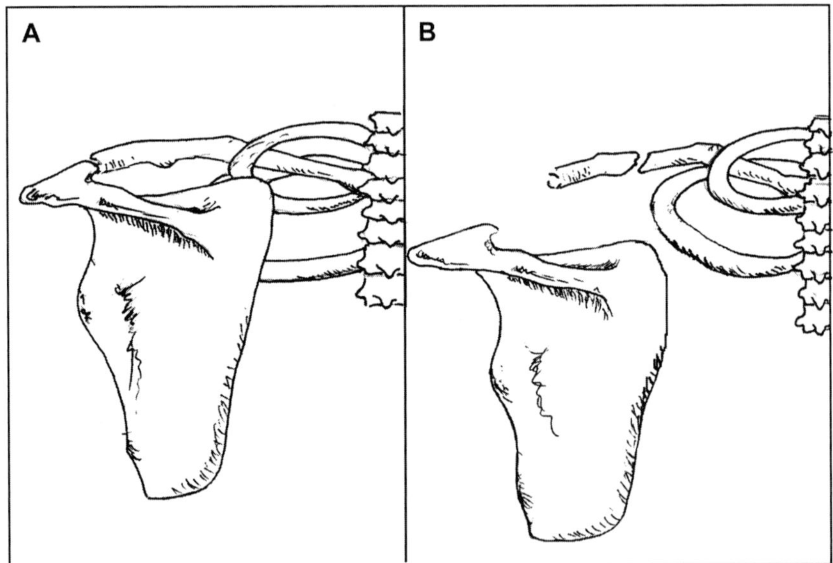

Scapulothoracic Dislocation
3/07

Fig. 1. (*A*) Normal scapula, posterior view. (*B*) Scapulothoracic dissociation.

symmetrically during the chest radiograph because it can affect scapular position. Common associated radiographic findings include complete acromioclavicular separation, distracted clavicular fracture, and a hematoma over the affected shoulder. Associated sternoclavicular dislocation is also reported [5].

Sternoclavicular dislocation

The sternoclavicular joint (SCJ) has strong ligamentous support and is rarely dislocated. The injury is difficult to diagnose solely on physical examination or plain radiograph. Typically, an SCJ dislocation occurs from a tremendous force. The most common scenarios include a motor vehicle accident or a collision sporting injury, particularly a football injury. The medial end of the clavicle lies in close proximity to several important mediastinal structures, including the trachea. A posterior SCJ dislocation can compress these vital structures, resulting in neurovascular or airway compromise and life-threatening emergency.

Mechanism of action

The injury can occur in either an anterior or a posterior direction. Anterior SCJ dislocations are far more common. Typically, the dislocation takes place after a strong lateral force is applied to the shoulder. Anterior-lateral forces result in an anterior SCJ dislocation. During the injury, the strong costoclavicular ligament acts as a fulcrum against the anterolateral force, prying the medial clavicle out of its articulation in an anterior direction.

Posterior dislocations can result from two different mechanisms. A force applied to the posterior lateral shoulder is the most common. Direct trauma over the medial clavicle, such as a high-speed motor vehicle accident causing the chest wall to impact the steering wheel, can also produce the injury. Rarely are atraumatic, spontaneous, SCJ dislocations reported [6]. Usually, the patient has other evidence of ligamentous laxity.

Clinical presentation

The patient will complain of marked pain at the SCJ. Typically, the affected arm is flexed at the elbow and positioned across the trunk. The patient's head is usually tilted toward the injured side.

Anterior dislocations create a palpable bony prominence over the SCJ. However, because of marked tissue swelling at the site, this physical examination finding cannot be relied on to confirm an anterior dislocation. A palpable hollow may be noted at the SCJ, with a posterior dislocation (Fig. 2).

Posterior SCJ dislocations can present with symptoms resulting from compression of mediastinal structures. The great vessels, trachea, esophagus, brachial plexus, and dome of the lung all lie in close proximity to the

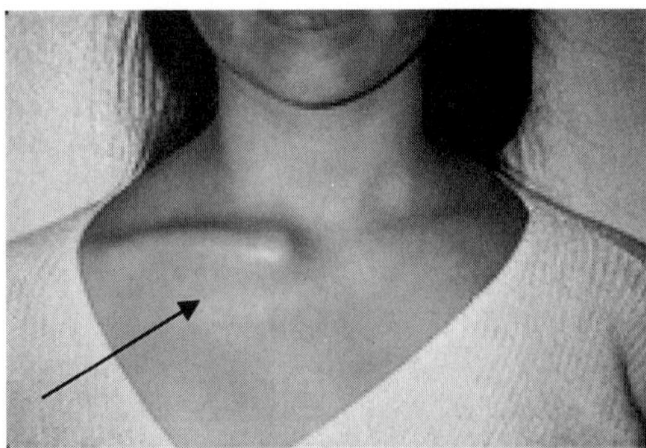

Fig. 2. Anterior sternoclavicular dislocation (*arrow*). (*From* Mandavia D, Newton E, Demetriades D. Atlas of emergency trauma. New York: Cambridge University Press; 2003.)

SCJ. Important signs and symptoms resulting from SCJ impingement include neck or extremity venous congestion, hoarseness, dyspnea, dysphagia, and extremity neurologic impairment. It is critical that the emergency physician recognize this spectrum of findings as a potential life-threatening emergency.

Radiographic findings

A CT scan that includes both clavicles is the best radiographic modality to determine the presence and type of SCJ dislocation (Fig. 3).

Intravenous contrast delineates mediastinal great vessel injury or impingement. A chest radiograph cannot reliably confirm or exclude the diagnosis. However, on comparison, subtle clues may include the appearance of superior or inferior medial displacement of the involved clavicle. The "serendipity" view is a plain radiographic technique specifically designed to visualize the clavicles. Comparing the medial clavicular position can help determine the type of SCJ dislocation. The medial clavicle appears superiorly displaced with an anterior dislocation, and conversely, inferiorly shifted

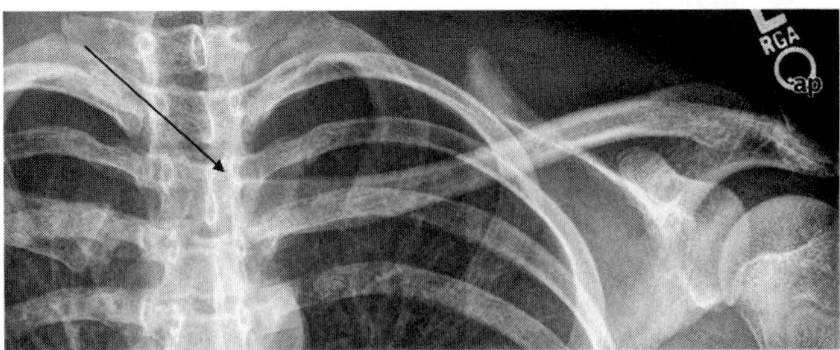

Fig. 3. Chest radiograph, revealing asymmetry of the clavicles with a posterior SCJ dislocation on the left (*arrow*).

from a posterior dislocation. The disadvantage of plain radiograph is that it does not provide anatomic detail regarding compression or injury to the mediastinum (Fig. 4).

Treatment

Most SCJ dislocations are treated by closed reduction. Irreducible posterior SCJ dislocations are managed in the operating room under general anesthesia.

Two different closed reduction techniques are described. Both methods involve similar initial positioning. The patient is placed supine, with a towel roll between the shoulder blades. The injured side is situated near the edge of the gurney.

The abduction traction technique is used to treat anterior and posterior SCJ dislocations with only a minor variation. The arm is straight, abducted to approximately 90°, placed in traction, and then brought into slight extension by moving the hand toward the floor. In anterior dislocations, direct pressure is then applied over the SCJ.

An audible snap and a loss of the bony prominence indicate a successful reduction. Most anterior dislocations are unstable. Frequently, the dislocation spontaneously reoccurs after reduction. This possibility should be explained to the patient before attempting closed reduction, to set reasonable expectations. In fact, "skillful neglect" is described as an acceptable alternative management option [7]. If the dislocation recurs or reduction is not attempted, the arm is placed into a sling and range of motion permitted as pain allows. The patient should be counseled that a bony prominence will persist, but full return of function is expected. Operative fixation for an anterior dislocation is not indicated [7].

In posterior dislocations the reduction procedure is the same, except, rather than pushing on the medial clavicle, it is grasped with fingers in an attempt to pull it anteriorly from behind the sternum (Fig. 5).

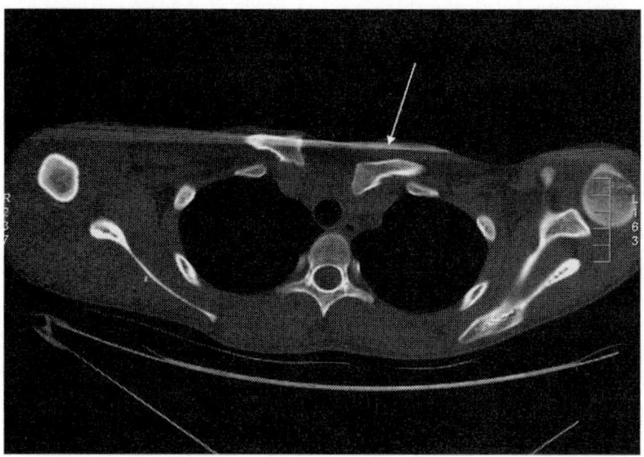

Fig. 4. CT scan of the chest, showing a left posterior SCJ dislocation (*arrow*) with mediastinal impingement.

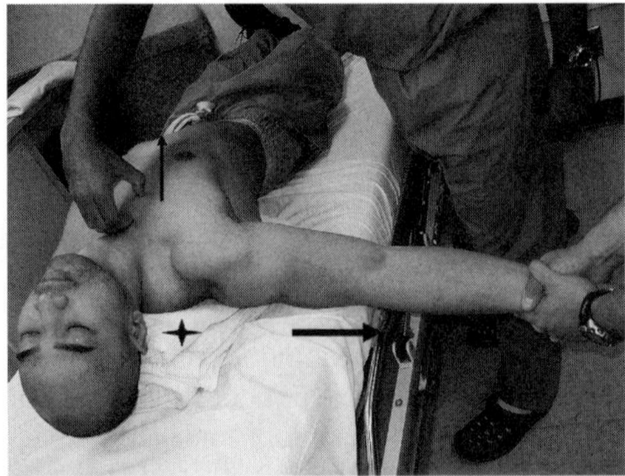

Fig. 5. Reduction technique for a posterior right SCJ dislocation. See text for details. Note the role of the towel in extending the SCJs bilaterally.

If the attempt is unsuccessful, a sterile towel clamp can be used to grasp the medial clavicle for greater leverage, using local anesthesia. Consultation with vascular and orthopedic surgery should be obtained before the addition of a towel clamp because of the close proximity to the great vessels. Sterile technique is required.

The adduction traction technique is an alternative method for posterior SCJ dislocations, and should be attempted if the first reduction technique is unsuccessful. The patient is placed into the same initial position, except that the arm is in adduction. Traction is applied to the arm while the shoulder is pushed posteriorly. Both reduction techniques are painful and the patient will require procedural sedation. Local anesthetic around the SCJ may be helpful.

A postreduction CT scan is recommended to confirm successful posterior SCJ reduction, and to evaluate for possible complications resulting from mediastinal impingement. Posterior SCJ dislocations are usually stable, once reduced. Postreduction management includes a figure-of-eight clavicle strap and serial neurovascular examinations.

Scapula fractures

Scapula fractures occur infrequently, and account for less than 1% of all fractures. The injury typically results from a high-energy trauma. Common mechanisms include significant falls and high speed motor vehicle and motorcycle accidents. All scapula fractures should serve as a warning sign for other possibly linked severe thoracic trauma. Scapular spine or body fractures are particularly associated with a high incidence of thoracic injuries. Less violent mechanisms, including ground level falls, can result in glenoid rim fractures and avulsion fractures of the coracoid process.

Clinical presentation and management

The affected arm is usually held in adduction across the chest wall. The patient will resist all arm movement, particularly abduction. Deep inspiration is typically painful because of associated scapular movement, rib fractures, or pneumothorax. Common linked injuries include pneumothorax, ipsilateral rib fractures, pulmonary contusion, and brachial plexus injuries [8]. Most scapula fractures are treated nonoperatively with a sling, pain control, and early range-of-motion exercises. A few exceptions include intra-articular displaced glenoid fractures, select coracoid fractures proximal to the coracoclavicular ligament, and displaced acromion fractures impinging on the subacromion space [8]. Early orthopedic consultation is indicated.

Radiographic findings

One case series reported that more than one half of scapula fractures are not visualized on a standard trauma anteroposterior (AP) chest radiograph, because of the overlying rib shadows [8]. Complete radiographic analysis includes true scapular AP, tangential lateral, axillary, and Stryker-notch views. A scapular CT scan is an excellent imaging modality for detecting fractures, especially those involving the glenoid fossa, and coracoid process. It also easily excludes subtle associated glenohumeral dislocation. All patients who have a scapular fracture involving a significant mechanism of injury should undergo a complete trauma evaluation, including a chest CT scan to evaluate for associated injuries.

Os acromiale is a radiographic finding that can easily be confused with an acromion fracture. The condition results from failure of the acromion ossification centers to close, and usually occurs at the midacromion. The reported frequency ranges between 1% and 15%, and bilateral involvement occurs in 41% to 62% of cases [9]. The condition is visualized most easily on a lateral axillary view (Fig. 6).

Helpful clues supporting the presence of os acromiale include a bilateral incidence and rounded cortical borders [9]. Another suggestion is the "double density" sign on an AP shoulder view, which is produced from the overlap of the two separate acromion cortical densities [10].

Shoulder dislocations

Acute and recurrent glenohumeral dislocations are the most frequently encountered joint dislocations in emergency medicine. Shoulder dislocations are categorized as anterior, inferior, or posterior, based on the position of the humeral head relative to the glenoid fossa. More than 90% of glenohumeral dislocations are anterior and are successfully reduced by several well-described techniques.

Inferior and posterior shoulder dislocations are comparatively rare and have a higher incidence of complications, and their diagnosis can be subtle. Complications resulting from a shoulder dislocation include extremity

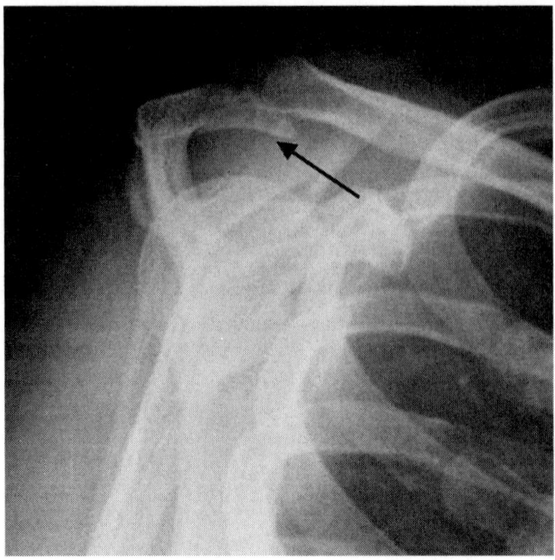

Fig. 6. Scapular Y radiograph, demonstrating os acromiale (*arrow*). The condition is easily confused with an acromion fracture.

neurovascular compromise, rotator cuff injuries, and impression fractures to the humeral head and glenoid rim.

The axillary (circumflex) nerve is the most frequently injured nerve from a shoulder dislocation because of its unique anatomic arrangement. The circumflex nerve originates from the posterior cord of the brachial plexus, and wraps around the proximal humerus. During the dislocation, tension is placed on the axillary nerve and a stretch injury can be produced. The circumflex nerve is responsible for lateral sensation to the proximal arm and motor function to the deltoid muscle.

A careful initial examination is important. A common mistake is to assess axillary nerve sensation through light touch only. Normal sensation does not rule out motor impairment. It is important to assess and document sensation and motor function pre- and postreduction. Ideally, an assessment of deltoid motor function would include shoulder abduction. However, the dislocation, possible associated rotator cuff injury, or postreduction pain often limits abduction. A simple alternative is to document static deltoid muscle contraction. One relatively painless method to test deltoid firing is to give the patient a strong handshake while your other hand is palpating the shoulder for deltoid contraction. If a neurapraxia is detected and does not completely resolve postreduction, then orthopedic, or possibly neuroloic, follow-up should be obtained. The patient is monitored with serial examinations, and electrodiagnostic testing is typically obtained within 4 weeks. Gradual complete recovery is the norm over a 3- to 6-month period. Observation, rather than early operative intervention, is favored. Injuries to the brachial plexus and the radial and ulnar nerves, are less common, but can occur.

Vascular injury is rare following a shoulder dislocation. Risk factors include advanced patient age and inferior dislocations. The axillary artery and vein are predominantly involved because of the close proximity to the humeral head. The shoulder has a rich collateral vascular network and the presence of a peripheral pulse does not completely exclude injury. Complications from unrecognized vascular injuries include delayed thrombosis, arterial-venous fistula, and aneurysm formation. All patients with diminished or absent pulses, enlarging or pulsatile hematomas, or a bruit require emergent vascular surgery consultation. More subtle arterial vascular injuries can occur. The arterial pressure index, comparing Doppler systolic blood pressure in both arms, is an easy bedside examination that can be used to screen for an arterial vascular injury. A (injured-to-uninjured) ratio of less than 0.9 calls for additional studies, such as color flow Doppler or angiography.

Rotator cuff injuries can be confused with circumflex nerve injuries because both conditions limit shoulder abduction. Also, acute postreduction pain limits standard examination techniques for detecting rotator cuff injury. Management of rotator cuff injury depends on the degree of tear, the presence of associated fracture, patient age, and lifestyle. In general, routine surgical repair is recommended for younger, active patients. Older individuals may be treated initially with immobilization followed by physical therapy. Routine orthopedic follow-up is indicated.

Radiography

The shoulder series should include an AP radiograph in the scapular plane, a scapular Y view, and an additional view to confirm humeral head position relative to the glenoid fossa. An axillary lateral radiograph is the preferred method for documenting humeral head position. However, the axillary lateral radiograph requires shoulder abduction, which is typically very painful after a shoulder dislocation. The Velpeau axillary lateral and trauma axillary lateral radiographs are two modified versions that require minimal shoulder abduction. The trauma axillary lateral radiograph is taken while the patient is supine. The Velpeau view requires a standing position. If plain radiographs leave doubt, a CT scan is excellent at detecting fractures and defining glenohumeral position.

Fractures following a shoulder dislocation or reduction procedure are relatively common. Impression fractures can occur to the humeral head as it compresses against the glenoid rim. Two well-described deformities associated with anterior shoulder dislocations are the Bankart lesion and the Hill-Sachs deformity. The Bankart lesion is a disruption to the anterior-inferior glenoid rim, and may predispose the patient to future recurrent dislocations. The Hill-Sachs deformity is an osteochondral impression fracture to the posterolateral humeral head. A reverse Hill-Sachs deformity is also described and can occur during a posterior shoulder dislocation. The defect is located on the anterior aspect of the humeral head. Two radiographs that provide excellent detail of the glenoid fossa are the West Point and the axial oblique views. The Stryker notch view is helpful at detecting a Hill-Sachs deformity. Fractures to the greater and lesser tuberosities can also occur.

Inferior shoulder dislocation (Luxatio erecta)

Luxatio erecta is rare, and accounts for less than 1% of all glenohumeral dislocations [11]. Direct and indirect forces can produce an inferior shoulder dislocation. The most common mechanism of injury is an indirect force, which occurs from a sudden, violent hyperabduction of the arm. While the arm is in an overhead position, the proximal humerus abuts against the acromion and levers the humeral head out of the joint capsule. The inferior support structure is damaged, and contraction of the teres major and latissimus dorsi muscle groups pulls the humeral head inferiorly. Simultaneous contraction of the pectoralis major pulls the humerus, medially locking the arm in an overhead position [12]. Conversely, a direct axial force applied to an overhead arm or elbow can drive the humeral head through the inferior joint capsule. An example includes bracing a head-first fall with an overhead arm.

The classic presentation is a patient holding an arm in an overhead position. The elbow is typically flexed, and the forearm pronated. The arm is locked in position, and any movement is extremely painful. The arm is already positioned for an axillary lateral radiograph (Fig. 7).

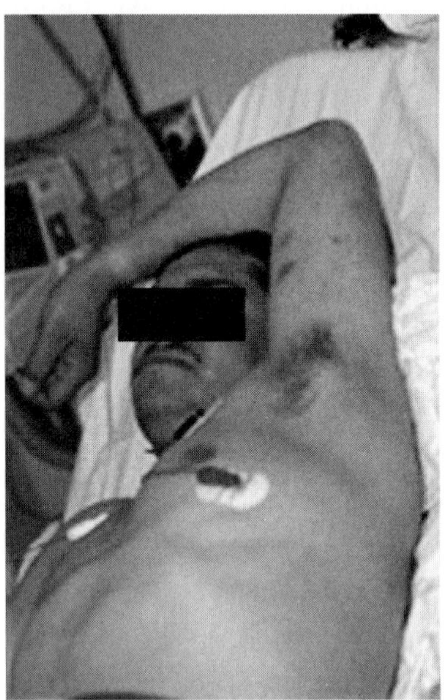

Fig. 7. Typical presenting arm position for luxatio erecta. See text for details. (*From* Mandavia D, Newton E, Demetriades D. Atlas of emergency trauma. New York: Cambridge University Press; 2003.)

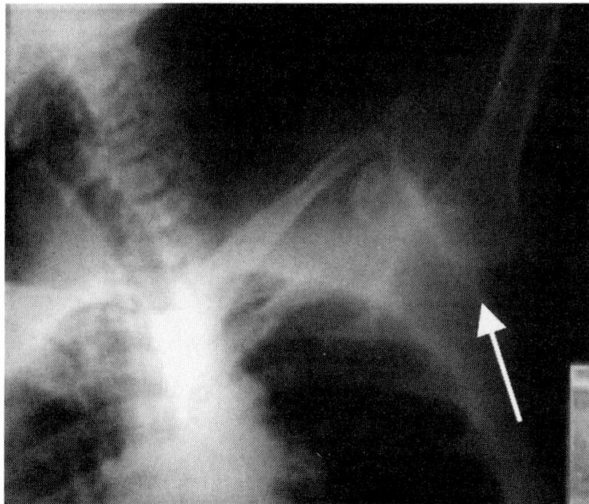

Fig. 8. AP radiograph of the shoulder, showing luxatio erecta (*arrow*). (*From* Mandavia D, Newton E, Demetriades D. Atlas of emergency trauma. New York: Cambridge University Press; 2003.)

Luxatio erecta has the highest complication rate of all shoulder dislocations. Rotator cuff injuries or greater tuberosity fractures occur in 80% of cases. Neurologic injury is reported in 60% of patients, and, although comparatively rare, vascular compromise still occurs in 3.3% of cases [11]. Osteochondral impression fractures are reported.

The reduction can usually be accomplished with a traction-countertraction technique. After appropriate procedural sedation, axial in-line traction is applied to the overhead humerus. An assistant can apply counter-traction with a sheet draped across the ipsilateral clavicle (Fig. 8).

After successful reduction, the arm is brought down across the chest to a position of adduction and internal rotation. A recently described alternative technique uses a two-step reduction maneuver. First, the luxatio erecta is converted to an anterior dislocation by simultaneously applying lateral axial traction to the humerus and pushing the humeral head into an anterior dislocation position. Once accomplished, the humerus is then adducted against the body. The anterior dislocation can then be reduced by the external rotation method or another common reduction technique [13]. Closed reduction in the emergency department is usually possible, unless the humeral head is pushed through an inferior joint capsule buttonhole deformity, in which case open reduction is required. Recurrent inferior dislocations are rare. Postreduction care includes placing the arm into a sling, careful neurovascular assessment, and orthopedic referral.

Posterior shoulder dislocation

Posterior shoulder dislocations account for 2% to 4% of all glenohumeral dislocations [14]. A careful clinical assessment is required because the condition is commonly missed. The delay or improper diagnoses are usually attributed to inadequate radiographs or impaired patient cognition. Delay in recognition and successful reduction are associated with significant long-term complications.

The mechanism of injury is interesting. The most common precipitating causes are seizure or electrocution. During these events, involuntary muscle contraction internally rotates the humerus and displaces the humeral head posteriorly. Combined contraction from the pectoralis major, subscapularis, and latissimus dorsi muscle groups is responsible. A less common mechanism is a direct violent axial load to the arm. The shoulder is at greatest risk when the arm is in a position of forward elevation, adduction, and internal rotation.

The patient usually holds the affected arm in a position of adduction and internal rotation. The osteochondral head defect is in a fixed position on the posterior glenoid rim. The shoulder is frequently described as frozen. Either passive or active attempts at external rotation are painful and unsuccessful. Physical examination may reveal an increased prominence of the coracoid process anteriorly and humeral head posteriorly.

The AP radiograph is frequently misinterpreted as normal because the humeral head is usually only in a subluxed position. Three subtle, easily missed radiographic clues in the AP view have been described. The "light bulb" sign is a frequent hint noticed on an AP shoulder radiograph. The humeral head appears as a light bulb stuck on the end of the humerus. The light bulb sign can also be seen on an AP chest radiograph (Fig. 9).

Careful comparison of each shoulder is important because a seizure or electrocution can produce bilateral posterior shoulder dislocations. Another clue is the "rim or ellipse sign." A normal AP shoulder radiograph produces

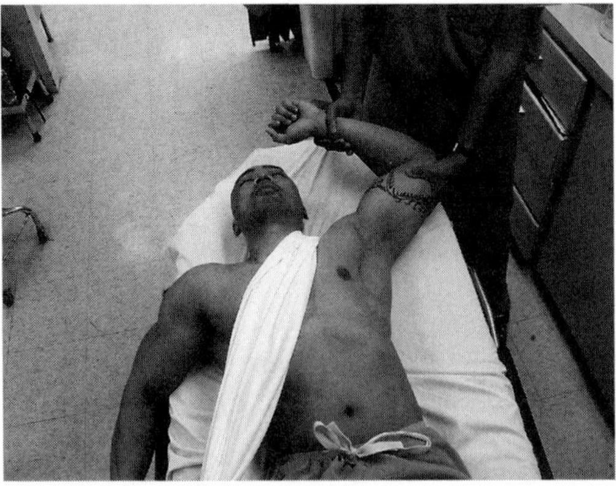

Fig. 9. Traction-countertraction reduction technique for luxatio erecta. An assistant maintains countertraction by securing the ends of the sheet. This technique is also used for anterior shoulder dislocations.

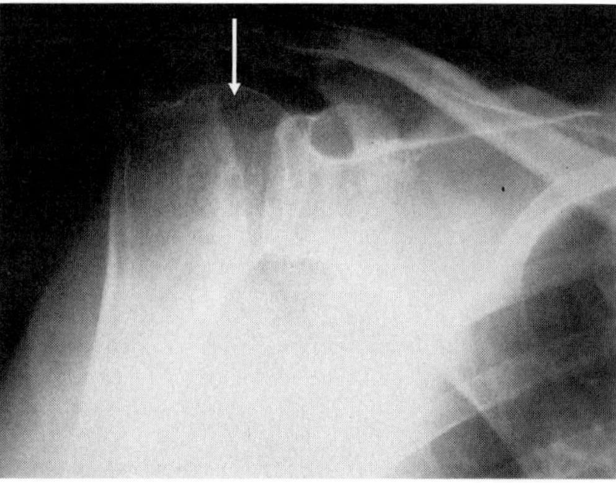

Fig. 10. AP shoulder radiograph, showing a posterior dislocation. A direct axial load applied to the arm can drive the humeral head posterior. The AP view can appear deceptively normal. The arrow is pointing to a relatively normal appearing glenohumoral joint in spite of the posterior dislocation.

an ellipse pattern from overlap of the humeral head and glenoid fossa. The posterior dislocation distorts the normal elliptic appearance (Fig. 10).

The "trough line" is a less common finding, but occurs from the reverse Hill-Sachs deformity. The appearance is a vertical line noted through the humeral head adjacent to the glenoid rim (Fig. 11).

The axillary lateral view is the key to proper diagnosis. The humeral head and glenoid fossa relationship is properly defined, and the anterior-medial osteochondral defect is visualized.

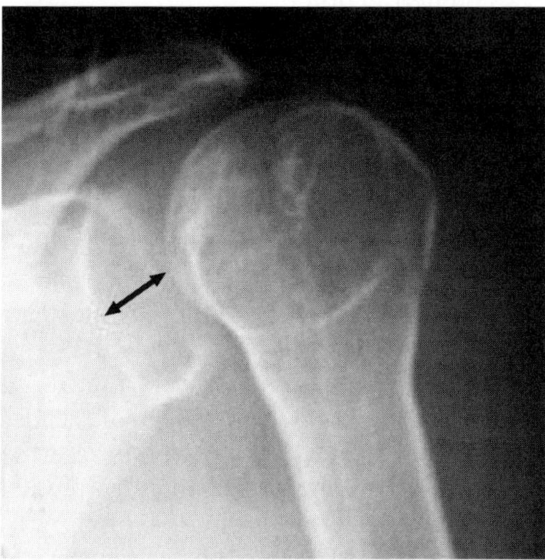

Fig. 11. The trough line is a sclerotic vertical line adjacent to the glenoid rim. See text for details.

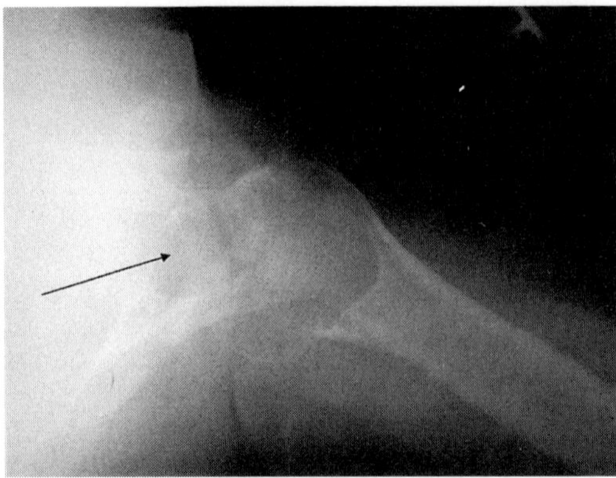

Fig. 12. AP radiograph of the shoulder, showing posterior shoulder dislocation and demonstrating the light bulb and rim signs (*arrow*). The rotation of the humeral head makes it appear as light bulb stuck onto the end of the humerus. The normal humeral head and glenoid fossa overlap, demonstrating the "rim or ellipse sign," is not present.

Treatment options are either closed or open reduction. The two factors that influence the probability of a successful closed reduction are the time since the dislocation and the size of the reverse Hill-Sachs deformity. Dislocations more than 3 weeks old, or humeral head articular surface defects greater than 25%, are very difficult to manage with closed reduction [14]. Orthopedic consultation is advised. The reduction technique combines in-line and lateral traction to the humerus, with simultaneous posterior pressure applied to the humeral head. Placing a folded sheet through the ipsilateral axilla provides countertraction.

Postreduction immobilization depends on shoulder stability. A stable shoulder is splinted in neutral rotation. If the examination reveals instability, the current recommendation is to immobilize in 20° of external rotation [14]. Standard postreduction radiographs and neurovascular examination are recommended.

Forearm

Fractures of the radius and ulna are among the most common fractures seen in the ED. This fracture is usually an isolated injury and occurs primarily in osteoporotic elderly patients as a result of a fall on an outstretched arm. The fracture of the radius is within 2 to 3 cm of the distal articular surface of the radius, and classically does not extend intra-articularly. An associated fracture of the ulnar styloid is commonly present. The fracture fragment is displaced dorsally and the radius is shortened, with loss of volar angulation. The wrist appears swollen, with a characteristic "dinner fork" deformity. Median and ulnar nerve injury can occur, and their functions in the hand should be assessed. Many Colles fractures are reduced and casted in the emergency department with acceptable results. Inability to restore the length and volar angulation of the distal radius may require open reduction and internal fixation (ORIF). Most patients suffer some residual disability, with chronic pain or limited range of motion at the wrist. A Smith fracture is often called a "reverse Colles" and occurs as a result of a fall on a flexed wrist. The fracture line is identical but the displacement is volar rather than dorsal.

Forearm fractures resulting from a fall on an outstretched arm can produce various radius and ulna fractures. A Galeazzi's fracture is important to detect because it requires ORIF to maintain reduction. This fracture involves a displaced fracture of the radius at the junction of the middle and distal thirds, and dislocation of the proximal radial head that may be subtle. These injuries can be missed if the elbow is not examined carefully for tenderness and swelling and if typical findings of an elbow effusion or misalignment of the radial head are not appreciated radiographically. Once detected, the arm is placed in a long arm splint and urgent orthopedic consultation is obtained (Fig. 12).

A Monteggia's fracture is sometimes referred to as a "reverse Galeazzi's" fracture. Several varieties of Monteggia's fracture have been described, but all involve a fracture of the proximal or midulnar shaft, with disruption of the distal radial ulnar joint (DRUJ). Clinically, tenderness to palpation at the DRUJ in the presence of an ulnar fracture should raise suspicion for a Monteggia's lesion. The ulna fracture is usually evident on plain radiographs. Disruption of the DRUJ may be subtle, and an increase in the width of the joint by as little as 2 mm may be significant. Comparison views of the other wrist may be helpful. Closed reduction can be attempted in children, with casting for 6 weeks in a long arm cast. ORIF is preferred in adults and generally produces a good outcome [15].

Barton's fracture is an intra-articular distal radius fracture that dislocates posteriorly with the carpus attached. The reverse fracture, in which the distal radial fragment and carpus dislocate volarly ("volar Barton's"), is actually more common. These fractures are clinically and radiographically obvious and both benefit from ORIF to avoid loss of reduction, degenerative arthritis, and limited wrist motion [16,17].

Lower extremity

Femur and hip

Hip dislocation

Hip dislocation is an orthopedic emergency because the incidence of complications increases directly with the time elapsed before relocation. The main complications of hip dislocation are avascular necrosis (AVN), osteoarthritis, and heterotopic bone deposition. The three clinical scenarios in which traumatic hip dislocation occurs are pediatric, adult, and dislocation of a prosthetic hip.

Adult native hip dislocation results primarily from high-energy traumatic mechanisms, chiefly frontal motor vehicle crashes (MVC), auto versus pedestrian accidents, major falls, and contact sports injuries. Motor vehicle–associated trauma accounts for 62% to 93% of adult hip dislocations [18]. Three main types of dislocation are seen: anterior, posterior, and central or acetabular. Posterior dislocations are 10 to 20 times more common than any other type of dislocation [18].

In the adult, the hip joint is formed by the articulation of the proximal head of the femur into the acetabulum. This relationship is supported by strong muscular and ligamentous attachments and the joint capsule, making the hip a very stable joint requiring significant force to dislodge. Despite the inherent stability of the joint, the wide range of motion of the hip renders it more susceptible to dislocation.

The most common mechanism for hip dislocation occurs when front seat passengers of a motor vehicle are involved in a frontal impact crash. The forward motion of the passengers causes the knee to strike the dashboard of the interior of the car, transmitting force to a flexed, adducted hip. Depending on the position of the hip at the time of impact, the hip dislocates posteriorly, often causing a posterior acetabular fracture.

Most patients who have hip dislocations have associated fractures of the acetabulum. Up to 95% have associated injuries, including other fractures and head and chest injuries [19]. Seat belts and air bags are effective in preventing impact of the knee against the dashboard in most cases, and in some series almost all hip dislocations occurred in patients who were not wearing seatbelts. This mechanism results in injuries to the "knee-thigh-hip complex" in approximately 30,000 patients per year in the United States, at a cost of $4.7 million in 2004 (Fig. 13A, B) [20].

Anterior hip dislocation occurs after a blow to the posterior aspect of the hip with the leg in abduction and the hip extended. The force pries the femoral head out of the acetabulum and it dislocates either anteriorly toward the obturator foramen or laterally toward the pubis.

Pediatric hip dislocation

The pediatric hip includes a relatively shallow and incompletely developed acetabulum, lax ligamentous support, and less powerful musculature to check excessive hip movement. Consequently, pediatric hip dislocations can occur after relatively minor trauma such as low-level falls or while simply running. Fractures of the acetabulum can occur but are much less common. Inferior dislocation is extremely rare and occurs almost exclusively in children.

Prosthetic hip dislocation

Dislocations of prosthetic hip joints occur fairly commonly and often after little force. Dislocation can occur while crossing one's legs or in rising from a sitting position. Some patients develop repeated dislocations and require revision of the prosthesis.

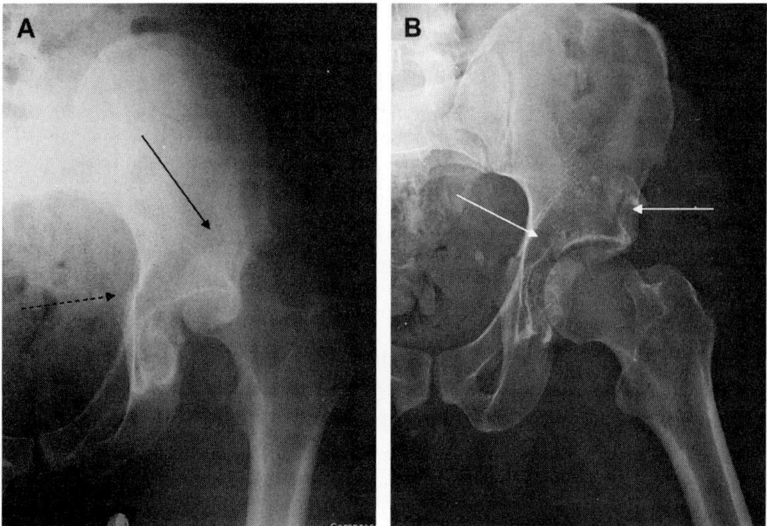

Fig. 13. (*A*) AP radiograph of the pelvis, showing a posterior dislocation of the femoral head (*solid arrow*). A subtle acetabular fracture is present (*dotted arrow*). (*B*) The hip is successfully reduced, but the comminuted acetabular fracture is more apparent (*arrows*).

Clinical presentation. Because most hip dislocations occur in the context of major motor vehicle–related trauma or significant falls, a standardized approach to trauma should be used to avoid missing associated major injuries. Patients who have posterior hip dislocation present with pain in the region of the hip and buttock on the affected side. The ipsilateral gluteal area may be more prominent, but the dislocated femoral head is usually not easily palpated. The leg is shortened and held in adduction with the hip flexed and internally rotated. Associated injury to the sciatic nerve is present in 10% of cases and should be specifically sought out [21].

With anterior dislocation, the leg is lengthened and the hip is held in abduction, external rotation, and slight flexion. The femoral head may be palpable inferior to the pubis. Fracture of the femoral head or neck is much more common in anterior dislocations. Associated injury to the femoral vessels can occur and the leg should be assessed for adequacy of perfusion. Central dislocation can result in variable position of the affected leg, but some degree of abduction is usually present and there is resistance to adduction and rotation of the hip.

Diagnosis. AP and lateral plain radiographs of the pelvis and hip are sensitive for the presence of dislocation and should be obtained either as part of a routine trauma assessment or when injury to the hip is suspected, depending on hospital policy. The lateral view of the pelvis may be required to confirm the nature of the dislocation. On the AP pelvic view, the integrity of

Shenton's line (the smooth contour of the line running from the inner aspect of the femur and femoral neck up to the inferior surface of the pubis) should be verified. Disruption of this line suggests either dislocation of the hip or fracture of the femoral neck. Any evidence of vascular injury mandates further investigation by Doppler or duplex ultrasound, angiography, or CT angiography. Once the patient is sufficiently stable, a CT scan of the hip and acetabulum is helpful in detecting acetabular fractures that are often unapparent on plain radiographs and in detecting bony fragments within the joint space that may prevent reduction or result in severe osteoarthritis in the long term.

Management. The outcome of hip dislocation is closely related to the rapidity of reduction and the presence of associated fractures of the femoral head or neck. Overall, 10% of children and 30% of adults develop AVN following hip dislocation [18]. Reductions that are accomplished within 6 hours of dislocation have a significantly better long-term outcome in terms of both AVN and osteoarthritis and this has become the standard of care for these injuries [22]. The reasons for delay in reduction include pre-emptive lifesaving surgery in an unstable patient, long transfers to a trauma center from centers without the expertise to reduce a hip, the presence of fracture/dislocation of the hip that makes closed reduction difficult or impossible, and failure to diagnose the condition in a timely manner.

Closed reduction of the dislocated hip is preferred over ORIF because the outcomes are somewhat better with closed reduction. Emergency physicians should be familiar with at least two methods of closed hip reduction in the event that an orthopedic specialist is unavailable in a timely manner. However, repeated attempts at reduction may result in a worse outcome and should be avoided. Procedural sedation and systemic analgesia greatly facilitate reduction but must be used judiciously in the multiple trauma patient to avoid hypotension.

Of the many techniques for closed hip reduction, the most commonly used are the Allis, the Stimson, and the more recently described Whistler techniques. In the Allis technique, the patient remains supine on the bed and the physician stands on the bed straddling the patient's pelvis. The affected leg is adducted slightly and gradually flexed to 90° at the hip. Traction is applied until the reduction is accomplished. An assistant can apply counterpressure to the pelvis. This technique is used commonly, but often requires two operators and some acrobatic ability on the part of the physician. At times, the combined weight of the patient and physician may exceed the capacity of the gurney (Fig. 14A–C) [23].

In the Stimson technique, the patient is placed prone, with the affected side hanging down over the lateral edge of the bed. Downward traction is applied to the leg, with an assistant applying stabilizing pressure to the pelvis. Although the weight of the patient's leg assists in the reduction, it may be impossible to move a multiply injured patient safely into the prone

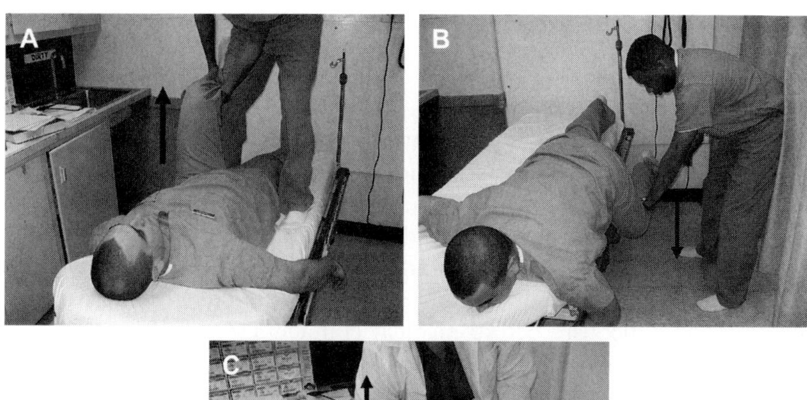

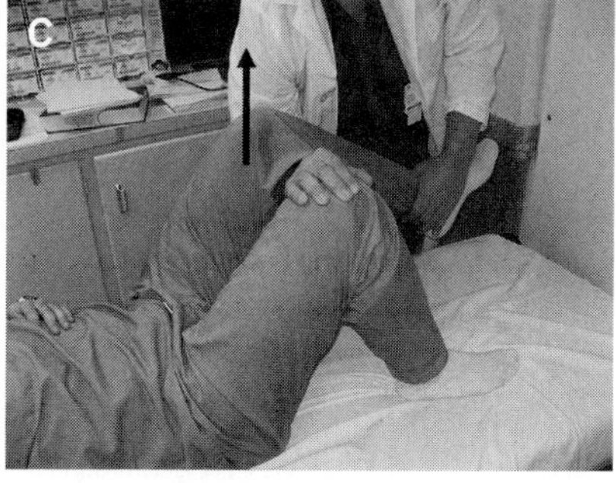

Fig. 14. (*A*) The Allis technique for reduction of a posterior hip dislocation. Anterior traction is applied to bring the femoral head into the acetabulum. An assistant is often required to stabilize the pelvis by applying downward counterpressure to the pelvis. (*B*) Stimson technique for reduction of a posterior hip dislocation. Alternatively, the patient can be positioned at the end of the bed with both hips over the edge of the bed. (*C*) Whistler technique for reduction of posterior hip dislocation. The operator raises his/her arm and shoulder, exerting upward traction on the hip while maintaining slight adduction of the leg.

position and it is difficult to monitor the patient's airway in this position if deep sedation is used [23].

The Whistler technique is a more recently described method of reducing posterior hip dislocation in skiers and snowboarders, but it is applicable in other scenarios as well and can be performed by a single operator. After appropriate procedural sedation, the patient is placed supine on the bed with the unaffected knee flexed and the foot placed firmly on the bed. The operator places his/her nondominant hand under the affected knee and places his/her hand on the unaffected knee. By straightening his/her arm or lifting his/her shoulder, the operator adducts the patient's leg and applies gradual traction to the hip until it reduces. The advantages of this technique are that it can be performed by a single operator and the patient's airway can be monitored during the procedure [24].

Following relocation of the hip, the neurovascular status of the leg should again be verified. An adductor splint can be applied to limit any motion that might dislocate an unstable reduction again.

Knee

Knee dislocation

Single ligament injuries and tears of a single meniscus are among the most common sports injuries. Disruption of more than one knee ligament can result in significant abnormal motion of the knee, and injury to popliteal vessels and nerves can occur. The clinical presentation ranges from those with obvious angulation, swelling, and pain in the knee, to subtle presentations that can be overlooked in a multiple trauma patient, especially if his/her consciousness is altered. Complete knee dislocations are notorious for relocating spontaneously before medical contact. In some cases the knee may not appear very swollen because a tear of the joint capsule allows bleeding in the joint to diffuse into the surrounding tissues. Assessment of a major trauma victim should always include palpating all the long bones and ranging the major joints to determine their stability. When examination reveals an unstable knee joint, assessment of the vascular status of the leg is imperative. Popliteal artery injury occurs in approximately 40% of high-energy knee dislocations [25]. Anterior dislocations (31%) and posterior dislocations (25%) account for most cases and are most likely to cause popliteal artery injury. Peroneal nerve injury occurs in 14% to 35% of cases and its sensory and motor function should always be assessed [25]. Anterior dislocations (50%–60% of cases) result from hyperextension injuries, such as when a car bumper strikes the femur above a firmly planted leg. Posterior dislocations most commonly occur when the knee strikes the dashboard in a frontal MVC (Fig. 15).

A knee dislocation may be diagnosed readily on physical examination in cases of gross deformity and instability. In less obvious cases, plain radiographs of the knee may show abnormal positioning of the femur and tibia. All cases require radiographic views of the femur, knee, and tibia, including the ankle joint, because associated injuries are common. CT and MRI are useful in delineating the exact nature of ligamentous tears, meniscal injury, and subtle fractures that may be missed on plain films. The main controversy with these injuries is how to detect injury to the popliteal vessels. Because vascular injury is so common with knee dislocation, some advocate angiography for all knee dislocations. Others favor a more selective approach based on the physical findings. Patients with hard findings of arterial injury need to undergo operative repair within 6 hours of injury. More prolonged warm ischemia leads to progressive permanent damage to nerves and muscles and can produce compartment syndrome. Delay of care beyond 8 hours results in an amputation rate of 85%, compared with 15% when repair is accomplished within 8 hours [25]. An intraoperative angiogram can be obtained to delineate the extent and nature of the vascular injury. If primary reanastamosis is not possible because of extensive soft tissue damage or the need to address other life-threatening injuries, a temporary vascular shunt can be placed to bypass the injury until definitive repair can be

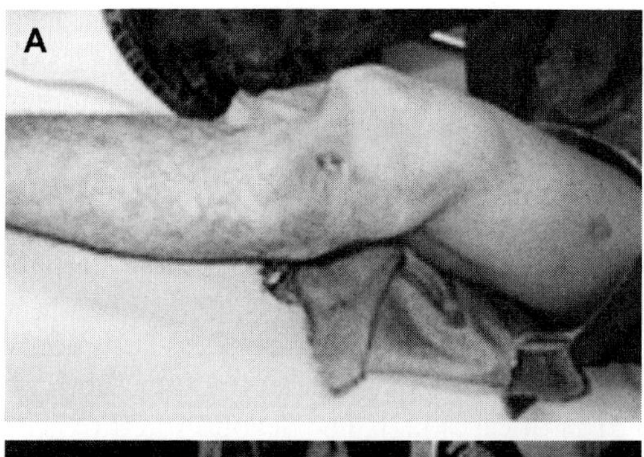

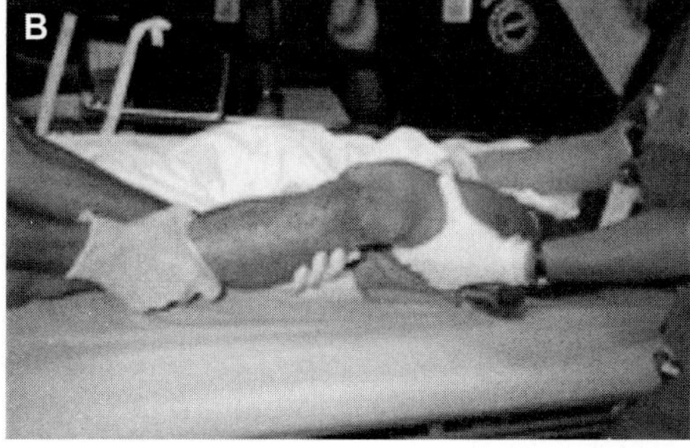

Fig. 15. (*A*) Auto versus pedestrian accident resulting in complete knee dislocation with loss of peripheral pulses. (*B*) Emergency reduction of the dislocation by longitudinal traction. (*From* Mandavia D, Newton E, Demetriades D. Atlas of emergency trauma. New York: Cambridge University Press; 2003.)

undertaken. In patients with soft signs of arterial injury, additional investigation is indicated. Controversy exists as to the relative merits of the ankle-brachial index (ABI), duplex ultrasound, CT angiogram, digital subtraction arteriography, and formal angiography, although angiography remains the gold standard in this situation. Patients who have normal ABI and Doppler studies after knee dislocation should still be admitted for repeated vascular assessment over 24 hours. Outcome is good in most cases if repair is accomplished expeditiously, although 10% of patients have permanent peroneal nerve palsy [26].

Tibia and fibula

The tibia is the second strongest bone in the body. Despite that, it is the most common long bone fracture. The principal situations that result in tibia fracture are auto versus pedestrian accidents, MVC, falls, and sports injuries. The mechanism of injury is important in determining the incidence of complications and the ultimate outcome. High-energy trauma with significant soft tissue damage and open fractures commonly result in poor outcomes.

Tibial plateau

The tibial plateau is composed of the medial and lateral tibial condyles forming the inferior articular surface of the knee. Fractures of the plateau are relatively common in elderly persons with osteoporosis and can occur with minor trauma. Fractures in younger persons are usually the result of high-energy motor vehicle trauma, falls, or contact sports injuries, and associated injuries are often present. The most common mechanism resulting in tibial plateau fracture is an abduction force applied to the leg with an axial load resulting in a lateral plateau fracture. Less commonly, an adduction force to the leg results in a medial plateau fracture. Both plateaus are fractured in 11% to 31% of cases [27]. The Segond fracture is important to recognize because it is associated with an anterior cruciate ligament tear in 75% to 100% of cases [28]. The fracture occurs as a result of forced internal rotation of the tibia with varus stress applied to the knee. The resultant tension on the lateral knee capsule avulses a small vertical fragment from the margin of the lateral tibial condyle. The fracture itself is unimpressive but it is a reliable sign of anterior cruciate ligament tear. A "reverse Segond" fracture has also been described, with bony avulsion from the medial condyle and a strong association with a posterior cruciate ligament tear [29]. Fracture of the tibial spines appears as an ossified fragment within the joint space. Although subtle, this finding is also commonly associated with avulsion by the cruciate ligaments at their insertion on the tibial spines.

Clinically, the patient presents with pain, knee effusion, and inability to bear weight. Neurovascular injury is uncommon, but compartment syndrome can occur. Ligamentous injury will render the knee unstable on examination. Diagnosis is usually apparent with plain radiographs of the knee, including a tunnel view that is taken perpendicular to the tibial plateaus and typically demonstrates depression of one or both plateaus. MRI is often obtained to detect associated ligamentous injury and to delineate the extent of the fracture more accurately. By definition, tibial plateau fractures are intra-articular, and near anatomic reduction is required to avoid late complications of arthritis and chronic knee pain. Fractures with less than 3 mm depression of the plateau can be managed, closed in a long leg nonweight-bearing cast. Fractures with more than 3 mm plateau depression require ORIF to restore joint congruity. Failure of the operative reduction is common, especially in patients over 60 years old. In a recent study by Heckler and colleagues [30], collapse of the tibial plateau was seen in 31% of young persons and 79% of patients over 60 years who underwent surgical repair of the plateau fracture (Fig. 16).

Tillaux fracture

A Tillaux fracture can occur in children (juvenile Tillaux) or adults (Tillaux fracture). In adolescents, the Tillaux fracture is a Salter III fracture that occurs vertically through the lateral distal tibial epiphysis after forced lateral rotation of the foot or medial rotation of the leg on a fixed foot. An avulsion

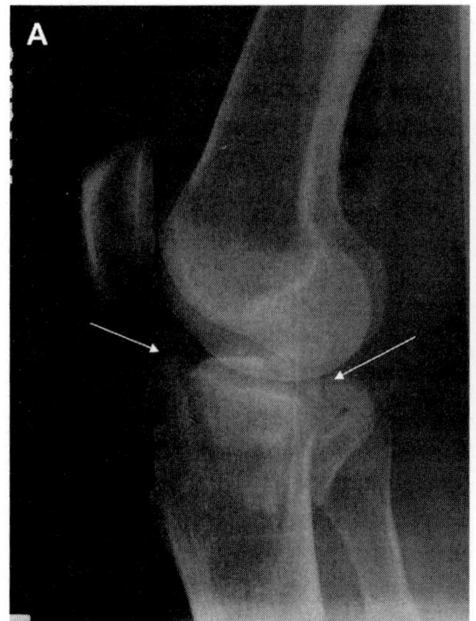

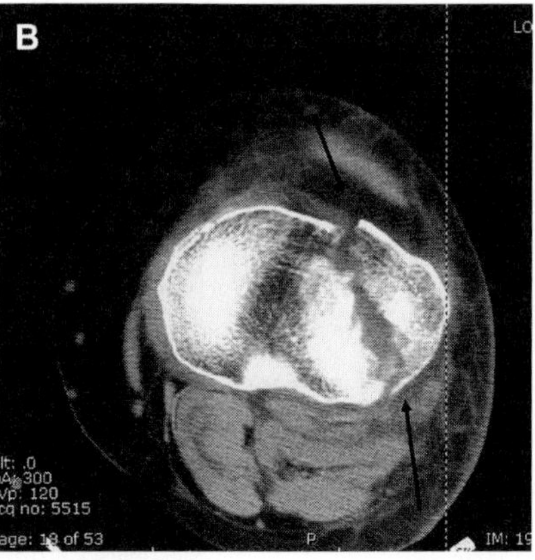

Fig. 16. (*A*) Lateral radiograph of the knee, showing a minimally displaced tibial plateau fracture (*arrows*). (*B*) CT scan of the knee, showing a fracture of the lateral tibial plateau of the tibia (*arrows*).

fracture occurs through the partially fused lateral tibial physis because of pull from the anterior tibiofibular ligament, which results in a fracture fragment in the center of the ankle that displaces anterolaterally. In children this is a Salter III injury and growth abnormalities are possible, although degenerative arthritis is the more common complication. ORIF is indicated if closed reduction cannot restore the position of the epiphyseal fragment (Fig. 17) [31].

The distal articular surface of the tibia is termed the plafond. A pilon fracture occurs during axial loading of the leg, such as a major fall or MVC, in which the talus is driven like a "pilon" into the tibial plafond. Fractures of the tibial plafond are almost always comminuted and often open. The fibula is fractured in 75% to 85% of cases [32]. Associated fractures of the calcaneus, hip, and vertebrae, and significant soft tissue injuries are relatively common. Because the plafond is a major weight-bearing surface, outcomes are often poor despite proper treatment and, at best, most patients cannot return to athletic activities. Clinically, the patient presents with pain, massive swelling, and deformity of the distal tibia. If the fibula is also fractured, the extremity will appear shortened. Open wounds are also common. Gentle longitudinal traction should be applied if there is evidence of neurovascular injury, in an attempt to restore perfusion. Definitive care is somewhat controversial, although most series report slightly better outcome with the application of an external fixation device, such as the Ilizarov fixator, compared with ORIF. Often, both techniques are needed to restore the articular surface and maintain the reduction.

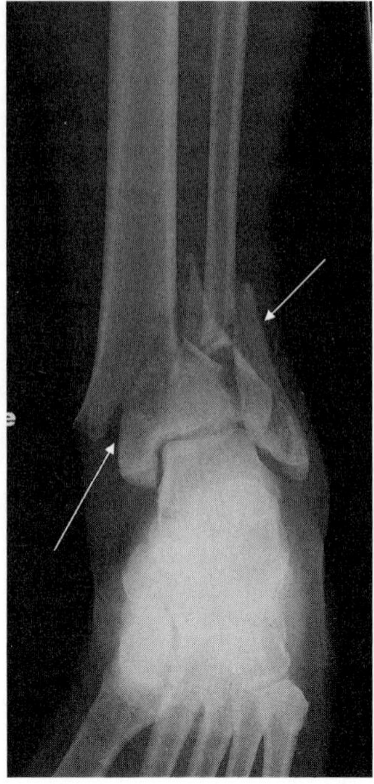

Fig. 17. AP radiograph of the foot, showing a pilon fracture of the distal tibia and fibula (*arrows*).

Ankle

Maisonneuve fracture

Maisonneuve fractures result from an external rotation force at the ankle in which there is either a complete tear of the deltoid ligaments or a horizontal avulsion fracture of the medial malleolus along with a higher oblique fibular shaft fracture (Fig. 18). The force is transmitted through the syndesmosis, which is torn also. This injury is unstable and often requires surgical repair involving screws through both bones. The diagnostic clue is a widened mortise joint or a medial malleolus fracture. When this is encountered, examination of the fibula will usually reveal tenderness in the area of the fibular fracture. Radiographs that include the entire lower leg will reveal the fracture and widened mortise.

Foot

Hindfoot

Calcaneus. Fracture of the calcaneus is a relatively common and often disabling injury. It represents 2% of all fractures, but two thirds of all tarsal fractures [33]. The most frequent mechanism for calcaneal fracture is

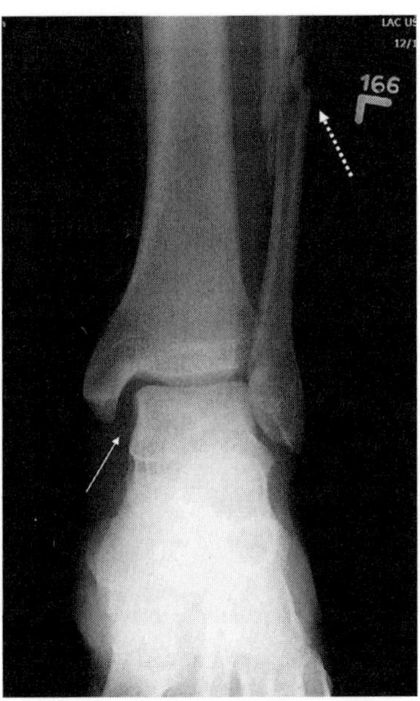

Fig. 18. AP radiograph of the ankle, showing a Maisonneuve-type fracture. The mortise is widened medially (*solid arrow*), indicating deltoid ligament disruption. An oblique fibular shaft fracture is also shown (*dotted arrow*). The fibular fracture is typically more proximal in a Maisonneuve fracture, but the mechanism is the same as with this fracture.

a fall from a height while landing on one or both feet, or a high-speed frontal MVC in which the foot is compressed against the floorboards. The mechanism of injury is an axial load in which the talus is driven through the calcaneus. Lawnmower injuries are responsible for many open calcaneal fractures, especially in children [34]. Patients who have calcaneal fracture often have severe associated injuries related to a major fall from height. Spinal fractures occur in 10% of patients and 20% have other extremity fractures. Calcaneal fractures are bilateral in 9% of cases (Fig. 19) [35].

Clinical presentation. Patients with significant falls often have multiple life-threatening injuries to the head, spine, abdomen, and aorta, and these injuries will dominate the clinical picture. Calcaneal fractures should be suspected and the heels carefully examined in patients who have sustained major falls. Fractures produce significant swelling and pain in the heel area, inability to bear weight, ecchymosis, and often fracture blisters on the skin of the hindfoot. Compartment syndrome occurs in 10% to 50% of cases [33]. The emergency physician should suspect compartment syndrome if there is pain out of proportion to the injury, tense swelling in the region of the heel, weak flexion of the toes, pain increased by dorsiflexion of the toes, the presence of fracture blisters, and hypesthesia on the plantar surface of the foot [33]. Compartment pressure is measured and

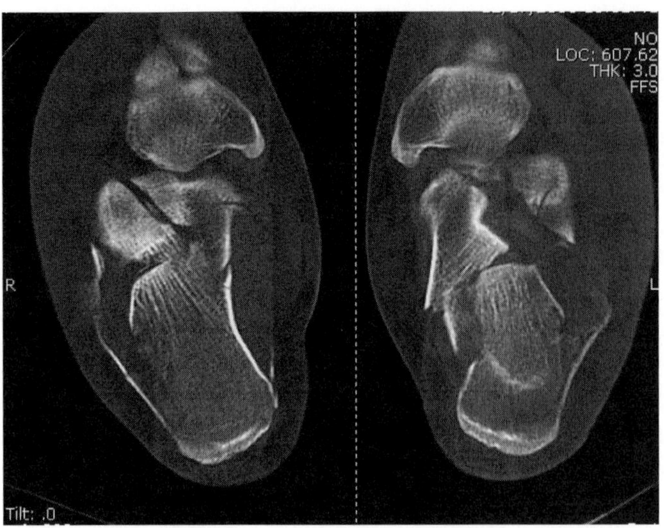

Fig. 19. CT scan of both feet, showing comminuted fractures of the calcanei in a patient who jumped from a building.

fasciotomy is indicated within 6 hours of the injury if the pressure reaches critical levels. Failure to reduce compartment pressure by fasciotomy in a timely manner can result in gangrene, flexion contractures of the toes ("claw toes"), persistent foot pain, or amputation. Measurement of Bohler's angle is traditionally used to detect calcaneal fracture, but it may be normal even with severely comminuted fractures. Its use is better reserved for predicting outcome, which is inversely related to the degree of collapse of the calcaneal arch and, hence, Bohler's angle (Fig. 20).

Management. The emergency physician's main role in managing calcaneal fracture is to diagnose the injury, provide adequate analgesia, detect the presence of neurovascular injury or compartment syndrome in the foot, and diagnose any associated injuries. The heel is placed in a bulky padded dressing, pending definitive treatment. The orthopedic management of these fractures is controversial, with various investigators advocating either ORIF or closed reduction. In either case, weight bearing is delayed for several months and recovery is a slow process. Complications include persistent heel pain and degenerative arthritis with conservative management and osteomyelitis, iatrogenic nerve injury, wound dehiscence, malunion, and arthritis with ORIF. More than 80% of patients have a "good" outcome, defined as regaining the ability to work and ambulate, but many of these patients experience ongoing heel pain and are not able to return to athletic activities [33,36]. Occasionally, subtalar fusion may be required in patients with incapacitating pain.

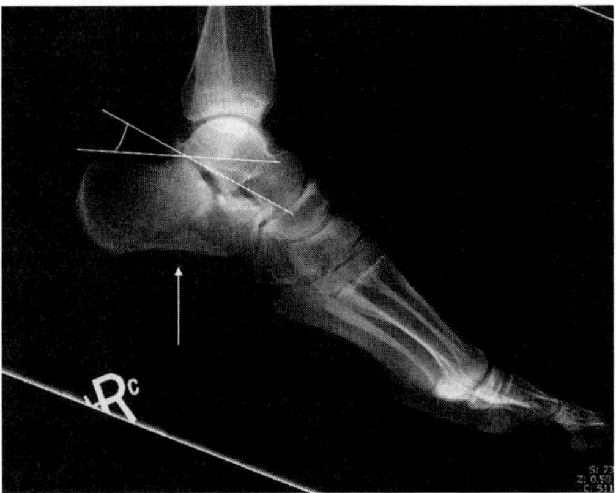

Fig. 20. A lateral radiograph of the foot, showing a comminuted calcaneal fracture (*arrow*). Bohler's angle is normal despite a severe fracture.

Talus fracture. The talus is the tenon that inserts into the mortise formed by the malleoli of the tibia and fibula. It also forms complex articulations with the calcaneus and tarsal navicular. The talus is divided into the anterior head, the body that forms the tenon, and the neck that bridges the head and body. The neck is the most commonly fractured part of the talus. The talus is fractured less often than the calcaneus but by similar mechanisms, primarily axial load from major falls and MVCs. Hyperdorsiflexion of the foot often results in fracture of the talar neck as it impacts against the anterior tibia [34]. Lateral process fracture most commonly results from snowboarding injury but is rare otherwise. More commonly, the medial and lateral processes sustain avulsion fractures by eversion or inversion ligamentous injuries of the ankle. The articular surface of the dome of the talus is commonly injured from crush injuries, resulting in an osteochondral defect and loose intra-articular fragments similar to osteochondritis dissecans in the knee. A CT scan is often needed to delineate the injury fully. Severe osteochondral injuries may require arthrodesis if they fail to respond to conservative measures [37]. Because of its precarious anastomotic blood supply, the head of the talus is susceptible to AVN following fractures of the neck.

The clinical presentation of talar fracture varies with the severity and displacement of the fragments. Avulsion fractures may be clinically and radiographically difficult to distinguish from ankle sprains. Major talar fractures are usually apparent on standard radiographs including a mortise view of the ankle, but the full extent of the fracture may require CT scan or MRI to be seen.

An initial attempt at closed reduction is indicated if there is evidence of neurovascular compromise. The os calcis is stabilized, and longitudinal traction is applied to the plantar flexed foot. If closed reduction is successful, the foot can be immobilized in a short-leg, nonweight-bearing cast for 6 to

8 weeks. In cases with severe displacement, ORIF is often required to restore anatomy and function. Recurrence of pain in healed talus fracture should raise suspicion of AVN of the talar head. MRI is diagnostic of this condition.

Forefoot fractures

Lisfranc fracture. The Lisfranc joint is the articulation of the midfoot and the forefoot and consists of the multiple strong ligaments on the plantar arch of the foot and ligaments joining the proximal metatarsal (MT) heads to each other. The second MT head acts as a keystone in its insertion between the first and second cuneiforms preventing medial and lateral movement of the MTs on the tarsal bones. Fracture of the base of the second MT therefore renders the joint unstable. Injury to this joint complex usually results from severe plantar flexion of the foot with an abduction force [34]. However, it can also occur with relatively minor trauma, as in the case depicted in Fig. 21, in which a massively obese man simply stepped off a sidewalk curb. Associated fracture of the navicular or cuboid may be seen as well.

Three types of Lisfranc injury are based on the congruity of the MTs. In Type A, the MTs dislocate or sublux as a unit in a single direction. In Type B, there is divergence between the first MT and the second through fifth

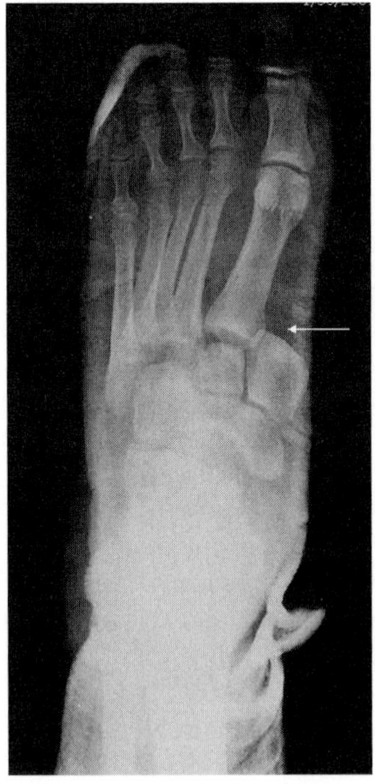

Fig. 21. AP radiograph of the foot, showing a type A Lisfranc fracture-dislocation in which all MTs are dislocated laterally (*arrow*).

MTs, which dislocate laterally. This divergence creates the typical radiographic pattern in which the space between the first and second MT is widened (> 5 mm, measured at the base between the first and second MTs). In Type C there is an assortment of patterns with lack of congruity of the MT dislocations. Usually, the first MT dislocates medially and the remaining MTs dislocate either medially or laterally in various combinations (see Fig. 21) [38].

Clinical presentation. The patient with Lisfranc injury is unable to bear weight on the affected foot. The dorsum of the midfoot shows swelling, ecchymosis, deformity, and tenderness. Pedal pulses may be difficult to palpate because of the swelling, but assessment of perfusion of the foot distal to the injury should still be made, based on warmth, color, and hand-held Doppler.

Diagnosis. Standard AP and lateral radiographs of the foot are usually sufficient to demonstrate the fracture. At times the fracture may reduce spontaneously and the only abnormality may be an innocuous-appearing fracture of the base of the second MT. This fracture should always be viewed with suspicion because it renders the Lisfranc joint unstable.

Management. The fracture should be reduced under procedural sedation and analgesia. Closed reduction is attempted and typically yields satisfactory results; however, further stabilization of the tarsometatarsal joints with percutaneous Kirschner wires is often needed. The foot is placed in a nonweight–bearing short-leg cast for 6 to 8 weeks. Outcome is good in 80% to 85%. Potential complications include forefoot ischemia, skin necrosis, foot instability, and degenerative arthritis [34].

References

[1] Johansen K, Sangeorzan B, Copass MK. Traumatic scapulothoracic dissociation. Case report. J Trauma 1991;31:147–9.

[2] Sampson LN, Britton JC, Eldrup-Jorgensen J, et al. The neurovascular outcome of scapulothoracic dissociation. J Vasc Surg 1993;17:1083–8.

[3] Damschen DD, Cogbill TH, Seigel MJ. Scapulothoracic dissociation caused by blunt trauma. J Trauma 1997;42:537–40.

[4] Althausen PL, Le M, Finkemeier CG. Scapulothoracic dissociation: diagnosis and treatment. Clin Orthop Relat Res 2003;416:237–44.

[5] Tsai DW, Swiontkowski MF, Kottra CL, et al. A case of sternoclavicular dislocation with scapulothoracic dissociation. AJR 1996;167:332.

[6] Martin SD, Altchek D, Erlanger S, et al. Atraumatic posterior dislocation of the sternoclavicular joint: a case report and literature review. Clin Orthop Relat Res 1993;292: 159–64.

[7] Gilot GJ, Worth MA, Rockwood CA. Injuries to the sternoclavicular joint. In: Bucholz RW, Heckman JD, Court-Brown C, et al, editors. Rockwood and Green's fractures in adults. 6th edition. Philadelphia: Lippincott William and Wilkins; 2005. p. 1365–400.

[8] Butters KP. Fractures of the scapula. In: Bucholz RW, Heckman JD, Court-Brown C, et al, editors. Rockwood and Green's fractures in adults. 6th edition. Philadelphia: Lippincott, Williams and Wilkins; 2005. p. 1257–84.

[9] Sammarco VJ. Os acromiale: frequency, anatomy, and clinical implications. J Bone Joint Surg Am 2000;82:394–400.

[10] Lee DH, Lee KH, Lopez-Ben R, et al. The double density sign: a radiographic finding suggestive of os acromiale. J Bone Joint Surg Am 2004;86A:2666–70.

[11] Mallon WJ, Bassett FH 3rd, Goldner RD. Luxatio erecta: the inferior glenohumeral dislocation. J Orthop Trauma 1990;4:19–24.

[12] Davids JR, Tallbott RD. Luxatio erecta humeri: a case report. Clin Orthop Relat Res 1990; 252:144–9.

[13] Nho SJ, Dodson CC, Bardzik KF, et al. The two-step maneuver for closed reduction of inferior glenohumeral dislocation (luxatio erecta to anterior dislocation). J Orthop Trauma 2006;20:354–7.

[14] Cicak N. Posterior dislocation of the shoulder. J Bone Joint Surg 2004;86:324–32.

[15] Ring D, Jupiter JB, Simpson NS. Monteggia fracture in adults. J Bone Joint Surg Am 1998; 80:1733–44.

[16] Lorenzo-Calderon SA, Doornberg J, Ring D. Fractures of the dorsal articular margin of the distal part of the radius with dorsal radiocarpal subluxation. J Bone Joint Surg Am 2006;88: 1486–93.

[17] Zoubos AB, Babis GC, Korres DS, et al. Surgical treatment of 35 Barton's fractures. No need for routine decompression of the median nerve. Acta Orthop Scand 1997;275:65–8.

[18] Sahin V, Karakas ES, Aksu S, et al. Traumatic dislocation and fracture-dislocation of the hip: a long-term follow-up study. J Trauma 2003;54:520–8.

[19] Hak DJ, Goulet JA. Severity of injuries associated with traumatic hip dislocation as a result of motor vehicle collisions. J Trauma 1999;47:60–3.

[20] Rupp JD, Scneider LW. Injuries to the hip joint in frontal motor vehicle crashes: biomechanical and real-world perspectives. Orthop Clin North Am 2004;35:493–504.

[21] Cornwall R, Radomisli TE. Nerve injury in traumatic dislocation of the hip. Clin Orthop Relat Res 2000;377:84–91.

[22] Pallia CS, Scott RE, Chao DJ. Traumatic hip dislocation in athletes. Curr Sports Med Rep 2002;1:338–45.

[23] Nordt WE III. Maneuvers for reducing hip dislocations. Clin Orthop Relat Res 1999;360: 260–4.

[24] Walden PD, Harner JR. Whistler technique to reduce traumatic dislocation of the hip in the emergency department setting. J Emerg Med 1999;17:441–4.

[25] Dickson KF, Galland MW, Barrack RL, et al. Magnetic resonance imaging of the knee after ipsilateral femur fracture. J Orthop Trauma 2002;16:567–71.

[26] Perron AD, Brady WJ, Sing RF. Orthopedic pitfalls in the ED: vascular injury associated with knee dislocation. Am J Emerg Med 2001;19:583–8.

[27] Lyn E, Pallin D, Antosia RE. Knee and lower leg. In: Marx JA, Hockberger RS, Walls RM, et al, editors. Rosen's emergency medicine: concepts and clinical practice. 6th edition. St. Louis (MO): Mosby Inc; 2006. p. 770–807.

[28] Campos JC, Chung CB, Lektrakul N, et al. Pathogenesis of the Segond fracture: anatomic and MRI imaging evidence of an iliotibial tract or anterior oblique band avulsion. Radiology 2001;219:381–6.

[29] Escobedo EM, Mills WJ, Hunter JC. The "reverse Segond" fracture: association with a tear of the posterior cruciate ligament and medial meniscus. AJR 2002;178:979–83.

[30] Heckler MW, Hatic SO II, DiCicco JD III, et al. Management of complications associated with fractures around the knee. J Knee Surg 2007;20:78.

[31] Kooury SL, Harrell G. La Charita DD recognition and management of Tillaux fracture in adolescents. Pediatr Emerg Care 1999;15:37–9.

[32] Mockford BJ, Ogonda D, Warnock RJ, et al. The early management of severe tibial pilon fractures using a temporary ring fixator. Surgeon 2003;1:104–7.
[33] Lim EVA, Leung JPF. Complications of intra-articular calcaneal fractures. Clin Orthop Relat Res 2001;391:7–16.
[34] Ribbans WJ, Natarajan R, Alavala S. Pediatric foot fractures. Clin Orthop Relat Res 2005; 432:107–15.
[35] Ricci WM, Bellabarba C, Sanders R. Transcalcaneal talonavicular dislocation. J Bone Joint Surg 2002;84A:557–61.
[36] Carr JB. Surgical treatment of the intra-articular calcaneus fracture. Orthop Clin North Am 1994;25:665–75.
[37] Baumhauer JF, Alvarez RG. Controversies in treating talus fractures. Orthop Clin North Am 1995;26:335–51.
[38] Hardcastle PH, Reschauer R, Kutcha-Lissberg E, et al. Injuries to the tarsometatarsal joint. J Bone Joint Surg 1982;64B:349–56.

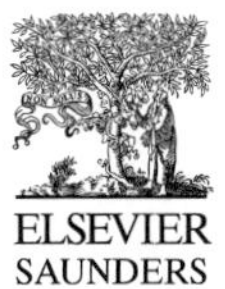
ELSEVIER
SAUNDERS

EMERGENCY
MEDICINE
CLINICS OF
NORTH AMERICA

Emerg Med Clin N Am 25 (2007) 795–802

Pelvic Fractures

Phillip L. Rice, Jr, MD[a,*], Melissa Rudolph, MD[b]

[a]*Brigham and Women's Hospital, 75 Francis Street, Boston, MA 02115, USA*
[b]*Harvard Affiliated Emergency Medicine Residency, Beth Israel Deaconess Medical Center, 330 Brookline Avenue, Boston, MA 02215, USA*

Pelvic fractures are associated with significant morbidity and mortality. Despite advances in emergency, radiologic, surgical, and ICU care that have improved survival during the past decade, the morbidity and the mortality remain significantly high [1]. The incidence of pelvic fractures in the United States is estimated to be more than 100,000 per year [2]. Motor vehicle collisions are the most common cause of pelvic fractures [3]. Nine percent of blunt abdominal trauma patients have pelvic fractures, with a mortality rate approaching 50% when associated with hemodynamic instability [4]. This article focuses on the recent developments in the initial management of pelvic fractures, including the use of external pelvic binders, radiographic imaging, interventional radiology, and operative management including the newer use of the technique of preperitoneal packing.

Anatomy of the pelvis

The pelvis consists of a massively constructed bony ring. If one fracture is identified on radiograph, there usually is an associated second fracture. The pelvic bones are located near many large blood vessels, including the internal iliac (or hypogastric) artery, the superior and inferior gluteal arteries, and the external iliac artery. The path of the venous system is similar to that of the arterial system but more posterior [5]. Most hemorrhage in pelvic fractures is caused by venous bleeding (90%); however, about 10% to 15% of patients have arterial bleeding [6].

Fractures are classified using two basic systems: Tile and Young. The Tile classification system helps predict the need for operative repair. Type A represents stable pelvic ring injuries that do not require operation. Type B fractures, which are rotationally unstable but vertically stable, and Type C

* Corresponding author.
E-mail address: price@partners.org (P.L. Rice).

doi:10.1016/j.emc.2007.06.011 *emed.theclinics.com*

fractures, which are both rotationally and vertically unstable, require intervention. Young's classification system is based on the mechanism of injury: lateral compression, anteroposterior compression, vertical shear, or a combination of these injury patterns [7]. This system helps predict the chance of associated injuries and mortality risk.

Predictors of mortality

A recent study by Lunsjo and colleagues [8] revealed that fracture stability was not a significant predictor for mortality. Injury Severity Score (ISS), and not the type of pelvic instability, was the most important predictor in defining mortality in patients who had pelvic fractures in their study [9]. The ISS increases markedly in patients who have injuries accompanied by pelvic fractures. Great force is needed to fracture a pelvis, and therefore intra-abdominal injuries often are associated with pelvic ring disruption because of the large forces absorbed [1]. Obviously the pelvic fracture contributes to the calculation of the ISS, so it is not completely independent.

Previous studies had the opposite conclusion: the more severe the fracture (Type C or vertical shear), the more common the associated injuries and blood loss, and thus the higher the ISS and mortality [4,10–14]. Others have noted that this finding holds true for younger patients but not for the elderly. Patients 60 years and older have a high likelihood of active retroperitoneal bleeding. Kimbrell and colleagues [15] noted in their study that 94% of patients older than 59 years who had pelvic fractures required arterial embolization, whereas only 52% of those age 59 years and younger required intervention. Additionally, Blackmore and colleagues [16] found that quantifying the amount of pelvic hemorrhage volume from pelvic CT scans predicts severity of injury (fracture with or without arterial bleeding) and the need for pelvic arteriography and transfusions.

Assessment

As with all trauma patients, a quick assessment following standard Advanced Trauma Life Support protocols should be made on arrival at the emergency department, addressing any life-threatening issues as they are found. If the patient is hemodynamically unstable, the goal is to identify quickly the cause of shock, which in most cases is active hemorrhage. As the initial resuscitation proceeds, the examination is tailored to finding the source of bleeding quickly and instituting measures to achieve hemostasis [16]. Obvious external bleeding, thoracic cavity bleeding, intraperitoneal bleeding, and retroperitoneal bleeding are the major sources of significant hemorrhage. The retroperitoneum is a closed space that usually can tamponade the bleeding from a pelvic fracture. This ability is lost in the case of the open pelvic fracture, leading to much greater hemorrhage. The finding of an open pelvic fracture should immediately raise the level of concern for high mortality and morbidity (70% mortality in the most recently published series) [17–19].

Diagnostic imaging

Focused Abdominal Sonography for Trauma

As part of the initial trauma assessment, a Focused Abdominal Sonography for Trauma (FAST) is performed looking for free intraperitoneal fluid. FAST is a poor indicator of retroperitoneal fluid and has been found to be less accurate in patients who have major pelvic injury than in patients who have sustained blunt trauma. The highest sensitivity and specificity of ultrasound, however, was in the subgroup of patients who had the most severe fractures, enabling emergent stabilization, embolization, or laparoscopy. Tayal and colleagues [20] suggest an algorithm in which a positive FAST examination coupled with a negative pelvic film leads to an emergent laparotomy, whereas an abnormal pelvic radiograph warrants diagnostic peritoneal lavage to differentiate between blood (suggesting immediate laparotomy) and urine (suggesting immediate embolization therapy for exsanguination and delayed laparotomy).

Pelvic radiograph

Additional imaging in the trauma bay traditionally included an anteroposterior view of the pelvis. This single film aids in the classification of pelvic fractures, but currently there is debate as to its routine use. It is an effective screening tool in hemodynamically unstable patients in whom a CT scan is not possible. In hemodynamically stable trauma patients, however, little may be gained by obtaining a plain pelvic radiograph [21]. The sensitivity of plain film for detecting fractures of the pelvis is less than 80%. Recent prospective data have shown that an acute anteroposterior radiograph of the pelvis is not useful in detecting a fracture specifically of the iliac wing or os sacrum. In this study, Lunsjo and colleagues [22] used CT scans of the pelvis as the reference standard for imaging. They found that CT scans allowed better evaluation of the bony injury as well as an evaluation of the associated organs in proximity to the pelvis. Three-dimensional reconstructions have replaced the traditional use of inlet and outlet views of the pelvis. Therefore the hemodynamically stable trauma patient should have a pelvic CT in place of a pelvic radiograph.

Stabilization

Various modalities can be used to stabilize the pelvis initially and to control hemorrhage. Most simply, a sheet can be tied around the greater trochanters to apply pressure and close the pubic symphysis in an open-book fracture. More recently, commercial devices have been developed to stabilize the pelvis that can be applied during the initial resuscitation. Both these mechanisms help reduce the pelvic volume and thus the space for accumulation of blood. Nunn and colleagues [23] explain that the immediate application of improvised pelvic binder should be the first step in extended resuscitation from life-threatening hypovolemic shock in conscious patients who have unstable pelvic injuries. In addition, pelvic binding minimizes the shearing of vessels during transport from stretcher to imaging tables and aids in tamponading the bleeding. Stabilization involving the use of pelvic binders or sheets also is successful in reducing pain and reducing the pelvic volume [24].

There are several commercial pelvic binders in use in both hospital and prehospital settings, but the most common is a plain sheet [25]. Both types are advantageous because of their easy application, noninvasive character, and general effectiveness. In the emergency department, sheets are most commonly used and are endorsed for use by the American College of Surgeons Committee on Trauma [26]. The Dallas Pelvic Binder and the Geneva Belt both use the iliac wings, whereas the London Pelvic Splint, TPOD, and plain sheets use the greater trochanters to reduce the pelvic volume and stabilize the pelvis. The use of the iliac wings to reduce the pelvic volume is best when there is an open-book fracture [27]. External pelvic fixation reduces transfusion requirements, length of stay, and mortality in patients with unstable pelvic fractures (Fig. 1) [28].

Treatment

After the initial stabilization, definitive management must be addressed. Interventional radiology and operative packing comprise the majority of the current methods, with the final outcome based on the nature of the fracture, stability of the patient, and institutional resources.

The present dominant paradigm for unstable patients who have pelvic fractures is interventional radiologic management [29]. Interventional radiology is a first choice for stabilization of pelvic fractures among the four places of acute care: the emergency department, operating room, interventional radiology, and surgical ICU. Dominant paradigms in the past included the use of external fixation devices as the primary modality accompanied by laparotomy and pelvic packing. Interventional radiology, if available, has shown tremendous utility and efficacy in many centers and is an integral part of the trauma milieu. Interventional radiology has tremendous sensitivity and specificity [29,30]. It is considered less invasive than operative management and is used in conjunction with hardware stabilization of the pelvis after the bleeders are embolized. Interventional radiology allows the selective embolization of bleeding arteries that external fixation cannot tamponade.

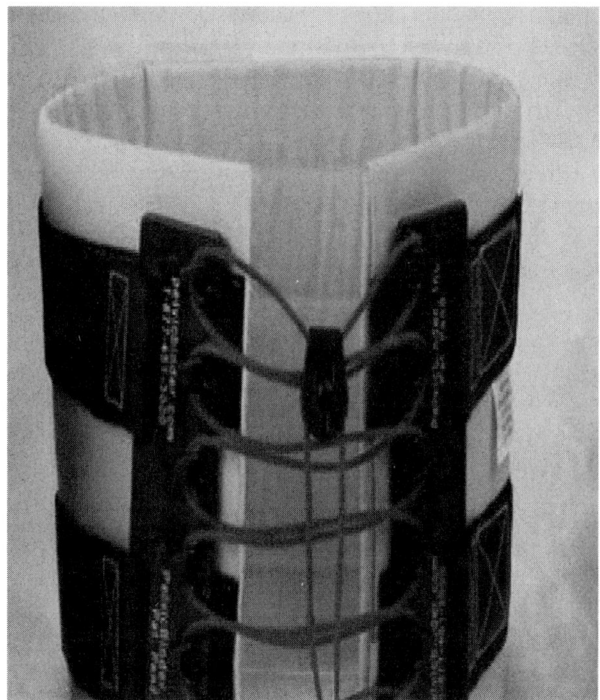

Fig. 1. A standard emergency room pelvic binder. (*Courtesy of* Pelvic Binder, Inc., Dallas, TX; with permission.)

According to the Pelvic Injury Symposium in 2000, physicians can use specific scenarios to determine if interventional radiology is the appropriate disposition for a pelvic injury:

Hemodynamic instability poorly responsive to fluid challenge, no hemoperitoneum, pelvic fracture

Hemodynamic stability, little hemoperitoneum, pelvic fracture, more than 4 units transfusion in 24 hours

Hemodynamic stability, little hemoperitoneum, pelvic fracture, more than 6 units transfusion in 48 hour

Large or expanding retroperitoneal hematoma encountered at laparotomy; or active bleed on CT scan (recent)

With these scenarios, angiography usually is performed in the first few hours, and the incidence of finding extravasation on angiography is about 90% [31].

Even with aggressive resuscitation, mechanical stabilization, and embolization, recent analysis shows 40% mortality in hemodynamically unstable patients who have a pelvic fracture. Most (85%–90%) pelvic bleeding associated with fractures is venous is origin. Therefore, this hemorrhaging will be stopped only by tamponade within the retroperitoneal space, not necessarily by embolization [32]. In these cases a new technique for stabilization has been developed recently. Extraperitoneal packing is an intervention that provides stabilization of the hemodynamically unstable patient in the operating room, allowing transport to the angiography suite for embolization.

European traumatologists have championed preperitoneal or extraperitoneal pelvic packing [32–34]. The intraperitoneal space is not entered. Again this procedure is used only when there is no intraperitoneal hemorrhage. It is described as follows:

> When the origin of bleeding can clearly be focused to the pelvic region, a midline incision of the lower abdomen is used, leaving the peritoneum intact. In the majority of cases all parapelvic fascias are already disrupted. After incision of the skin a large paravesicle cavity filled with hematoma and blood clots is usually present. A direct manual access through the right or left paravesicle space down to the presacral region is therefore possible without further dissection.
>
> In external type injuries the sources of bleeding is generally located close to the anterior pelvic ring. In this region control of bleeding by surgical hemostasis, closure of the pelvic ring and paravesicle packing is relatively easy. With a higher degree of pelvic instability, especially in C-type injuries, the origin of bleeding is most frequently located in the paravesicle region. With all compartment borders disrupted this space is generally easy to be manually accessed. The presacral and paravesicle region is packed using standard surgical lap packs. An amount of 4–8 packs will be necessary for sufficient compression in the small pelvis. After pelvic bone reduction the definitive packing is applied and the fascia is closed. With stabilized hemodynamics the packing is left in place for 24–48 hours [35].

This procedure is followed by interventional radiologic embolization [36]. All methods of management involve stabilization of the pelvis with orthopedic hardware [37]. The advantages of extraperitoneal packing are that it is quick and easy to perform, and the packing remains in the pelvis and does not dislocate intra-abdominally [32]. In a recent retrospective study by Totterman, and colleagues [34], extraperitoneal packing provided a significant increase in systolic blood pressure. Eighty percent of patients who had extraperitoneal packing were found to have arterial injury requiring embolization. Therefore, extraperitoneal packing functions well as part of a multi-interventional resuscitation protocol functioning as damage control to elevate blood pressure followed by angiography for subsequent intervention.

Summary

Pelvic injuries account for nearly 10% of the injuries obtained from blunt trauma [6]. The mortality rate of these injuries approaches 10% but has been decreasing in recent years in response to new interventions and diagnostic algorithms. In the emergency department, rapid assessment and stabilization of the pelvis with a sheet, a commercial binder, or an external fixation device followed by a FAST examination should occur. Hemodynamic stability determines the subsequent management pathway of these patients. In the hemodynamically stable patient, a routine pelvic radiograph probably is not needed; instead, a CT of the pelvis with cystography should be obtained if the patient has a pelvic fracture. For the unstable patient who has a pelvic fracture, the anteroposterior view of the pelvis, although not exquisitely sensitive or specific, is used to detect gross deformity or obvious fractures. With this information, the emergency physician and trauma surgeon must determine the next course of action: to the operating room for laparotomy versus retro-/preperitoneal packing for stabilization and/or to the angiography suite for embolization.

References

[1] Demetriades D, Karaiskakis M, Toutouzas K, et al. Pelvic fractures epidemiology and predictors of associated abdominal injuries and outcomes. J Am Coll Surg 2002;195:1–10.
[2] Gray's anatomy. 20th edition. Philadelphia: Lea & Febiger; 1918. New York: BARTLEBY.COM; 2000. p. 171–85.
[3] The EAST Practice Management Guidelines Work Group. Practice management guidelines for hemorrhage in pelvic fracture.
[4] Gilliland M, Ward R, Barons RM, et al. Factors affecting mortality in pelvic fractures. J Trauma 1982;22:691.
[5] Geeraerts T, Chhor V, Cheisson G, et al. Clinical review: initial management of blunt pelvic trauma patients with homodynamic instability. Crit Care 2007;11(1):204.
[6] Huittinen VM, Slatis P. Postmortem angiography and dissection of the hypogastric artery in pelvic fractures. Surgery 1973;73:454–62.
[7] Rosen P, Barkin R, Wolfe R, et al. Rosen and Barkin's 5-minute emergency medicine consult. Philadelphia: Lippincott Williams and Wilkins; 2003. p. 810–1.
[8] Lunsjo K, Tadros A, Hauggaard A, et al. Associated injuries and not fracture instability predict mortality in pelvic fractures: a prospective study of 100 patients. J Trauma 2007;62(3):687–91.
[9] Maurer E, Morris J. Injury severity scoring. In: Moore E, Feliciano D, Mattox K, editors. Trauma. 5th edition. New York: McGraw-Hill; 2004. p. 87–91.
[10] Poole G, Ward E, Muakkassa F, et al. Pelvic fracture from major blunt trauma. Outcome is determined by associated injuries. Ann Surg 1991;213:532–9.
[11] Riemer B, Butterfield S, Diamond D, et al. Acute mortality associated with injuries to the pelvic ring: the role of early patient mobilization and external fixation. J Trauma 1993;35:671–5.
[12] Association for the Advancement of Automotive Medicine. Abbreviated Injury Scale (AIS) 1990—update 98. Chicago: Association for the Advancement of Automotive Medicine; 1998.
[13] Dalal S, Burgess A, Siegel J, et al. Pelvic fracture in multiple trauma: classification by mechanism is key to pattern of organ injury, resuscitative requirements, and outcome. J Trauma 1989;29(7):981–1002.
[14] Smith W, Williams A, Agudelo J, et al. Early predictors of mortality in hemodynamically unstable pelvis fractures. J Orthop Trauma 2007;21(1):31–7.
[15] Kimbrell BJ, Velmahos GC, Chan LS, et al. Angiographic embolization for pelvic fractures in older patients. Arch Surgery 2004;139(7):728–32 [discussion: 732–3].
[16] Blackmore CC, Jurkovich GJ, Linnau KF, et al. Assessment of volume of hemorrhage and outcome from pelvic fracture. Arch Surg 2003;138(5):504–8 [discussion: 508–9].

[17] Dente D, Feliciano D, Rozycki G, et al. The outcome of open pelvic fractures in the modern era. Am J Surg Vol 2005;190(6):830–5.
[18] Grotz M, Allami M, Harwood P, et al. Open pelvic tractures epidemiology, current concepts of management and outcome [abstract]. Injury 2005;36:1–13.
[19] Perry J. Open pelvic fractures. Clin Orthop 1980;151:41–5.
[20] Tayal V, Neilsen A, Jones A, et al. Accuracy of trauma ultrasound in major pelvic injury. J Trauma 2006;61:1453–7.
[21] Obaid AK, Barleben A, Porral D, et al. Utility of plain film pelvic radiographs in blunt trauma patients in the emergency department. Am Surg 2006;72(10):951–4.
[22] Lunsjo K, Tadros A, Hauggaard A, et al. Acute plain anteroposterior radiograph of the pelvis is not useful in detecting fractures of iliac wing and os sacrum: a prospective study of 73 patients using CT as gold standard. Australas Radiol 2007;51(2):147–9.
[23] Nunn T, Cosker TD, Bose D, et al. Immediate application of improvised pelvic binder as first step in extended resuscitation from life-threatening hypovolaemic shock in conscious patients with unstable pelvic injuries. Injury 2007;38(1):125–8 [E-pub Sep 22, 2006].
[24] Bottlang M, Krieg JC, Mohr M, et al. Emergent management of pelvic ring fractures with use of circumferential compression. J Bone Joint Surg 2002;84-A:43–7.
[25] Ramzy AI, Murphy D, Long WB. The pelvic sheet wrap. Initial management of unstable fractures. JEMS 2003;28:68–78.
[26] American College of Surgeons. Advanced Trauma Life Support for doctors, ATLS. Instructor course manual. Chicago: American College of Surgeons; 1997. p. 206–9.
[27] Bottlang M, Simpson TS, Sigg J, et al. Noninvasive reduction of open-book pelvic fractures by circumferential compression. J Orthop Trauma 2002;16:367–73.
[28] Croce MA, Magnotti LJ, Savage SA, et al. Emergent pelvic fixation in patients with exsanguinations pelvic fractures. J Am Coll Surg 2007;204(5):935–9.
[29] Velmahos G, Toutouzas K, Vassilu P, et al. A prospective study on the safety and efficacy of angiographic embolization for pelvic and visceral injuries. J Trauma 2002;53:303–8.
[30] Piotin M, Herbereteau D, Guichard J, et al. Percutaneous transcatheter embolization in multiply injured patient with pelvic ring disruption associated with sever hemorrhage and coagulopathy. Injury 1995;25:677–80.
[31] OTA-AAST Combined Annual Meeting. 2000. Pelvic injury symposium. Available at: http://hwbf.org/ota/s2k/panel/pelvic.htm.
[32] Cothren CC, Osborn PM, Moore EE, et al. Preperitoneal pelvic packing for hemodynamically unstable pelvic fractures: a paradigm shift. J Trauma 2007;62(4):834–9.
[33] Taller S, Lukas R, Sram J, et al. Urgent management of the complex pelvic fractures. Rozhl Chir 2005;84(2):83–7.
[34] Tötterman A, Madsen J, Skaga N, et al. Extraperitoneal pelvic packing: a salvage procedure to control massive traumatic pelvic hemorrhage. J Trauma 2007;62(4):843–52.
[35] Hannover T, Pohlemann A, et al. Early management of polytraumatized patients with pelvic fracture. Unfallchirurgische Klinik der Medizinischen Hochschule. Symposium on Exsanguinating Pelvic Injury. Presented at the combined OTA/AAST meeting. April 25, 2007.
[36] Panetta T, Sclafani S, Goldstein A, et al. Percutaneous transcatheter embolization for massive bleeding from pelvic fractures. J Trauma 1985;25(11):1021–9.
[37] Thannheimer A, Woltmann A, Vastmans J, et al. The unstable patient with pelvic fracture. Zentralbl Chir 2004;129(1):37–42.

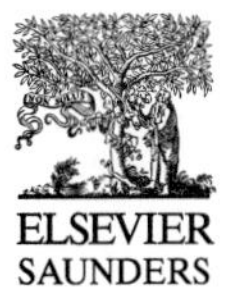

ELSEVIER
SAUNDERS

Emerg Med Clin N Am 25 (2007) 803–836

EMERGENCY
MEDICINE
CLINICS OF
NORTH AMERICA

Pediatric Major Trauma: An Approach to Evaluation and Management

Jahn T. Avarello, MD, FAAP[a,*], Richard M. Cantor, MD, FAAP, FACEP[a,b]

[a]*Department of Emergency Medicine, SUNY Upstate Medical University, 750 East Adams Street, Syracuse, NY 13210, USA*
[b]*Central New York Poison Center, 750 East Adams Street, Syracuse, NY 13210, USA*

More than 45% of all deaths in children from 1 to 14 years are the result of trauma. Over 5000 traumatic deaths per year occur within this age group; 80% of these mortalities were unintentional and 47% directly related to motor vehicle collisions (MVCs). Injury accounts for approximately 5% of infant deaths as well [1,2]. Nationwide estimates of mortality for children hospitalized after injury are uniformly low; however, most fatalities occur in the field before arrival at a health care facility. This contributes to an underestimation of the magnitude of overall mortality figures.

The most common single organ system injury associated with death in injured children is head trauma [3,4]. Rates of 80% have been reported in patients with combined thoracoabdominal injuries [1,5]. Because multiple injury is common in children, the emergency physician (EP) must evaluate all organ systems in any injured child, regardless of the actual mechanism of injury.

Within the subset of MVC, death rates begin to climb steeply in children 13 years of age and beyond. MVC mortality statistics demonstrate that the youngest occupant in the vehicle is the most vulnerable to injury. Within the school-age group of 5 to 9 years old, pedestrian injuries and bicycle crashes predominate. Submersion injury accounts for 10% to 15% of injury, burns 5% to 10%, and falls from heights approximately 2% [5–7]. Nationwide, the number of children who are victims of violent acts has decreased by 39% from 1994 to 2004. Even with this significant decline, 13% of all traumatic deaths in the age group of children 1 to 14 years old were a result of

* Corresponding author.
E-mail address: avarellj@upstate.edu (J.T. Avarello).

doi:10.1016/j.emc.2007.06.013 **emed.theclinics.com**

homicide in 2004 [2,8]. The leading causes of traumatic death in the United States are listed in Table 1.

Principles of disease

There are major anatomic, physiologic, and psychological differences in the pediatric and adult patients that play a significant role in the evaluation and management of the pediatric trauma patient. A summary of overall anatomic differences and their implications in the pediatric trauma patient are listed in Box 1. Anatomic differences in the pediatric and adult airway and their implication in the pediatric trauma patient are listed in Table 2.

Compared with adults, in children, any given force is more widely distributed though the body, making multiple injuries significantly more likely to occur. The proportionately large surface area of an infant or child relative to weight predisposes them to greater amounts of heat loss as a result of evaporation. Maintenance requirements for free water, trace metals, and minerals are therefore magnified to a greater degree. All these factors contribute to a significantly higher energy and caloric requirement for the injured child when compared with an injured adult. Physiologically, children respond to injury quite differently than adults, depending on the age and maturation of the child and the severity of the injury. Unlike adults, children have a great capacity to maintain blood pressure despite significant acute blood losses (25% to 30%). Subtle changes in heart rate, blood pressure, and extremity perfusion may indicate impending cardiorespiratory failure and should not be overlooked. Finally, children may not cope well outside of their usual environment. They are often disproportionately irritable relative to their degree of injury, making assessment all the more difficult. Recent evidence suggests that 25% of children involved in road traffic accidents will show signs of posttraumatic stress disorder after discharge [9]. They need to be approached in a calming and sometimes unconventional manner so as to lessen their anxiety.

Table 1
Leading causes of traumatic deaths in children 1 to 14 years of age in the United States—2004

Etiology	No.	%
Motor Vehicle Accidents	2,026	38.2
Homicide	706	13.3
Drowning[a]	699	13.2
Fire/Burn[a]	484	9.1
Suicide	285	5.4
Suffocation[a]	238	4.5
Other	860	16.3

[a] Unintentional.

Box 1. Anatomic difference in adults and children—implications for pediatric trauma management

- The child's body size allows for a greater distribution of traumatic injuries, therefore multiple trauma is common.
- The child's greater relative body surface area also causes greater heat loss.
- The child's internal organs are more susceptible to injury based on more anterior placement of liver and spleen and less protective musculature and subcutaneous tissue mass.
- The child's kidney is less well protected and more mobile, making it very susceptible to deceleration injury.
- The child's growth plates are not yet closed, leading to Salter-type fractures with possible limb-length abnormalities with healing.
- The child's head-to-body ratio is greater, the brain less myelinated, and cranial bones thinner, resulting in more serious head injury.

From Marx JA, Holberger RS. Rosen's emergency medicine: concepts and clinical practice. 5th edition. Mosby; 2002. p. 267–81; with permission.

Clinical features

Initial assessment priorities/primary survey

The highest priority in the approach to the injured child is ruling out the presence of life- or limb-threatening injury. Treatment of these injuries must occur before proceeding with the rest of the physical examination. This initial assessment (the primary survey) and necessary initial resuscitation efforts must occur simultaneously. In general, they should be addressed within the first 5 to 10 minutes of evaluation.

Any infant or child with a potentially serious or unstable injury requires continual reassessment. Vital signs should be repeated every 5 minutes during the primary survey and every 15 minutes thereafter until the patient is considered stable.

The International Liaison Committee on Resuscitation (ILCOR) pediatric task force is a multinational team of expert reviewers that was assigned to review resuscitation science and develop an evidence-based consensus to guide resuscitation practices. In January of 2005, the ILCOR presented the evidence at the International Consensus Conference on Cardiopulmonary Resuscitation and Emergency Cardiovascular Care Science With Treatment Recommendations, hosted by the American Heart Association (AHA). By the end of the conference some major changes to the Pediatric Advanced Life Support (PALS) guidelines were established and simultaneously

Table 2
Anatomic differences in the pediatric airway—implications in pediatric trauma management

Differences	Implications
Relatively larger tongue, which can obstruct the airway	Most common cause of airway obstruction in children May necessitate better head positioning or use of airway adjunct (oropharyngeal [OP] or nasopharyngeal [NP] airway)
Larger mass of adenoidal tissues may make nasotracheal intubation more difficult	NP airways may also be more difficult to pass in infants <1 year of age
Epiglottis is floppy and more Ω-shaped	Necessitates use of a straight blade in young children
Larynx more cephalad and anterior	More difficult to visualize the cords; may need to get lower than the patient and look up at 45-degree angle or greater while intubating
Cricoid ring is the narrowest portion of the airway	Provides natural seal and allows for use of uncuffed tubes in children up to size 6 mm or about 8 years of age
Narrow tracheal diameter and distance between the rings, making tracheostomy more difficult	Needle cricothyrotomy for the difficult airway versus a surgical cricothyrotomy for the same reason
Shorter tracheal length (4 to 5 cm in newborn and 7 to 8 cm in 18-month-old)	Leading to intubation of right mainstem or dislodgement of the endotracheal tube
Large airways are more narrow	Leads to greater airway resistance ($R = 1/\text{radius}^4$)

From Marx JA, Holberger RS. Rosen's emergency medicine: concepts and clinical practice. 5th edition. Mosby; 2002. p. 267–81; with permission.

published in *Circulation* and *Resuscitation* in November 2005. A summary of these changes can be found in the winter 2005 to 2006 issue of AHA-published *CURRENTS in Emergency Cardiovascular Care*.

Primary survey

Airway. Indications for endotracheal intubation of the pediatric trauma patient include (1) any inability to ventilate by bag-valve-mask (BVM) methods or the need for prolonged control of the airway; (2) Glasgow Coma Scale (GCS) score of $\leq$ 8 to secure the airway and provide controlled hyperventilation as indicated; (3) respiratory failure from hypoxemia (eg, flail chest, pulmonary contusions) or hypoventilation (injury to airway structures); (4) any trauma patient in decompensated shock resistant to initial fluid administration; and (5) the loss of protective laryngeal reflexes. With these indications in mind, it is also important to know that endotracheal intubation may not be the most effective means of ventilation in the prehospital setting. In 2000, Gausche and colleagues [10] published data in *JAMA* presenting good evidence that BVM is as effective and may be safer than endotracheal intubation in the prehospital setting. Patients were randomized to receive either BVM or endotracheal intubation. Of the 830 pediatric patients enrolled, there was a 4% better survival rate and a 3% better neurologic outcome rate in the BVM group with even more significance in the subgroups of respiratory arrest and child maltreatment. The AHA included these findings in their PALS updates stating to "ventilate and oxygenate infants and children with a bag-mask devise, especially if transport time is short" [10].

Intubation of the pediatric patient involves special considerations. Cuffed endotracheal tubes have recently been considered as safe as uncuffed tubes for infants beyond the newborn period and in children when in the hospital setting. The 2005 update by the AHA states "In certain circumstances (eg, poor lung compliance, high airway resistance, or a large glottic air leak) a cuffed tube may be preferable provided that attention is paid to endotracheal tube size, position, and cuff inflation pressure" [11]. On the contrary, in patients younger than 8 years who do not fit those circumstances, uncuffed tubes should be used, as the narrowest portion of the pediatric airway in this age group is at the level of the cricoid cartilage (Table 2). For children 1 to 10 years of age, the following formulas may be used for estimation of proper endotracheal tube size (ID, internal diameter):

- Uncuffed endotracheal tube size (mm ID) = (age in years + 16)/4
- Cuffed endotracheal tube size (mm ID) = (age in years + 12)/4

In general, the orotracheal approach is recommended. Problems associated with nasotracheal intubation include inherent difficulties in children, impairment of tube passage by the acute angle of the posterior pharynx, and the probability of causing or worsening bleeding within the oral cavity and causing increases in intracranial pressure (ICP) with insertion.

Breathing/ventilation. Assess for adequacy of chest rise. In a young child this will occur in the lower chest and upper abdomen. Also assess respiratory rate. Rates that are too fast or slow can indicate impending respiratory failure. Treatment is assisted ventilation. If ventilation is necessary, a BVM device is recommended initially. Be careful to provide only the volume necessary to cause the chest to rise, because excessive volume or rate of ventilation can increase the likelihood of gastric distention and further impair ventilation. Once an advanced airway is placed, ventilations should be given at a rate of 1 breath every 6 to 8 seconds (8 to 10 breaths per minute). Cricoid pressure may be useful to decrease the amount of air entering the esophagus during positive-pressure ventilation. With regard to assessment of ventilation, early monitoring with pulse oximetry is very useful; however, pulse oximetry will measure adequacy of oxygenation only. There are many limiting factors that compromise ventilatory function in the injured child, including depressed sensorium, occlusion of the airway itself, painful restriction of lung expansion, and direct pulmonary injury. Determination of adequate ventilation is possible only in the face of airway patency and adequate air exchange. The diaphragm plays a special role in the maintenance of proper ventilatory status in children. It is easily fatigued in the young child and is often displaced by any process that promotes distention of the stomach. In this regard, it is advisable to consider early placement of a nasogastric tube to facilitate decompression of the stomach.

Circulation and hemorrhage control. Assessment of circulation in a child involves a combination of factors, namely the pulse, skin color, and capillary refill time. In a child, maintenance of systolic blood pressure does not ensure that the patient is not in shock, a direct effect of the ability of the pediatric vasculature to constrict and increase systemic vascular resistance in an attempt to maintain perfusion. Therefore skin signs such as cool distal extremities, decreases in peripheral versus central pulse quality, and delayed capillary refill time are signs of pediatric shock, even when blood pressure is maintained. The lowest acceptable blood pressures for age (5th percentile) are as follows [11]:

- 60 mm Hg in term neonates (0 to 28 days)
- 70 mm Hg in infants (1 month to 12 months)
- 70 mm Hg + (2 × age in years) in children 1 to 10 years of age
- 90 mm HG in children ≥ 10 years of age

In general, a palpable peripheral pulse correlates with a systolic blood pressure greater than 80 mm Hg and a palpable central pulse with a pressure greater than 50 to 60 mm Hg [12]. Normal capillary refill times are less than 2 seconds. Alteration in a child's response to the environment or interaction with caregivers may also indicate respiratory failure or shock. External hemorrhage should be sought for and controlled with direct pressure.

All pediatric patients involved in major trauma should be placed on a cardiac monitor, receive supplemental oxygen, and have constant reassessment of vital signs and oximetry. Vascular access is best obtained by accessing the upper extremity for the establishment of two large-bore intravenous (IV) lines. In the absence of available upper extremity peripheral sites, lower extremity sites could be used, and many clinicians favor the femoral vein as a safe site for insertion of a central line, by use of a guide wire technique. If cutdowns are necessary, the antecubital or saphenous sites will suffice. If access is needed emergently or if there is no success in the first 5 minutes of an urgent scenario, intraosseous access may be obtained at the proximal medial tibia 1 cm below and medial to the tibial tuberosity, the distal tibia 1 to 2 cm proximal to the medial malleolus, or the lower third of the femur at the midline 3 cm above the lateral condyle (Fig. 1) [13]. The intraosseous route serves as an appropriate venous access site; however, delivery rate of large amounts of crystalloid solutions is limited based on maximum flow rates of approximately 25 mL/min [14–16]. Intraosseous placement in a fractured extremity is contraindicated.

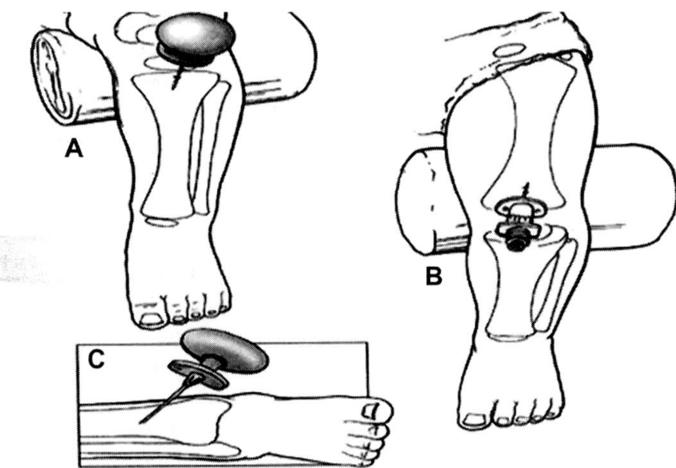

Fig. 1. (*A–C*) Preferred locations for intraosseous needle placement. (*Reprinted from* Fleisher GR, Ludwig S, Henretig FM. Textbook of pediatric emergency medicine. 5th edition. Philadelphia: Lippincott Williams and Wilkins; 2006. p. 1879; with permission.)

Most hypovolemic pediatric trauma patients respond to infusions of 20 mL/kg of isotonic crystalloid solutions. If 40 mL/kg has already been given and a third bolus is still required to reverse systemic signs of hypoperfusion, an infusion of packed blood cells at 10 mL/kg should be considered [17]. In patients who present in decompensated shock or cardiopulmonary failure, and occult bleeding is a potential cause for the shock, administer crystalloid and blood products simultaneously.

In contrast to the adult, cardiogenic shock is a rare event in the face of childhood injury [3,18]. However, any degree of chest trauma associated with the presence of shock must alert the clinician to the possibility of concomitant myocardial contusion or rupture. The classic presentation of neurogenic shock, involving hypotension without an increase in heart rate or compensatory vasoconstriction, should be considered in patients with head or neck injuries.

With regard to cardiopulmonary resuscitation (CPR) in the infant and child, the guidelines have been recently updated. The chest compression-ventilation ratio for one lay rescuer and one lone health care provider is now 30:2, and 15:2 for health care providers performing two-rescuer CPR. Although these recommendations come mostly from theoretical data and rational conjecture, the thought is that, besides less fatigue of the rescuer(s), more interruptions in chest compressions will prolong the duration of low coronary perfusion pressures reducing the likelihood of a return of spontaneous circulation. High-dose epinephrine has been removed from the recommendation with the exceptions being if it is administered by the endotracheal route or in exceptional circumstances such as β-blocker overdose.

Disability assessment (thorough neurologic examination). To assess patient disability, there is need for a rapid neurologic evaluation. The GCS (Boxes 2 and 3) and the AVPU System (Box 4) are used for a rapid neurological evaluation. It is important to rule out hypoglycemia in any patient with altered mental status. This is particularly important in younger children since their glycogen stores are easily depleted, predisposing them to hypoglycemia.

Exposure. The final component of the primary survey involves fully undressing the patient to assess for hidden injury. Maintenance of normothermia is of paramount importance in the toddler and infant during the exposure phase because metabolic needs are greatly increased by hypothermia.

Family. In the management of children, the family could be added to the primary survey. Rapidly informing the family of what has happened and the evaluation that is proceeding will help lessen the stress of the caregivers. Allowing family presence during resuscitations is acceptable and often preferred by families. Some caregivers will choose not to be present, but that choice should be given to them. If a caregiver is present, it is advisable to assign a staff member to be with them during the trauma resuscitation to explain the process [19].

Box 2. Glasgow Coma Scale

Eye opening response (1–4 points)

4. Spontaneous
3. To verbal stimuli
2. To painful stimuli
1. None

Verbal response (1–5 points)

5. Oriented
4. Confused
3. Inappropriate words
2. Nonspecific sounds or incomprehensible
1. None

Motor response (1–6 points)

6. Normal spontaneous movements
5. Localizes painful stimuli
4. Withdraws from painful stimuli
3. Abnormal flexion (decorticate rigidity)
2. Abnormal extension (decerebrate rigidity)
1. None

Box 3. Modified GCS

Modified GCS for infants
Eye opening response (1–4 points)
4. Spontaneous
3. To verbal stimuli
2. To painful stimuli
1. None

Verbal response (1–5 points)
5. Coos and/or babbles
4. Irritable and continuous crying
3. Cries to painful stimuli
2. Moans to painful stimuli
1. None

Motor response (1–6 points)
6. Spontaneous purposeful movements
5. Withdraws to touch
4. Withdraws to painful stimuli
3. Abnormal flexion (decorticate rigidity)
2. Abnormal extension (decerebrate rigidity)
1. None

Secondary survey

The secondary survey is designed to assess the patient and treat additional injury not found on the primary survey and also to obtain a more complete and detailed history. Features of the detailed history that need to be obtained can be remembered by the mnemonic *AMPLE* (Box 5). During the secondary survey the EP should attend to the tasks outlined in Box 6.

Specifics of the head examination include pupillary size and reactivity, funduscopic examination, and palpation of the skull itself. Assessment of the cervical spine must be done carefully, with the patient in full c-spine immobilization.

Assessment of the chest and internal structures involves inspection for wounds and flail segments, palpation for tenderness and crepitance, and

Box 4. The AVPU system

A = ***A***lert
V = Responds to ***V***erbal stimuli
P = Responds to ***P***ainful stimuli
U = ***U***nresponsive

Box 5. The AMPLE history

A, ***A***llergies
M, ***M***edications
P, ***P***ast medical history
L, ***L***ast meal
E, ***E***nvironments and events

auscultation for asymmetry or poorly transmitted breath sounds or cardiac impulses.

Examination of the pediatric abdomen is most reliable when performed on a cooperative patient and should be considered an insensitive screening process for the presence of an injury when the patient has an associated head injury or a GCS $\leq$ 13 [20].

A rectal examination provides information concerning sphincter tone, prostatic position, and the presence of blood in the stool. Although urethral injury is rare in children, all trauma patients should be assessed for a perineal or lower abdominal hematoma and blood from the urethral meatus. Examination of the extremities is directed toward the evaluation of any deformities, penetrations, and interruptions of perfusion. Most fracture sites may be stabilized with splinting until surgical intervention can be performed. Early orthopedic consultation is advisable.

As mentioned previously, the pediatric patient is at great risk for the development of hypothermia. This is based on the large amount of surface area relative to body weight. Careful attention to core temperatures in these vulnerable patients is required, with early intervention as needed, with supplemental external warming techniques.

An overview of recommended interventions for the multiply traumatized child is contained in Tables 3–8.

Box 6. Tasks to be completed after the secondary survey

- Complete head-to-toe examination
- Appropriate tetanus immunization
- Antibiotics as indicated
- Continued monitoring of vital signs
- Ensure urine output of 1 mL/kg/hr

From Marx JA, Holberger RS. Rosen's emergency medicine: concepts and clinical practice. 5th edition. Mosby; 2002. p. 267–81; with permission.

Table 3
Airway: assessment and treatment

Assessment priorities	Interventions
Airway patency	Jaw thrust, suction, airway adjuncts
Level of consciousness	Cervical spine immobilization
Maxillofacial injury	Apply 100% O_2 by mask
Stridor or cyanosis	Intubate for: Glasgow Coma Scale ≤ 8 or absent gag reflex or $Po_2 < 50$ or $Pco_2 > 50$
	Needle cricothyrotomy if intubation impossible

Laboratory

Blood sampling for the pediatric trauma patient is no different from that of the adult trauma patient; however, use of smaller blood collection tubes and microtechnique by laboratory staff may be necessary in infants and small children. All older children and adolescent trauma patients should be assessed for the possible use of drugs or alcohol as contributing factors to the traumatic event. In patients with hypovolemic shock, the hemoglobin alone is not sensitive because equilibration may not have occurred upon presentation to the emergency department (ED) [21,22].

Radiology

The most important "traditional" radiographs to obtain on a moderately to severely injured child are of the chest and pelvis to assess for sites of blood loss or potential causes of shock. In stable, alert children without

Table 4
Breathing: assessment and treatment

Assessment priorities	Interventions
Respiratory rate	Oxygen 100% by nonrebreather mask or intubate if in respiratory failure; fast rates may indicate shock (fluid resuscitation) or pain (parenteral analgesics)
Chest wall movements	For pneumo- or hemothorax: place chest tube
	Transfer to operating room if initial drainage >20 mL/kg or output >2 mL/kg/hr
Percussion note	Open pneumothorax: seal with occlusive dressing (vaseline gauze) followed by tube thoracostomy
Paradoxical breathing	Contusion/flail chest: intubate if tachypneic or $Po_2 < 50$ mm or $Pco_2 > 50$ mm Hg
Tracheal deviation	Tension pneumothorax: needle decompression at second intercostal space, midclavicular line, followed by placement of chest tube
Flail segments	Oxygen by nonrebreather mask or intubate if in respiratory failure
Open wounds	Compress bleeding sites and cover as indicated

From Marx JA, Holberger RS. Rosen's emergency medicine: concepts and clinical practice. 5th edition. Mosby; 2002. p. 267–81; with permission.

Table 5
Circulation: assessment and treatment

Assessment priorities	Interventions
Open wounds	Compress bleeding sites and cover as indicated
Capillary refill	Oximeter and cardiac monitor, oxygen and fluid resuscitation 20 mL/kg
Heart rate	Monitor vital signs every 5 minutes
Peripheral pulses	Two large-bore intravenous sites
Sensorium	Bolus with 20 mL/kg lactated Ringer's or normal saline solution (warm all intravenous fluids)
Pulse pressure	Repeat fluid bolus 2 times if necessary
Skin condition/perfusion	Packed red blood cells, 10–20 mL/kg for decompensated shock secondary to blood loss

distracting injuries, the pelvic film may be eliminated. The radiographs of the cervical spine may be delayed until after further diagnostic studies are obtained depending on the clinical presentation of the patient.

The diagnostic test of choice to assess intra-abdominal injury in stable trauma patients is rapid abdominal CT scanning [23]. The role of diagnostic peritoneal lavage (DPL) and Focused Abdominal Sonography for Trauma (FAST) is somewhat more limited although the FAST exam is gaining more acceptance [24,25]. As with all of these tests, the finding of intraperitoneal hemorrhage alone is not an indication for surgery in the pediatric patient (Box 7).

Other radiographs will be obtained based on the physical examination. For patients sustaining minor trauma, radiographs may not be needed. Finally, children younger than 2 years of age with injuries consistent with child abuse will need a skeletal survey including skull, chest, abdomen, and long-bone radiographs.

Table 6
Disability: assessment and treatment

Assessment priorities	Interventions
Level of consciousness	Maintain blood pressure and oxygenation and ventilation
AVPU system or GCS	If head injury with GCS $\leq$ 8: RSI and intubate; head CT, neurosurgical consult
	If normotensive, consider mannitol 0.25–1 g/kg
Pupil size and reactivity	Hyperventilate Pco_2 to 30–35 mm Hg with signs of herniation
Extremity movement and tone	Stabilize spinal column
	If blunt cord trauma: methylprednisolone (See Table 9 for dosing recommendations)
Posturing	Hyperventilate Pco_2 to 30–35 mm Hg
Reflexes	Assess for signs of respiratory failure

Abbreviation: RSI, rapid sequence intubation.

Table 7
Exposure: assessment and treatment

Assessment priorities	Interventions
Undress	Trauma examination including rectal examination
Look under collar and splints	Keep patient warm:
Log roll and examine back	• Remove wet clothes
	• Place under heater
	• External warming devices
	• Warm blanket
	• Warm fluids

Specific disorders/injuries

Head injury

Perspective

Head trauma is the leading cause of death among injured children and is responsible for 80% of all trauma deaths [3]. Each year, 29,000 children younger than 19 years old suffer permanent disability from traumatic brain injury. In children younger than 14 years old, there are 475,000 hospital visits, 37,000 hospitalizations, and nearly 3000 deaths each year related to traumatic brain injury [4,26].

Falls account for 39% of pediatric head injuries, and MVCs are responsible for 11% [4,27,28]. In addition, pedestrian injuries account for 17% and falls from bicycles 10%. On an age-related basis, infants and toddlers are more prone to falls from their own height, school-age children are involved in sports injuries and MVCs, and all ages are subject to the sequelae of abuse [26].

Clinical features

In most cases it is important to establish whether there was loss of consciousness at the time of the injury event. With playground trauma, the history may be vague and the interpretation of any change in consciousness of the child may be regarded as an actual loss of consciousness. The behavior of the child after the event should include questions related to the presence or absence of irritability, lethargy, abnormal gait, or alterations in behavior. Most importantly, establishment of a timeline from the point of insult is helpful in determining whether there have been changes in the mental status of the patient. A caretaker present to establish the child's baseline behavior, mental status, and neurologic function is very useful.

The prognostic significance of vomiting after pediatric head trauma is uncertain [26,29]. There is no adequate study defining an acceptable time frame in which vomiting after head injury is benign in nature. The development of seizures after head trauma, in contrast to vomiting, has been well studied [30]. A brief seizure that occurs immediately after the insult (with rapid return of normal level of consciousness) is commonly called "an impact seizure" and is usually unassociated with intracranial parenchymal injury

Table 8
Emergent management of increased intracranial pressure

Therapy	Dose	Mechanism of action
Head evaluation (30 degrees)		Lowers intracranial venous pressure
Head in midline		Prevents jugular vein compression
Hyperventilation	Reduces $Paco_2$ to 30–35 mm Hg	Promptly decreases cerebral blood volume and thus intracranial pressure Caution: too much ventilation can ↓ cerebral blood flow
Lidocaine	1–2 mg/kg IV	↓ airway reflex's that may ↑ intracranial pressure
Mannitol	0.25–1 g/kg IV	↓blood viscosity → improved cerebral blood flow Contraindicated in hemodynamically unstable patients
Thiopental	3–5 mg/kg IV	Decreases cerebral metabolism reducing cerebral ischemic risk Caution with hypotensive patients
Etomidate	0.3 mg/kg IV	Decreases cerebral metabolism reducing cerebral ischemic risk
Emergent burr hole: Only in the rapidly deteriorating patient when all medical interventions have failed, a neurosurgeon is unavailable, and the patient will not likely survive transport		Temporary decompression to ameliorate herniation
Hypothermia (27°C–31°C)		Thought to decrease cerebral blood flow and metabolic rate; can cause cardiac dysrhythmias

From Marx JA, Holberger RS. Rosen's emergency medicine: concepts and clinical practice. 5th edition. Mosby; 2002. p. 267–81; with permission.

and in no way mandates the institution of anticonvulsant therapy. Seizures that occur later (longer than 20 minutes after the insult) portend the greater possibility of both internal injury and the development of seizures at a later date. Patients who experience seizures later in the course of the posttraumatic event are best evaluated by the neurosurgical service. As in all instances of trauma, a careful history related to the possibility of substance abuse must be obtained.

Table 9
Corticosteroid treatment recommendations in acute spinal trauma

Indications	Acute spinal cord injury presenting within 8 hours of injury
Contraindications	(1) Patient presents >8 hrs postinjury (2) Gun shot injury (3) Pregnancy (4) Involvement of nerve root/cauda equina only (5) Other life threatening illness (6) Receiving maintenance steroids for other reasons (7) <13 years of age (relative contraindication)
Treatment	Methylprednisolone 30 mg/kg IV over 15 minutes then a 45-minute pause, then (1) 5.4 mg/kg/hr IV over 23 hrs if <3 hrs since injury OR (2) 5.4 mg/kg/hr IV over 47 hrs if 3–8 hrs since injury

Data from Refs. [17,65,81].

There are several methods for evaluating head-injured patients. These include AVPU and the GCS. The GCS has been modified for pediatric patients as illustrated in Box 3.

The GCS more reliably predicts outcome of traumatic brain injury in children than in adults. In a study involving 80 children with traumatic brain injuries admitted to an intensive care unit (ICU), initial GCS scores were compared with eventual outcome. Both ICU lengths of stay and time to cognition relative to GCS scores indicated that scores greater than or equal to 6 were associated with favorable outcomes and neurologic status. While the numbers in this study are small, the important message is that no matter

Box 7. Potential uses for the FAST examination

- Rapidly identify the source of hypotension in the hemodynamically unstable patient
- Assist in decision making in the child with head and abdominal trauma (head and abdominal CT versus laparotomy and/or craniotomy)
- Evaluate the stable and alert trauma patient without finding on physical exam who would not routinely undergo radiology imaging
- Help prioritize imaging studies in the multiple-trauma patient
- Help avoid additional imaging in a child with an already low likelihood of intra-abdominal injury

From Marx JA, Holberger RS. Rosen's emergency medicine: concepts and clinical practice. 5th edition. Mosby; 2002. p. 267–81; with permission.

how the patient presents neurologically, all efforts should be generated to ensure survival and maintain stable neurologic status within the ED [31].

Examining the brain-injured child involves cranial nerve testing and motor and sensory testing. The evaluation of cranial nerve function is essentially no different from that of the adult. The most important aspect of both motor and cranial nerve evaluation involves ruling out the presence of increased ICP. Common symptoms and signs of increased ICP in infants and children are described as follows:

Infants

- Full fontanel
- Split sutures
- Altered states of consciousness
- Paradoxical irritability
- Persistent emesis
- The "sun-setting" sign (inability to open eyes fully)

Children

- Headache
- Stiff neck
- Photophobia
- Altered states of consciousness
- Persistent emesis
- Cranial nerve involvement
- Papilledema
- Cushing's triad (Hypertension, bradycardia and irregular respirations)
- Decorticate or decerebrate posturing

Minor injury to the scalp of infants and children involves the development of three possible injury complexes: caput succedaneum, injury to the connective tissue itself; subgaleal hematoma, injury to the tissue surrounding the skull; and cephalohematoma, a collection of blood under the periosteum.

Skull fractures in children occur in many different configurations [27,30,32]. Linear fractures, the most common type of skull fracture, rarely require therapy and are often associated with good outcomes. Factors favoring a poor outcome include the presence of the fracture overlying a vascular channel, a diastatic fracture, or a fracture that extends over the area of the middle meningeal artery. Diastatic fractures, or defects extending through suture lines, are unlike linear fractures, in that leptomeningeal cysts (growing fractures) may develop at these sites. Fractures of the basilar portions of the occipital, temporal, sphenoid, or ethmoid bones commonly occur in children [33]. The presence of cerebrospinal fluid (CSF), rhinorrhea, and otorrhea has been associated with these injuries. Signs of basilar skull fractures in children are similar to adults and include hemotympanum, seventh and eighth nerve dysfunction, posterior auricular ecchymosis, or Battle's sign, and raccoon eyes, or the presence of periorbital subcutaneous bleeding [17,26]. As a basic rule, serial examinations are the most reliable indicators of clinical deterioration [26,29,30,32]. The presence of focality is a reliable indicator of a localized insult, whereas the absence of focality may be misleading. Although there may be few or subtle signs and symptoms of intracranial injury, the following independent predictors have been identified [29]:

- Altered mental status
- Focal neurologic deficits
- Signs of a basilar skull fracture
- Seizure
- Skull fracture

Concussion

Strictly speaking, *concussion* is defined as a brain insult with transient impairment of consciousness. Amnesia is often involved and patients who suffer from concussive insults frequently demonstrate anorexia, vomiting, or pallor soon after the insult. This transitional period is followed by rapid recovery to baseline and if a CT scan of the head is obtained, it is most often normal. Following the Second International Symposium on Concussion in Sport November 2004, concussion was reclassified as simple or complex [34].

- **Simple concussions** are those where loss of consciousness (if any) was less than 1 minute, and symptoms resolve without complication within 7 to 10 days. In such cases, apart from limiting playing and other activities while symptomatic, no further intervention is required during the period of recovery.
- **Complex concussions** include those where there is prolonged loss of consciousness, symptoms or cognitive impairment last longer than 7 to 10 days, or there is a history of multiple concussions. In these cases, return to play should be managed by a multidisciplinary team, and formal neuropsychological testing (testing of attention, memory, and so forth) should be considered.

Since Saunders and Harbaugh [35] first described it in 1984, second-impact syndrome has gained much attention and has led to strict "return-to-play" guidelines for athletes who have suffered a head injury. Second-impact syndrome has been defined as an injury in which "an athlete who has sustained an initial head injury, most often a concussion, sustains a second head injury before symptoms associated with the first have fully cleared" [36]. Given that this can ultimately lead to death, the return-to-play guidelines require strict adherence. When a player shows ANY symptoms or signs of a concussion:

1. The player should **NOT** be allowed to return to play in the current game or practice.
2. The player should not be left alone, and regular monitoring for deterioration is essential over the initial few hours following injury.
3. The player should be medically evaluated following the injury.
4. Return to play must follow a medically supervised stepwise process.

In contrast to concussions, contusions are often the result of coup and contrecoup forces at work. They may not be associated with any loss of consciousness at the time of insult. Patients often present with associated symptoms such as altered level of consciousness, severe headache, vomiting, or focal deficits on neurologic assessment. These injuries are clearly demonstrable on CT.

Traditional teaching regarding the development of epidural hematomas involves the typical triad of head injury followed by a lucid interval, followed by rapid deterioration as intracranial hemorrhage worsens. Unfortunately, in contrast to the adult, pediatric epidural hematomas may be the result of venous bleeding, which predisposes them to a subtle and more subacute presentation over days. In any event, epidural hematomas are associated with a high incidence of overlying skull fractures (60% to 80% of cases).

Special attention to the infant or toddler should be made to rule out the presence of subdural hematomas [26,30]. This clinical scenario is most often secondary to rupture of bridging veins and is rarely associated with the presence of overlying fractures (<30%). Subdural hematomas most commonly occur in patients younger than 2 years of age, with 93% of cases involving children younger than 1 year. Chronic subdural hematomas are most often encountered in patients who have been subjected to what has been named "shaken baby syndrome." This clinical complex involves forcible shaking of the child with acceleratory and deceleratory forces impacting the cranial vault. Twenty-two percent of abused children have central nervous system (CNS) injuries. Patients will present with nonspecific findings, such as vomiting, failure to thrive, change in level of consciousness, or seizures. Retinal hemorrhages are present in 75% of cases, and all patients should have careful funduscopic examinations to rule out the presence of these pathognomonic findings. Left to their own development, the worst cases may actually present with signs of increased ICP. Retinal hemorrhages are not observed in children with mild-to-moderate trauma from other causes and are not associated with a prior history of CPR; the presence of retinal hemorrhages suggests child abuse.

Radiology

Skull films. With the advent of multislice CT scanners, the number of skull radiographs being done to rule out skull fractures in children has decreased dramatically. That being said, the presence of a skull fracture on a plain radiograph is one of the strongest predictors for intracranial injury in children younger than 2 [29,37]. Because of this, skull films still may play a role in the evaluation of head trauma in the infant and young child. This is not to say that skull radiography should take the place of CT scanning, but that under the right circumstances the higher radiation and sedation complications that come with CT scans could be avoided without compromising patient outcome [37]. Brenner and colleagues [38] estimated that for every 1500 head CTs done in children younger than 2, one lethal malignancy is directly related to the radiation from the CT. Previous studies have evaluated the utility of skull radiography versus CT scanning in the evaluation of pediatric head injury. It is universally understood that in any patient with signs and/or symptoms of intracranial injury, CT is the test of choice. In 2001, it was proposed that in a child younger than 2 without symptoms of brain injury but at some risk for skull fracture (eg, presence of scalp swelling), skull radiography may be of some utility [37]. Most clinicians agree that at present, firm indications for skull films alone include the skeletal survey involved with the evaluation of child abuse, establishment of a functioning ventricular peritoneal shunt, penetrating wounds of the scalp, the suspicion of foreign bodies underlying scalp lacerations, or for screening a child younger than 2 thought to have a fracture in the absence of signs or symptoms of brain injury.

CT of the head. There has been a considerable amount of research on the indications and relative value of CT scanning in the pediatric head-injured patient. A large study evaluated children between the ages of 2 and 17 years with loss of consciousness and GCS scores of 15 after mild head injury [39]. The children were grouped according to physical examination findings, neurologic status, and whether the head injury was isolated or nonisolated. Patients with obvious skull fractures were excluded. Two variables were highly associated with the presence of intracranial hemorrhage: the presenting neurologic status and presence of multiple injuries. None of the 49 neurologically normal children with isolated head injury had intracranial hemorrhages. All patients with intracranial hemorrhages were noted to have other traumatic insults on physical examination. The authors concluded that after isolated head injury with loss of consciousness, children older than 2 years who were neurologically normal may be discharged without a CT scan after careful physical examination alone. Other studies contradict these findings, establishing a clear association with parenchymal injury and loss of consciousness [29,37,40,41]. At present, recommendations for CT scanning include altered mental status, focal neurologic deficit, signs of a basilar skull fracture, seizure, and a skull fracture or injury patterns that are the result of major forcible insults [29,37]. Special consideration must be taken with children younger than 1 year. These patients challenge the clinician since their neurologic milestones are harder to evaluate. Within this age group any loss of consciousness, protracted vomiting, irritability or poor feeding, or suspicion of abuse would mandate CT scanning.

The infant with minor closed head injury has recently been studied. In a series of 608 children younger than 2 years who underwent CT scanning, a subset of 92 infants younger than 2 months was further scrutinized. The presence of a significant scalp hematoma was highly correlative (77% of subjects with intracranial injury) with underlying parenchymal brain injury. The authors recommend that radiographic imaging not only be directed at asymptomatic infants, but also at those asymptomatic infants with significant scalp hematomas [42].

Recently, the Pediatric Emergency Care Applied Research Network prospectively enrolled 42,495 children who had head trauma and a GCS of 14-15 [43]. The goal was to derive and validate clinical decision rules for obtaining head CT in children less than 2 years old and children greater 2 years with mild head trauma. The results should be available by late 2007–2008.

Cervical spine injury

Perspective

In the United States more than 1100 children sustain spinal injury annually, leading to an annual cost exceeding $4 billion [44,45]. Cervical injury patterns vary with the age of the patient. It has been reported that 1% to 10% of all spine injuries are in the pediatric age group and that 60% to 80% of all pediatric vertebral injuries are in the cervical spine [46–48]. Fractures below the C3 level account for only 30% of spinal lesions among children younger than 8 years, dramatically different from those patterns seen in the adult population. Likewise, spinal cord injury without radiographic abnormality (SCIWORA) has been found in 30% to 40% of spinal cord injuries in this same age group [48–51].

Imaging the pediatric cervical spine

A prospective study done in 3065 patients younger than 18 proved that when using their criteria for obtaining cervical spine imaging in pediatric blunt trauma, there was a 100% sensitivity and a 100% negative predictive value. Criteria for obtaining imaging included midline cervical tenderness, altered level of alertness, evidence of intoxication, neurologic abnormality, and the presence of a painful distracting injury. The authors urged caution in using the criteria in children younger than 2 years old, as this age group was not well represented (88 of 3065) [52]. Caution should also be used in patients with congenital or acquired abnormalities (eg, Down syndrome, juvenile rheumatoid arthritis, prior fracture) [50]. When indicated, radiographic evaluation should routinely consist of three views: a cross-table lateral view, an anteroposterior view, and an open-mouth view to help visualize the odontoid process of C1. With these three plain film views of the cervical region, the sensitivity for detecting cervical fractures is 89% and the negative predictive value of these three views adequately done is nearly 100% [53]. Interpretation of plain cervical spine films in children may be challenging because of the anatomic changes that occur with growth (Box 8). In addition, pseudosubluxation of C2 on C3 is common in children up to adolescence, occurring in approximately 40% of patients [54]. The EP distinguishes between pseudosubluxation and true subluxation by the posterior cervical line or spinolaminar line, also known as the *line of Swischuk*. A line is drawn from the anterior cortical margin of the spinous process of C1 down through the anterior cortical margin of C3. If this line at C2 crosses the anterior cortical margin of the

Box 8. Anatomic differences in the pediatric cervical spine

- Relatively larger head size, resulting in greater flexion and extension injuries
- Smaller neck muscle mass with ligamentous injuries more common than fractures
- Increased flexibility of interspinous ligaments
- Infantile bony column can lengthen significantly without rupture
- Flatter facet joints with a more horizontal orientation
- Incomplete ossification making interpretation of bony alignment difficult
- Basilar odontoid synchondrosis fuse at 3 to 7 years of age
- Apical odontoid epiphysis fuse at 5 to 7 years of age
- Posterior arch of C1 fuses at 4 years of age
- Anterior arch fuses at 7 to 10 years of age
- Epiphyses of spinous process tips may mimic fractures
- Increased preodontoid space up to 4 to 5 mm (3 mm in an adult)
- Pseudosubluxation of C2 on C3 seen in 40% of children
- Prevertebral space size may change because of variations with respiration

spinous process at C2 or is off by less than 2 mm and no fractures are visualized, then the patient has pseudosubluxation versus true subluxation of the ligaments at that level (Fig. 2) [55,56].

An important criterion for radiographic clearing of the cervical spine is complete visualization of all seven cervical vertebral bodies down to, and including, the C7 to T1 interface. The predental space should not exceed 4 to 5 mm in children younger than 10 years, and the prevertebral soft-tissue space should not be greater than normal. The 4 cervical radiographic lines should be evaluated, and the atlanto-occipital alignment should be assessed for dislocation in this region (see Fig. 2).

Other imaging modalities that can be used to delineate cervical fractures include thin-section CT and MRI.

Cardiothoracic injury

Perspective

The vast majority of serious chest injuries in children (83%) are the result of blunt trauma [8,57]. Most are the result of MVCs with the remainder secondary to bicycle crashes. Isolated chest injury is a relatively infrequent occurrence when considering the typical mechanisms of blunt trauma in the pediatric patient. The presence of significant chest injury greatly enhances

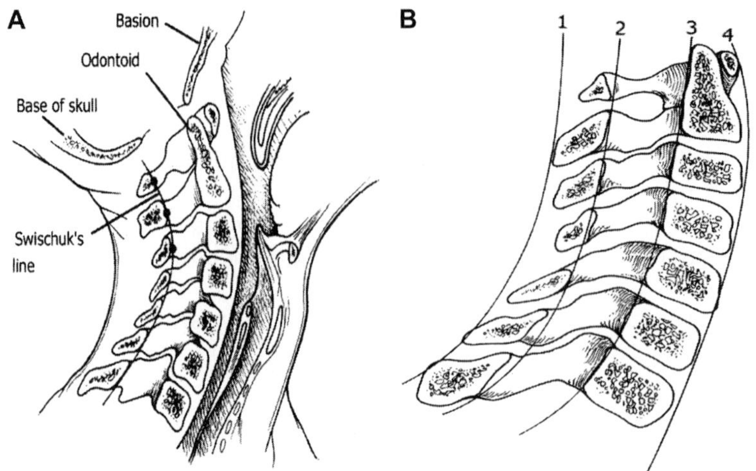

Fig. 2. (*A*) The spinolaminar line (Swischuk's line) used to determine the presence of pseudo-subluxation of C2 on C3. (*B*) Normal relationships in the lateral aspect of the cervical spine. 1 = spinous processes, 2 = spinolaminar line, 3 = posterior vertebral body line, and 4 = anterior vertebral body line. (*Reprinted from* Copley LA, Dormans JP. Cervical spine disorders in infants and children. J Am Acad Orthop Surg 1998;6:207; with permission.)

the potential for multisystem trauma mortality by a factor of 10. Sequelae of blunt injury include rib fractures and pulmonary contusion (50%), pneumothorax (20%), and hemothorax (10%).

Overall mortality is nearly equivalent for blunt versus penetrating trauma. Children subjected to penetrating trauma, unlike the injuries associated with blunt trauma, will often die from the primary insult itself. Penetrating trauma accounts for only 15% of thoracic insults in children [58–60]. Our nationwide fascination with the use of firearms has resulted in an increasing incidence of penetrating trauma with the child as victim. Specific clinical patterns should alert the clinician to the potential for concurrent abdominal and thoracic injury. Any patient with penetrating trauma at or below the level of the sixth rib will fall into this category.

Principles of disease

It is important to understand the physiology of pediatric respiration when considering the potential for early decompensation. Infants and young children are preferential diaphragm breathers and any impairment of diaphragmatic mobility will compromise ventilation. The presence of gastric distention will elevate the diaphragm and severely lessen the vital capacity of a child. In addition, the particular types of muscle fibers involved in the diaphragm of infants and young children predispose to the sudden development of apnea when fatigued. Most importantly, the presence of adequate oxygenation in the pediatric patient does not always ensure sufficiency of ventilation. It is important to rely upon auscultatory and other physical findings rather than simple measurements of oximetry.

Infants and children are anatomically protected against blunt thoracic cage trauma because of the compliance of the rib cage [61]. Compressibility of the rib cage will dissipate the force of impact, which will lessen the likelihood of bony injury. These protective mechanisms may also mask fairly complex pediatric thoracic insults. The compliance of the rib cage will allow significant injury to occur with little apparent external signs of trauma. Multiple rib fractures are a marker of serious injury in children, with child abuse being the most likely etiology and the mortality rate exceeding 40%. In addition, the pediatric mediastinum is mobile, which favors the development of rapid ventilatory and circulatory collapse in the presence of a tension pneumothorax.

Pneumothorax

The development of a traumatic pneumothorax is commonly associated with significant pulmonary injury [58]. In contrast to spontaneous pneumothoraces, these insults will not resolve spontaneously and are often associated with the presence of a hemothorax.

Signs and symptoms include external evidence of chest trauma such as abrasion, contusion, or ecchymosis; tachypnea; respiratory distress; hypoxemia; and chest pain. Decreased breath sounds may not be appreciated in children with pneumothoraces because of the wide transmission of breath sounds in the chest and upper abdomen.

Management of a simple pneumothorax noted on chest radiograph includes the placement of a large-caliber, laterally placed chest tube or close observation. Chest tube size can be estimated as 4 times the endotracheal tube size or can be found on a length-based resuscitation tape. Also, any patient with a pneumothorax who will be undergoing mechanical ventilation requires the placement of a chest tube. In the most conservative of scenarios, small (<20%), simple pneumothoraces that are not under tension, and in children who will not be mechanically ventilated, may be observed carefully for extended periods, with treatment of 100% oxygen supplementation and reassessment by repeat chest radiographs at selected intervals.

Tension pneumothorax

The development of pulmonary air leaks that occur in a one-way valve arrangement favors the development of a tension pneumothorax. Increasing amounts of free air within the pleural cavity will cause the mediastinal structures to shift toward the opposite side, compromising cardiac output. The final common pathway involves hypoxia, hypotension, and refractive cardiogenic shock. Most patients will present with severe respiratory distress, decreased breath sounds, and a shift in the point of maximal cardiac impulse. In the worst scenario, the mediastinum shift will force contralateral tracheal deviation and distention of the neck veins. In pediatric patients, signs of tension pneumothorax are often subtle. A short neck and increased soft tissue may make detection of tracheal deviation difficult. Therefore, the evaluation of pediatric patients for tension pneumothorax should consider skin signs and profound tachycardia, suggesting shock. The EP should consider the diagnosis of tension pneumothorax, and if detected or strongly suspected, should immediately treat the patient. Without adequate decompression, circulatory collapse and hypotension will occur.

The treatment for a tension pneumothorax involves rapid evacuation of the trapped air. In the out of hospital setting treatment includes needle thoracostomy placed in the second intercostal space within the midclavicular line or possibly in the fourth intercostal space anterior to the axillary line (nipple line). The needle should be placed above the rib margin to avoid injuring the intercostal vessels. In the ED, definitive treatment involves the use of a large-caliber thoracostomy tube that will favor drainage of the tension pneumothorax and any accompanying hemothorax.

Hemothorax

Significant bleeding may occur when injury is directed toward the intercostal, internal mammary vessels or lung parenchyma. Without an upright chest film, it is difficult to quantify the degree of bleeding on plain radiographs. Development of a massive hemothorax is rare in children and is most associated with severe impact, such as seen in high-velocity MVCs, falls from extreme heights, or the use of high-powered firearms. These injuries must undergo rapid evaluation and treatment. Clinically, patients will present with decreased breath sounds and dullness to percussion on the affected side. A pneumothorax may coexist with a hemothorax. The pediatric patient may present with early or late signs of hypovolemic shock.

Any alteration in cardiovascular sufficiency should be treated with rapid replacement of fluids with isotonic crystalloid solutions. One must also prepare for transfusion with the institution of red blood cell (RBC) replacement as necessary. Patients who present with profound shock may receive either type-specific or O-negative blood, while cross-matched blood may be used for more stable patients. The amount of blood that is salvaged from the chest tube should be quantified to help determine the need for RBC replacement. Many centers have the capability to salvage blood from hemothoraces and reinfuse, using an autotransfuser. As in all cases of trauma, initial measurement of the hemoglobin is often unreliable for estimating the amount of blood loss, since an adequate time interval for equilibration may not yet have passed.

The treatment of hemothorax includes a tube thoracostomy. The tube needs to be large enough to occupy most of the intercostal space and should be placed laterally and directed posteriorly. As in all interventions, repeat chest radiographs should be obtained to confirm positioning and document improvement in lung expansion. Indications for thoracotomy include evacuated blood volumes exceeding 10 to 15 mL/kg of blood, blood loss that exceeds 2 to 4 mL/kg/hr, or continued air leak. ED thoracotomy is reserved for patients suffering penetrating trauma who deteriorate to cardiopulmonary failure despite maximal resuscitation in the out of hospital setting or

ED. The EP will often be able to stabilize the patient with RBC replacement until surgical intervention is achieved [59–61].

Cardiac and vascular injuries

Fortunately, injuries to the heart and large vessels are uncommon in children [62–65]. The most common traumatic cardiovascular injury sustained by children is myocardial contusion. Patients will often present with chest wall tenderness or may have a complaint of generalized chest pain. Tachycardia is the most common finding. Elevation of myocardial enzymes may be diagnostic. Patients with myocardial contusions should be monitored closely for the development of both dysrhythmias and impaired myocardial function; however, in most cases of myocardial contusion, there are no long-term sequelae. The most life-threatening scenario involving the cardiac structures is the development of cardiac tamponade. Extravasated blood will fill the pericardial space and impair cardiac filling during diastole. Tamponade is most often the result of a penetrating wound. Firearm insult will often cause sudden death, and blunt trauma rarely results in the development of cardiac tamponade. Clinically, patients will present with tachycardia, distant heart sounds, narrow pulse pressure, jugular venous distention, and pulsus paradoxus. In the scenario of profound hypovolemia, venous distention will be absent. The final common pathway involves the development of pulseless electrical activity (PEA).

In cardiac and vascular injuries, the ECG may demonstrate anything from tachycardia with low voltage (pericardial tamponade) to findings consistent with acute myocardial infarction (ST elevation). In the subacute scenario, echocardiography will often make the diagnosis. Bedside transthoracic echocardiography will clearly define the degree of pericardial effusion present, as well as the significance of any diastolic dysfunction present. A simple single subxyphoid view during the FAST exam provides the EP with an excellent view of the pericardial sac and heart. Pericardiocentesis may be both diagnostic and therapeutic. Definitive treatment involves drainage of the fluid from the pericardial sac. In certain situations, the amount of pericardial blood and clot will necessitate the performance of a thoracotomy to adequately evacuate the pericardium.

Commotio cordis

Commotio cordis is a disorder described in the pediatric population that results from sudden impact to the anterior chest wall (such as seen in baseball injuries) that causes cessation of normal cardiac function [57,65,66]. The patient may have an immediate dysrhythmia or ventricular fibrillation that is refractory to resuscitation efforts.

Significant morbidity and mortality are associated with this disorder, and, although most recover completely, some patients require extended treatment with antiarrhythmic agents, cardiac pacemaker placement, inotropic agents, or intra-aortic balloon pumps. Cardiogenic shock and death are often frequent outcomes of patients, despite maximal therapeutic interventions [57,66].

Abdominal injuries

Serious abdominal injury accounts for approximately 8% of admissions to pediatric trauma centers [67]. Abdominal trauma is the third leading cause of pediatric traumatic death after head and thoracic injuries and is the most common cause of unrecognized fatal injury in children. Pediatric abdominal trauma results from blunt causes in 85% of cases, and penetrating trauma accounts for the remaining 15%. Of patients presenting primarily for other associated injuries, 9% die from abdominal trauma associated with these injuries.

Blunt trauma related to MVCs causes more than 50% of the abdominal injuries in children and is also the most lethal. "Lap-belt" injury including small bowel injury and Chance fractures occurs in approximately 5% to 10% of restrained children involved in MVCs [68–70]. Another common cause of abdominal injury involves bicycle crashes. Handlebar injuries represent a serious cause of injury and subsequent hospitalization for the pediatric population, with those requiring admission having a mean hospital stay exceeding 3 weeks. Often the effects of bicycle injuries may not be seen on initial presentation, with the mean elapsed time to onset of symptoms being nearly 24 hours.

Sports-related injuries are another common cause of pediatric abdominal trauma. Sports-related injuries are most commonly associated with isolated organ injury as a result of a blow to the abdomen. At particular risk are the spleen, kidney, and intestinal tract in children [71]. Finally, significant abdominal injury occurs in only about 5% of child abuse cases, but it is the second most common cause of death in these cases.

The anatomy of the child lends special protection from some abdominal injury patterns and predisposes the patient to other types of injuries in both blunt and penetrating abdominal trauma [71]. Children have proportionally larger solid organs, less subcutaneous fat, and less protective abdominal musculature than adults and therefore relatively more solid organ injury from both blunt and penetrating mechanisms. Children also have relatively larger kidneys with fetal lobulations that predispose them to renal injury. The child has a fairly flexible cartilaginous ribcage that allows for significant excursion of the lower chest wall, permitting compression of the internal organs. The combination of these factors provides the basis for the differences in abdominal injury patterns seen between children and adults.

Blunt abdominal trauma often presents as a part of the multitraumatized pediatric patient. In the child, history is often limited, traditional signs of decompensation seen in adults are often not as evident, and physical examination can be difficult [71]. Therefore, subtle, early abdominal findings may be overlooked, leading to significant morbidity and mortality. The history and examination of young children who have suffered trauma is challenging, as it may be difficult to know if the child hurts "all over" or has focal findings. The EP may use distraction with toys, lights, or keys to get the child's mind off the examiner and onto the distraction; in this way, areas of tenderness may be located.

Signs and symptoms of abdominal injury in children include tachypnea from impaired diaphragmatic excursion, abdominal tenderness, ecchymosis, and signs of shock. Abdominal distension is a common nonspecific later finding, often the result of air swallowing subsequent to a painful event. Children with hepatic and splenic injuries may have trouble localizing their pain. Thus, any abdominal tenderness on examination should prompt evaluation of the abdomen. Vomiting is usually a late sign or one associated with duodenal hematoma or traumatic pancreatitis. Signs of small bowel injury may be delayed and only noted clinically with serial examinations. Pelvic bone stability and a rectal examination looking for signs of urethral injury (rare) in boys or blood in the stool (both girls and boys) needs to be performed in all cases of serious trauma.

Even minor falls can result in significant splenic injury, but with only minimal findings on examination. Repeated examination, prolonged observation, and close attention to vital signs are warranted. Any child with a clinically suspicious abdominal examination should be evaluated further with additional radiologic and laboratory studies.

In patients with suspect abdominal injury or with mechanisms of possible injury, management and resuscitation must be rapid. Children, because of fear and pain, can compound the difficulties in the management of serious penetrating or blunt abdominal trauma. Children tend to distend the stomach greatly with ingested air that can then decrease the diaphragmatic excursion related to overdistention of the abdomen. This can compromise respiratory efforts, and therefore early decompression via nasogastric or orogastric tube insertion should be considered. Children with a stable pelvis and who are not at risk of urethral trauma should have a urinary catheter inserted to decompress the bladder, evaluate for the presence of urinary retention, and examine for the presence of blood in the urine [72]. Also, before any invasive evaluation of the abdomen, such as DPL, the bladder should be decompressed to prevent accidental laceration during the procedure.

Radiology

Because pediatric patients suffer more from injury to the spleen, liver, kidneys, and the gastrointestinal tract, CT of the abdomen can provide high sensitivity and specificity for identification of these injuries while being relatively noninvasive [23]. That being said, there are adverse effects related to CT in pediatric patients. Because of delays in evaluation, difficulty with administration, and risk for aspiration, the necessity of using oral contrast media in CT is often criticized. The radiation that accompanies CT is also of great concern. Brenner and colleagues [38] estimated that the total number of deaths attributable to 1 year of CT examinations in individuals who were less than 15 years of age at the time of examination is approximately 170 from head CT's and 310 from abdominal CT's [38]. In a 1 year-old child, the lethal malignancy risk from 1 abdominal CT is approximately 1 in 550. It is clear that CT-related malignancy is a major issue. Finding other modalities for predicting and evaluating the pediatric abdomen are needed to reduce that risk.

Another useful procedure in the acutely traumatized pediatric patient is the FAST exam. When used by a properly trained EP, the FAST evaluation has the potential to provide sensitive and specific identification of intraperitoneal hemorrhage without invasive measures. The FAST exam does not have the ability to reliably detect specific organ injuries. Holmes and colleagues [73] conducted a prospective, observational study of children with a mean age of 9.5 (± 4.7 years) with blunt trauma who underwent abdominal ultrasound in the ED (n = 224). They found that of the 13 patients who presented with hypotension, ultrasound had 100% sensitivity, specificity, positive predictive value and negative predictive value for detecting intra-abdominal injury-related hemoperitoneum. The sensitivity and specificities for all 224 patients were 82% and 95% respectively [73]. Soudack and colleagues [74] retrospectively reviewed the medical records and sonographic examinations of 313 patient ages 2 months to 17 years (mean, 7.1 years) who sustained multiple traumatic injuries and had FAST as their initial screening examination. There were 275 patients who had a negative FAST result; 73 subsequently had clinical signs of intra-abdominal injury and underwent CT evaluation. Only 3 of the 73 were positive for parenchymal injury and were managed nonoperatively. They concluded that in their institution, the sensitivities and specificities of the FAST evaluation for the pediatric age group was 92.5% and 97.2%, respectively [74]. The aforementioned studies do have some limitations but prove that the use of the FAST shows promise as an initial screening tool in the pediatric age group.

Although radiological evaluation can provide important diagnostic information in the pediatric patient with possible abdominal trauma, any patient with unstable vital signs should not be delayed in receiving operative intervention. Children with persistent or recurrent hypotension, continued abdominal pain, or persistent abdominal distention should have expedient evaluation by a surgeon [73,75,76].

Traumatic diaphragmatic hernia

Children involved in MVCs who are wearing lap belts are predisposed to the development of diaphragmatic herniation [68,77]. Mechanisms of traumatic diaphragmatic hernia involve sudden compressive forces exerted over the abdomen causing an increase in the intra-abdominal pressure and resulting in tearing of the diaphragm. Patients may initially present in stable condition with the degree of respiratory distress directly proportional to the amount of abdominal contents that protrude into the pulmonary space. Presence of ecchymosis across the abdomen and flanks, which may be secondary to lap belt compression, should alert the clinician to the possibility of diaphragmatic hernia, other intra-abdominal injuries (small bowel injury), and the possibility of associated thoracic spinal insults, such as Chance fractures [68,70]. Unfortunately, traumatic diaphragmatic herniation is one of the most commonly missed injuries and has been reportedly missed in 12% to -66% of cases [78].

Diagnosis is often difficult and although various imaging modalities are available to assist in making the diagnosis, there is no one highly sensitive test. In a retrospective chart review of a mostly adult population, Mihos and colleagues [78] reported an 80% sensitivity in diagnoses using CT alone. That same article reported that the sensitivity of CT ranges from 33% to 83%. This injury can be missed even after undergoing a laparotomy, stressing the difficulty in making the diagnosis.

Initial management for these patients involves placement of a nasogastric tube to decompress the stomach and augment diagnostic imaging. In cases of severe respiratory distress, intubation is indicated. Surgery will be required for repair of the injury.

Splenic injury

Injuries to the spleen are in the largest proportion of pediatric abdominal trauma. Children involved in MVCs, sudden deceleration injuries, and contact sports-related injuries may suffer from splenic trauma. Typical findings include left upper quadrant abdominal pain radiating to the left shoulder. The abdominal examination may show evidence for peritoneal irritation in the left upper quadrant of the abdomen. Patients may be hemodynamically stable or, after significant splenic rupture or laceration, may be persistently hypotensive or in fulminant cardiovascular collapse. A surgeon should evaluate all patients with suspected splenic injury. Stable patients may undergo CT for radiologic evaluation. A FAST exam may reveal associated intraperitoneal hemorrhage, but does not rule out a splenic injury if negative. Most often, with minor splenic trauma, bleeding will spontaneously be controlled without operative intervention. Because of the desire for splenic salvage to maintain immuncompetency, an injured spleen is often left in place as long as the patient can be adequately resuscitated with crystalloid and blood products. In cases with a contained splenic subcapsular hematoma, bleeding may present days later. Patients with splenic injury should be admitted to the hospital for close observation and repeated examinations.

Liver injury

The liver is the second most commonly injured solid organ in the pediatric patient with abdominal trauma. It is the most common cause of lethal hemorrhage, carrying a mortality of 10% to 20% in severe liver injury. Mechanisms of injury causing splenic injury may also cause liver trauma. Tenderness on palpation of the right upper quadrant of the abdomen along with the complaint of abdominal pain in this region or in the right shoulder are signs of possible liver injury. Patients managed conservatively often do well; however, those that are initially treated as such and then go on to require delayed laparotomy often have significant morbidity and mortality. Therefore, close observation in the hospital, serial abdominal examinations, and serial hemoglobin should be performed.

Renal injury

The kidney is less susceptible to trauma from forces applied to the anterior abdomen, but is often injured in the multitrauma pediatric patient [7]. Because this organ is retroperitoneal, complaints of abdominal pain are often less obvious and are more diffuse. Often dull back pain, ecchymosis in the costovertebral region, or hematuria are the only clues to renal injury. Renal ultrasound and CT may be used in the stable patient to assess the degree of renal involvement [41,79,80]. Other organs such as the pancreas and gastrointestinal tract are less frequently injured in the pediatric patient.

Penetrating injury

Penetrating wounds to the abdomen usually require rapid evaluation by a surgeon and in some cases, operative intervention. The role of DPL in the management of pediatric trauma is controversial and seems to be fading out of practice as the FAST exam continues to gain acceptance. DPL provides a rapid, nonspecific evaluation of possible intraperitoneal hemorrhage. Certainly patients who remain unstable despite fluid resuscitation may be candidates for DPL if they are too unstable for CT and there are multiple potential sites of blood loss. An important role for DPL is in the setting of an underlying small bowel injury (SBI). In some patients with SBI, CT findings of free fluid may be improperly ascribed to underlying splenic bleeding. Finally, DPL may be considered in the operating room for patients undergoing emergent craniotomy, when adequate evaluation of the abdomen cannot take place because of the time urgency required for intervention for head injury. If the wound appears superficial and does not appear to travel below the abdominal musculoaponeurotic layer, local exploration by an experienced surgeon may be useful [17].

Disposition

Finally, the EP must decide to admit the pediatric trauma patient, transfer the patient to a tertiary care facility, or discharge the patient. The decision for admission should be based on consultation with the surgeon and the patient's primary care physician. Infants and children who are moderately to severely injured have improved outcomes in a pediatric intensive care unit (PICU) versus an adult ICU; therefore, the primary role of the EP

Box 9. Indications for surgery

- Hemodynamic instability despite maximal resuscitative efforts
- Transfusion of greater than 50% of total blood volume
- Radiographic evidence of pneumoperitoneum, intraperitoneal bladder rupture, grade V renovascular injury
- Gunshot would to the abdomen
- Evisceration of intraperitoneal or stomach contents
- Signs of peritonitis
- Evidence of fecal or bowel contamination on diagnostic peritoneal lavage

would be to evaluate and stabilize the patient before admission to a PICU or before transfer to a tertiary care facility. Before transport, it is vital that the child be appropriately stabilized and that the EP communicates directly with the accepting physician at the transfer facility.

Indications for admission are many, but the main principle is to admit patients requiring ongoing monitoring for deterioration or complications of their injuries. Indications for surgery are outlined in (Box 9). Whatever the surgical preference within a health care facility, it is most important to establish a protocol for approaching these challenging patients. Of course, patients who remain hypotensive after adequate crystalloid infusion are candidates for early operative exploration. In addition, children with suspected physical injury from child abuse may be admitted for their protection as well as for medical treatment.

Summary

Trauma remains the leading cause of death in children nationwide. Proper management of the pediatric trauma patient involves most of the components of standard trauma protocols. By paying strict attention to the anatomic and physiologic differences in children, the clinician will be ensured the best patient outcomes.

References

[1] Jaffe D. Emergency management of blunt trauma in children. N Engl J Med 1991;324: 1477–82.

[2] Miniño A, Heron M, Smith B, et al. Deaths: final data for 2004. National vital statistics reports. Hyattsville (MD). National Center for Health Statistics.

[3] King DR. Trauma in infancy and childhood: initial evaluation and management. Pediatr Clin North Am 1985;32:1299–310.

[4] Langlois JA, Rutland-Brown W, Thomas KE. Traumatic brain injury in the United States: emergency department visits, hospitalizations, and deaths. Atlanta (GA): Centers for Disease Control and Prevention, National Center for Injury Prevention and Control; 2006.
[5] Peclet MH, Newman KD, Eichelberger MR, et al. Patterns of injury in children. J Pediatr Surg 1990;25:85–90.
[6] Sieben RL, Leavitt JD, French JH. Falls as childhood accidents: an increasing urban risk. Pediatrics 1971;47:886.
[7] Ablu-Jaude WA. Indicators of genitourinary tract injury or anomaly in cases of pediatric blunt trauma. J Pediatr Surg 1996;31:86.
[8] Corey TS. Infant deaths due to unintentional injury: an 11-year autopsy review. Am J Dis Child 1992;146:968–71.
[9] Schafer I, Barkmann C, Riedesser P, et al. Posttraumatic syndromes in children and adolescents after road traffic accidents—a prospective cohort study. Psychopathology 2006;39(4):159–64.
[10] Gausche M, Lewis RJ, Stratton SJ, et al. Effect of out-of-hospital pediatric endotracheal intubation on survival and neurological outcome: a controlled clinical trial. JAMA 2000;283:783–9.
[11] Part 12: Pediatric Advanced Life Support Circulation 112: IV-167-187IV-; published online before print as doi:10.1161/CIRCULATIONAHA.105.166573.
[12] Waltzman ML, Mooney DP. Major trauma. In: Fleisher GR, Ludwig S, Henretig FM, editors. Textbook of pediatric emergency medicine. 5th edition. Philadelphia: Lippincott Williams & Wilkins; 2006. p. 1339–48.
[13] Kanter RK, Zimmerman JJ, Strauss RH, et al. Pediatric emergency intravenous access. Evaluation of a protocol. Am J Dis Child 1986;140:132–4.
[14] Hodge D, Delgado-Paredes C, Fleisher G. Intraosseous infusion flow rates in hypovolemic "pediatric" dogs. Ann Emerg Med 1987;16:305–7.
[15] Fiser DH. Intraosseous infusion. N Engl J Med 1990;322:1579–81.
[16] Banerjee S, Singhi SC, Singh S, et al. The intraosseous route is a suitable alternative to intravenous route for fluid resuscitation in severely dehydrated children. Indian Pediatr 1994;31:1511–20.
[17] American college of surgeons. Advanced Trauma Life Support (ATLS) student course manual. 7th edition. Chicago: American College of Surgeons; 2004.
[18] Furnival RA. Delayed diagnosis of injury in pediatric trauma. Pediatrics 1996;98:56–62.
[19] Brown K, Bocock J. Update in pediatric emergecy resuscitation. Emerg Med Clin North Am 2002;20(1):1–26.
[20] Holmes JF, Sokolove PE, Brant WE, et al. Identification of children with intraabdominal injuries after blunt trauma. Ann Emerg Med 2002;39:500–9.
[21] Isaacman DJ. Utility of routine laboratory testing for detecting intra-abdominal injury (IAI) in the pediatric trauma patient. Pediatrics 1993;92:691–4.
[22] Zehtabchi S, Sinert R, Goldman M, et al. Diagnostic performance of serial haematocrit measurements in identifying major injury in adult trauma patients. Injury 2006;37:46–52.
[23] Stanescu LA, Gross JA, Bittle M, et al. Imaging of blunt abdominal trauma. Semin Roentgenol 2006;41(3):196–208.
[24] Saladino RA, Lund DP. Abdominal trauma. In: Fleisher GR, Ludwig S, Henretig FM, editors. Textbook of pediatric emergency medicine. 5th edition. Philadelphia: Lippincott Williams & Wilkins; 2006. p. 1339–48.
[25] Rose JS. Ultrasound in abdominal trauma. Emerg Med Clin North Am 2004;22(3):581–9.
[26] Theissen ML, Woolridge DP. Pediatric minor closed head injury. Pediatr Clin North Am 2006;53:1–26.
[27] Lescholier I. Blunt trauma in children: causes and outcomes of head vs extracranial injuries. Pediatrics 1993;91:721–5.

[28] Agran RA, Dunkle DE. Motor vehicle occupant injuries to children in crash and non crash events. Pediatrics 1982;70:993.
[29] Quayle KS, Jaffe DM, Kuppermann N, et al. Diagnostic testing for acute head injury in children: when are head computed tomography and skull radiographs indicated? Pediatrics 1998;99(5):1–8.
[30] Ghajar J. Management of pediatric head injury. Pediatr Clin North Am 1992;39:1093–125.
[31] Lieh-Lai MW. Limitations of the Glasgow Coma Scale in predicting outcome in children with traumatic brain injury. J Pediatr 1992;120:195–9.
[32] Hennes H. Clinical predictors of severe head trauma in children. Am J Dis Child 1988;142: 1045–7.
[33] Kadish HA. Pediatric basilar skull fracture: do children with normal neurologic findings and no intracranial injury require hospitalization? Ann Emerg Med 1995;26:37–41.
[34] McCrory P, Johnston K, Meeuwisse W, et al. Summary and agreement statement of the 2nd international conference on concussion in sport, Prague 2004. Clin J Sport Med 2005;15(2): 48–55.
[35] Saunders RL, Harbaugh RE. The second impact in catastrophic contact-sports head trauma. JAMA 1984;252:538–9.
[36] Cantu RC. Second impact syndrome. Clin Sports Med 1998;17(1):37–44.
[37] Schutzman SA, Barnes P, Dunhaime A, et al. Evaluation and management of children younger than two years old with apparently mild head trauma: proposed guidelines. Pediatrics 2001;107:983–93.
[38] Brenner D, Elliston C, Hall E, et al. Estimated risks of radiation-induced fatal cancer from pediatric CT. AJR Am J Roentgenol 2001;176(2):289–96.
[39] Davis RL. Cranial CT scans in children after minimal head injury with loss of consciousness. Ann Emerg Med 1994;24:640–5.
[40] Davis RL. The use of cranial CT scans in the triage of pediatric patients with mild head injuries. Pediatrics 1995;95:345.
[41] Livingston DH. The use of CT scanning to triage patients requiring admission following minimal head injury. J Trauma 1991;31:483–7.
[42] Greenes DS. Clinical indicators of intracranial injury in head-injured infants. Pediatrics 1999;104:861–7.
[43] Kupperman N, Holmes J, Dayan P, et al. Blunt head trauma in the pediatric emergency care applied research network (PECARN). Acad Emerg Med 2007;14(5):Suppl. 1.
[44] Apple JS, Kirks DR, Merten DF, et al. Cervical spine fractures and dislocations in children. Pediatr Radiol 1987;17:45–9.
[45] Chen LS, Blaw ME. Acute central cervical cord syndrome caused by minor trauma. J Pediatr 1986;108:96–7.
[46] Cirak B, Ziegfeld S, Knight V, et al. Spinal injures in children. J Pediatr Surg 2004;39:607–12.
[47] Reynolds R. Pediatric spinal injury. Curr Opin Pediatr 2000;12:67–71.
[48] Pang D. Spinal cord injury without radiologic abnomality in children, 2 decades later. Neurosurgery 2004;55:1325–43.
[49] Hadley MN, Zabramski JM, Browner CM, et al. Pediatric spinal trauma: review of 122 cases of spinal cord and vertebral column injuries. J Neurosurg 1988;68:18–24.
[50] Hill SA, Miller CA, Kosnik EJ, et al. Pediatric neck injuries: a clinical study. J Neurosurg 1984;60:700–6.
[51] Pang D, Wilberger JE. Spinal cord injury without radiographic abnormalities in children. J Neurosurg 1982;57:114.
[52] Viccellio P, Simon H, Pressman BD, et al, NEXUS Group. A prospective multicenter study of cervical spine injury in children. Pediatrics 2001;108(2):E20.
[53] Mower WR, Hoffman JR, Pollack CV Jr, et al, NEXUS Group. Use of plain radiography to screen for cervical spine injuries. Ann Emerg Med 2001;38(1):1–7.
[54] Cattell HS, Filtzer DL. Pseudosubluxation and other normal variations in the cervical spine in children. J Bone Joint Surg Am 1965;47:1295–309.

[55] Strange GR, editor. APLS: The pediatric emergency medicine course. Elk Grove (IL): American academy of pediatrics and American college of emergency physicians; 1998.
[56] Copley LA, Dormans JP. Cervical spine disorders in infants and children. J Am Acad Orthop Surg 1998;6:204–14.
[57] Maron BJ. Blunt impact to the chest leading to sudden death from cardiac arrest during sports activities. N Engl J Med 1995;333:337–42.
[58] Bender TM. Pediatric chest trauma. J Thorac Imaging 1987;2:60.
[59] Meller JL, Little AG, Shermeta DW. Thoracic trauma in children. Pediatrics 1984;74:813.
[60] Eichelberger MR. Trauma of the airway and thorax. Pediatr Ann 1987;16:307.
[61] Cooper A. Thoracic trauma. In: Barkin RM, editor. Pediatric emergency medicine: concepts in clinical practice. St Louis (MO): Mosby; 1992.
[62] Eshel G. Cardiac injuries caused by blunt chest trauma in children. Pediatr Emerg Care 1987;3:96–8.
[63] Fishbone G, Robbins DI, Osborn DJ, et al. Trauma to the thoracic aorta and great vessels. Radiol Clin North Am 1973;11:543–54.
[64] Tellez DW. Blunt cardiac injury in children. J Pediatr Surg 1987;22:1123–8.
[65] Abrunzo TJ. Commotio cordis: the single most common cause of traumatic death in youth baseball. Am J Dis Child 1991;145:1279–82.
[66] Amerongen RV. Ventricular fibrillation following blunt chest trauma from a baseball. Pediatr Emerg Care 1997;13:107–10.
[67] Schafermeyer RW. Pediatric trauma. Emerg Med Clin North Am 1993;11:187.
[68] Sivit CJ. Safety-belt injuries in children with lap-belt ecchymosis. AJR Am J Roentgenol 1991;157:111–4.
[69] Angran PF, Dunkle DE, Winn DG. Injuries to a sample of seat belted children evaluated and treated in a hospital emergency room. J Trauma 1987;27:58.
[70] Sturm PF. Lumbar compression fractures secondary to lap-belt use in children. J Pediatr Orthop 1995;15:521–3.
[71] Saladino R. The spectrum of liver and spleen injuries in children: failure of the PTS and clinical signs to predict isolated injuries. Ann Emerg Med 1991;20:636–40.
[72] Stalker HP. The significance of hematuria in children after blunt abdominal trauma. AJR Am J Roentgenol 1990;154:569–71.
[73] Holmes JF, Brant WE, Bond WF, et al. Emergency department ultrasonography in the evaluation of hypotensive and normotensive children with blunt abdominal trauma. J Pediatr Surg 2001;36(7):968–73.
[74] Soudack M, Epelman M, Maor R, et al. Experience with Focused Abdominal Sonography for Trauma (FAST) in 313 pediatric patients. Journal of Clinical Ultrasound 2004;32:53–61.
[75] Thourani VH, Pettitt BJ, Schmidt JA, et al. Validation of surgeon-performed emergency abdominal ultrasonography in pediatric trauma patients. J Pediatr Surg 1998;33(2):322–8.
[76] Ong AW, McKenney MG, McKenney KA, et al. Predicting the need for laparotomy in pediatric trauma patients on the basis of the ultrasound score. J Trauma 2003;54:503–8.
[77] Wiencek RG, Wilson RF, Steiger Z. Acute injuries of the diaphragm. J Thorac Cardiovasc Surg 1986;92:989–93.
[78] Mihos P, Potaris K, Gakidis J, et al. Traumatic rupture of the diaphragm: experience with 65 patients. Injury 2003;34:169–72.
[79] Bass DH. Investigation and management of blunt renal injuries in children. J Pediatr Surg 1991;26:196–200.
[80] Stein JP. Blunt renal trauma in the pediatric population: indications for radiographic evaluation. Urology 1994;44:406.
[81] Bracken MB, Shepard MJ, Holford TR. Administration of methyprednisolone for 24 or 48 hours or tirilazid mesylate for 48 hours in the treatment of acute spinal cord injury. JAMA 1997;277(20):1597–604.

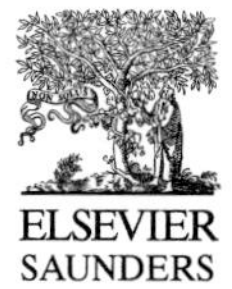

ELSEVIER
SAUNDERS

Emerg Med Clin N Am 25 (2007) 837–860

EMERGENCY
MEDICINE
CLINICS OF
NORTH AMERICA

Geriatric Trauma

David W. Callaway, MD*, Richard Wolfe, MD

Department of Emergency Medicine, Beth Israel Deaconess Medical Center, One Deaconess Road, W/CC-2, Boston, MA 02215, USA

The growth of the elderly population has greatly exceeded that of the remainder of the population. From 1900 to 1994, the elderly experienced an 11-fold increase, whereas the rest of the population only grew threefold [1]. Elderly patients today have an increased risk for trauma from an increasingly active life style and from impaired motor and cognitive functions. The elderly require far less mechanism to produce injuries. For all of these reasons the dramatic growth experienced in the number and severity of geriatric trauma patients can be expected to continue.

The elderly often require greater health care resources than younger patients who have similar injuries. Assessing the cost/benefit ratios of aggressive testing and interventions can be much more difficult in this group. Subsequent quality of life is also a key factor in decision making. Aggressive care and resuscitation have a dramatic effect in improving outcome in these patients. Because they are more challenging in underlying risk and occult presentations and because they benefit from resuscitation, they actually deserve a more aggressive approach than younger patients who have similar mechanism during their initial emergency management.

Triage

Advanced age clearly correlates with elevated mortality in trauma [2–4]. The largest trial evaluating the relationship between age and trauma mortality, the MTOS study, demonstrated that patients older than 65 years of age had elevated mortality across matched Injury Severity Score (ISS), mechanism of trauma, and body region injured [3]. Although age correlates with both early (<24 hours) and late (>24 hours) mortality across the geriatric trauma population, no literature clearly delineates a specific age above which trauma predicts increased in-hospital mortality [5]. Most studies on

* Corresponding author.
E-mail address: dcallawa@bidmc.harvard.edu (D.W. Callaway).

doi:10.1016/j.emc.2007.06.005 *emed.theclinics.com*

age and mortality are retrospective and may be affected by institutional biases toward or away from aggressive care in the elderly. With aggressive resuscitation, some studies suggest that up to 85% of elderly trauma patients return to independent living [5]. Advanced age should therefore heighten a physician's concern and prompt more aggressive care; it should not be used as a triage tool to limit care. Despite these recommendations and observations, studies indicate that undertriage of elderly trauma patients occurs twice as frequently as with younger patients [6,7].

In triaging the trauma patient, the physicians must balance the benefits of medical or surgical intervention with prognosis, resource use, and patient wishes. In the elderly, universally higher mortality, preexisting medical conditions, and a paucity of randomized prospective control trials complicate the triage process. Further, traditional triage tools, such as mechanism of trauma and vital signs, may be misleading in the elderly trauma patient. Physicians cannot use injury mechanism to reliably triage patients because the elderly are particularly susceptible to significant trauma from low-energy mechanisms. For example, 30% of the population older than 65 fall each year—the most common mechanism of trauma in the elderly. More than 6% of these falls result in fractures and 10% to 30% result in significant trauma [8] with a mortality rate approaching 7% [9].

Trauma severity scores seem to correlate with mortality in the elderly [5]. In the emergency department, the two most useful scores are the Trauma Score (TS) and Revised Trauma Score (RTS). The TS assesses blood pressure, respiratory rate, respiratory effort, Glasgow Coma Score (GCS), and capillary refill to produce a minimum score of zero and maximum score of 16. The RTS is similar, but does not account for respiratory effort or capillary refill (scores 0–8). Although studies are mixed, the RTS and TS seem to be useful tools in the triage of elderly trauma patients. Several studies demonstrated a universal mortality for elderly patients who had TS less than 7 to 9 [10,11]. These studies suggested an inverse relationship between TS or RTS and mortality, with patients having a TS from 7 to 14 benefiting most from aggressive resuscitation (Table 1). These studies also demonstrated that each component of the TS or RTS independently predicts mortality. For example, in Knudson's study [10] the geriatric trauma patient who had a respiratory rate less than 10 beats per minute (bpm) had

Table 1
Trauma score predicts mortality

Trauma score	Mortality
15–16	5%
12–14	25%
<12	65%

Data from Knudson MM, Lieberman J, Morris J, et al. Mortality factors in geriatric blunt trauma patients. Arch Surg 1994;129:448.

a 100% mortality. The ISS also seems to predict mortality in the elderly [12,13]. Within each category (ie, mild, moderate, and severe) the elderly demonstrated higher mortality than younger patients, with the most dramatic disparity in the moderately injured (ISS 16–24) who had a mortality of 30%, five times that of the younger cohort [3,10]. Unfortunately, the ISS may not represent the full potential for mortality in elderly trauma patients and its use in the emergency department is limited by a lack of timely availability of critical score components.

The exact relationship between TS, RTS, ISS, and mortality in the geriatric trauma patient is debated. These scoring systems represent clinical decision-making tools that can assist the physician in the initial trauma assessment. Geriatric trauma patients are extremely susceptible to adverse outcome from even minor trauma. The clinician's pretest probability for significant occult injury should be high. The most appropriate triage approach seems to use a combination of TS and RTS, clinical impression, age, and physiologic parameters to quickly classify patients as "unstable" or "apparently stable." The apparently stable patients are the most challenging and warrant exhaustive investigation to ensure a lack of occult pathology.

The American College of Surgeons currently recommends that emergency medical services transport trauma patients older than 55 years to a designated trauma center regardless of apparent injury severity [14]. Automatic trauma team activation should be considered for trauma patients older than 75 years regardless of mechanism or prehospital physiologic status [15].

Assessment and resuscitation

Several unique considerations are relevant during the primary and secondary survey of the elderly trauma patient. Physicians should be aware of the basic physiologic and anatomic change associated with aging and the potentially complicating role of medications and prosthetic devices. The principles of advanced trauma life support remain vital guidelines during the initial assessment and treatment. Of critical importance is prompt, aggressive resuscitation in the unstable elderly trauma patient and expedient directed evaluation of the apparently stable patient [16].

Attention to vital signs is particularly important in the elderly. Although abnormal vitals signs clearly warrant further investigation and direct resuscitation, normal vital signs should not necessarily reassure the physician. A normal blood pressure for a younger patient can constitute frank hypotension in an elderly patient who has a hypertensive history. Vital sign trends are critical in the severely injured elderly trauma patient. Nursing staff should to obtain and track vital signs, reporting any changes during the emergency department course. On arrival intravenous access should be obtained, supplemental oxygen given, and the patient should be placed on a cardiac monitor.

Airway

Supplemental oxygen should be placed on all elderly trauma patients. This practice provides the needed oxygen reserves if rapid sequence intubation is needed and contributes to cellular oxygenation. Early airway adjuncts, such as nasopharyngeal and oropharyngeal airways, are useful with the obtunded trauma patient. Elderly often have friable nasal mucosa and care should be taken when using the nasal passage for airway support or gastric decompression. Nasal hemorrhage from vigorous tube insertion can result in hemorrhage that is difficult to control and may complicate further airway management. Ventilation with a bag-valve mask can be complicated by an edentulous airway. The oral cavity should always be examined and poorly fitting or loose dental appliances should be removed (well-fitting dentures should be left in place when using bag-valve mask but must be removed before attempts at intubation).

Endotracheal intubation should be considered early in patients who have demonstrable signs of shock, significant chest trauma, or mental status changes [14]. Securing the airway in the elderly trauma patient can be challenging. Loss of the kyphotic curve, spondylolysis, arthritis, and spinal canal stenosis decrease cervical spine mobility. Inability to hyperextend the neck limits adequate visualization of the vocal cords. In addition to limiting range of motion, age-related arthritic and osteoporotic changes increase the incidence of cervical spine injury during instrumentation [17]. Maintenance of in-line stabilization is critical, but further impedes visualization of landmarks and placement of the endotracheal tube. Microstomia from systemic sclerosis and temporomandibular joint arthritis may limit access to the oral cavity and mandate use of a smaller laryngoscopic blade. Finally, delicate pharyngeal tissue in the elderly is more susceptible to trauma with subsequent bleeding that can obscure visualization of the vocal cords. The physician must take great care when inserting the laryngoscope blade to avoid traumatizing the soft palate and posterior pharynx.

Rapid sequence induction medication doses often require adjusting in the elderly trauma patient (Table 2). Relative contraindications to succinylcholine, such as hyperkalemia and prolonged immobility, are more frequent in the elderly patient. If uncertain, rocuronium or another nondepolarizing neuromuscular agent can be substituted. Priming doses of nondepolarizing agents should be avoided given the significant risk for completely abolishing airway and ventilatory reflexes [18,19]. Age-related decline in renal clearance and hepatic function increases sensitivity to opioids, benzodiazepines, and sedatives, such as etomidate. Resultant hypotension is the primary adverse outcome. The adrenal axis remains largely intact in the elderly and the potential transient adrenal suppression from etomidate is unlikely to have

Table 2
Rapid sequence induction medications and suggested dose adjustments

Medication	Adjustment
Succinylcholine 1.5 mg/kg IV	No change
Etomidate 0.1–0.2 mg/kg IV	Decreased from 0.3 mg/kg IV
Versed	Decrease 20%–40%
Fentanyl	Decrease 20%–40%
Ketamine	Should be avoided secondary to cardiac effects

Abbreviation: IV, intravenous.

clinically significant adverse effects [20]. In general, these medications are safe and appropriate at reduced doses.

Breathing

Aging has a myriad of effects on pulmonary function. Primarily, these changes can be classified as anatomic changes that increase susceptibility to trauma and physiologic changes that diminish protective responses to injury. Osteoporosis decreases rib durability and increases incidence of rib fractures. These changes create a brittle chest wall that is highly susceptible to rib fracture, sternal fracture, and pulmonary contusions even from seemingly low-energy trauma. Weakened respiratory muscles and degenerative changes decrease chest wall compliance and diminish maximum inspiratory and expiratory force by up to 50% [19]. Baseline age-related reductions in vital capacity, functional residual capacity and forced expiratory volume limit the elderly patient's ability to compensate for these injuries and dramatically increases mortality compared with younger patients. Increased splinting leads to hypoventilation, atelectasis, and subsequent pneumonia. As a result, apparently minor chest injuries frequently result in significant thoracic complications and patient morbidity.

Rib fractures and flail chest result in significantly higher morbidity and mortality in the elderly. Elderly blunt trauma patients also seem more susceptible to sternal fractures [21]. Physical examination findings, such as paradoxical chest wall movement, chest wall tenderness, crepitus, or ecchymosis, should prompt immediate action. The elderly have blunted responses to hypoxia, hypercarbia (response to hypoxia and hypercarbia declines by 50% and 40%, respectively, in the elderly), and acidosis that may delay the onset of clinically apparent signs of impending distress. Arterial blood gas measurements are therefore also an important component of the trauma assessment in geriatric patients.

Circulation

Elderly patients are particularly susceptible to the untoward effects of shock. Catecholamine insensitivity, atherosclerosis, myocyte fibrosis, and conduction abnormalities attenuate the elderly patient's chronotropic response to hypovolemia. Common medications, such as beta blockers and calcium channel blockers, can further limit the normal tachycardic response to shock. Baseline hypertension is more frequent in the elderly patient; thus normal blood pressure readings may actually indicate significant hypovolemia in the elderly patient. Resuscitation with intravenous fluid or blood should not be delayed during the assessment of the unstable patient.

The first critical step is to quickly identify and control life-threatening bleeding. External bleeding is usually obvious. Internal bleeding must be rapidly diagnosed in the elderly. As in most blunt trauma patients, the abdomen is a frequent culprit in hemorrhagic shock in the elderly. The general indications for Focused Assessment with Sonography for Trauma (FAST) and diagnostic peritoneal lavage (DPL) are similar in elderly trauma patients. In hemodynamically unstable patients, the FAST has a reported sensitivity of 90% to 98% and specificity of 99.7% for detecting clinically significant hemoperitoneum [22,23]. In particular, the FAST examination has sensitivities of 98% for detecting hemoperitoneum associated with grade III or greater liver injuries [24]. In hemodynamically stable trauma patients, ultrasound may lack sensitivity for detecting small amounts (less than 400 mL) of intraperitoneal fluid.

Patients who have hypotension and a positive FAST examination require prompt laparotomy [25]. In patients who have hypotension and an initially negative FAST, further evaluation is indicated, including either DPL or frequent repeated FAST examinations. Secondary or serial examinations dramatically increase the sensitivity and negative predictive value of the FAST [26].

Disability and exposure

Poor nutrition, loss of lean muscle mass, microvascular changes, and blunted hypothalamic function increase the elderly trauma patient's risk for hypothermia and pressure sores. Hypothermia drastically increases mortality in the hemorrhaging trauma patient. Rectal temperature should be obtained on major trauma patients. External rewarming with forced air warming systems (eg, Bair Hugger warming unit), heating blankets, and increased ambient temperature can decrease rates of hypothermia-induced coagulopathy. Additionally, intravenous fluid and blood products should be warmed by standard protocols. All efforts should be made to quickly clear the spine and remove patients from the hard backboard. Several orthopedic and wound-management studies have shown that in the elderly, the pathologic process of pressure sores begins early in the hospital course [27]. Pressure sores increase hospital length of stay, patient morbidity, and subsequent mortality. Action taken in the emergency department could thus significantly reduce length of stay, hospitalization costs, and patient morbidity.

In the emergency department, the patient's hemodynamic status determines the depth of the secondary examination. In the unstable patient, the physician should perform a rapid secondary survey that focuses on the neurologic examination. Three key components are GCS, pupil responsiveness, and gross motor examination. GCS predicts mortality and may influence treatment or disposition decisions [28]. Although the literature does not support a specific GCS on which to make triage decisions, the elderly have uniformly poor outcomes with scores less than 8 [29,30]. Altered pupil response and motor function may raise suspicions of intracranial hemorrhage that requires intracranial pressure monitoring before other operative intervention. Glaucoma, prior cataract surgery, and systemic medications can confuse the geriatric ophthalmologic examination.

Diagnostic imaging

Chest radiography

Chest radiographs are a standard component of nearly all trauma resuscitation protocols and are useful for rapid identification of life-threatening conditions, such as tension pneumothoraces. Plain film chest radiography fails to identify up to 50% of rib fractures, however, and has significantly lower sensitivity for aortic dissection [31,32]. In the elderly trauma patient, these limitations carry obvious clinical significance. Multidetector CT (MDCT) is superior to plain films for detecting rib fractures and concomitant torso injuries. Chest radiographs are useful in the unstable patient. MDCT should generally be considered the imaging modality of choice, however, in the elderly patient who has torso trauma.

Pelvic radiography

Several studies suggest a diminishing role for a routine plain radiograph of the pelvis in the alert, hemodynamically stable blunt trauma patient [33,34]. When clinical decision rules that identify low-risk patients (ie, no altered mental status, no pelvic pain or tenderness, no intoxication, and absence of distracting injury) are applied to stable patients, physical examination has a sensitivity of 98% for all pelvic fractures and 100% for clinically significant injuries [34]. In contrast, physical examination alone misses up to 20% of significant pelvic fractures in unstable patients [35]. Similar guidelines seem reasonable in the elderly trauma patient. Unstable patients should have routine pelvic plain films between the primary and secondary survey to rule out major pelvic fractures. In the stable patient, plain films may be useful to identify hip fractures in the polytrauma patient. A thorough clinical examination should suffice, however, even in the elderly [36].

Computed tomography torso

Computed tomography is a highly sensitive and specific diagnostic tool and is the primary mode of evaluation for most elderly abdominal trauma victims. The threshold to use CT in elderly victims of blunt abdominal trauma should be low.

The CT torso allows accurate assessment of the aorta, heart, bowel, pulmonary parenchyma, solid viscera, chest wall, pelvis, and spine. In adult blunt trauma patients, administration of oral contrast is rarely necessary on initial examination [37]. Oral contrast delays imaging and disposition of the patient while adding only minimal clinically relevant information on the general trauma patient. Noncontrast CT accurately detects pulmonary contusions, rib fractures, and significant pericardial effusions and has sensitivity and specificity up to 82% and 99% for detecting bowel or mesenteric injuries that require surgical repair [37].

The administration of intravenous contrast does provide useful clinical information. CT with intravenous (IV) contrast can delineate aortic injuries, reliably identify and grade solid organ injury, and further delineate injuries to the bowel and mesentery. The American Association for the Surgery of Trauma classification system for solid organ injury has been shown to correlate relatively well with mortality and the need for operative intervention [38]. Abnormal vascular patterns on CT (ie, contrast extravasation or contrast blush) correlate highly with the need for operative intervention or angiographic embolization of splenic and hepatic injuries. Contrast "blush" often corresponds to pseudoaneurysms of the splenic artery or its branches. The natural history of the lesions is not well studied, but may relate to delayed bleeding and subsequent failure of nonoperative management (NOM) [39]. Contrast extravasation is more vague and represents any pooling of contrast material outside of the splenic parenchyma. Active contrast extravasation has been shown to predict failure of NOM of splenic and hepatic injuries [40]. Recent evidence suggests that delayed-phase CT scans may better differentiate active hemorrhage from contained vascular leakage in adult solid organ injuries [41].

Intravenous contrast is not without risk. Preexisting renal insufficiency, diabetes mellitus, dehydration, hypotension, heart failure, and age greater than 75 years are well-identified risk factors for contrast-induced nephropathy (CIN) [42]. CIN is defined as an acute increase in serum creatinine of greater than 25% [43]. The elderly trauma patient is at particularly high risk for developing CIN. Strategies to reduce the incidence of CIN include extracellular volume expansion, premedication with bicarbonate or *N*-acetylcysteine, minimizing the dose of contrast media, using low-osmolar nonionic contrast media, stopping the intake of nephrotoxic drugs, and avoiding short intervals between procedures [44]. Ultimately, the clinician must weigh the risks and benefits of using intravenous contrast.

Computed tomography of the torso has the added advantage of allowing three-dimensional reconstruction imaging of the thoracic and lumbar spine. The incidence of vertebral fractures increases with age. Osteoporosis and calcific changes to supporting ligaments increase bone fragility and decrease the energy required to produce fractures. The clinician must have high clinical suspicion of vertebral fractures in all elderly trauma patients, especially those who have apparently minor injuries. All patients who have pain, tenderness, palpable deformity, or neurologic deficit should have imaging of the entire spine given high rates of polytrauma. Physical examination is notoriously inaccurate in identifying vertebral fractures [45,46]. In the asymptomatic patient, plain film radiography may be considered, but is often limited by normal age-related changes in the spine.

CT, especially spiral CT, is the imaging modality of choice for evaluation of the spine in the elderly trauma patient. Sensitivity and specificity of CT scans for thoracolumbar fractures are 100% and 97%, respectively, with a negative predictive value (NPV) of 100% [46,47]. Plain film radiographs are approximately 70% sensitive and 100% specific with NPV rates of 92% [46]. Admission torso CT with reconstructions is rapid and accurate and provides other critical information in the polytrauma patient (eg, evaluation of the aorta, solid organs, retroperitoneum, and so forth). The speed of CT evaluation is an additional advantage. Several studies have shown that CT-based protocols decrease patient manipulation, reduce per-patient cost, and improve time to definitive diagnosis.

Cranial computed tomography

Despite lower Glasgow outcome scale, functional independence measures, and longer rehabilitation for the elderly, some studies estimate that 82% of elderly patients hospitalized with traumatic brain injury (TBI) return to independent living if properly treated [48]. Early diagnosis and treatment of significant injuries is therefore critical. Multiple studies show that clinical variables are insufficient to reliably predict all cases of significant intracranial lesions following mild or minor head trauma in the elderly trauma patient [49]. Although loss of consciousness has a strong positive predictive value (PPV) for identifying clinically relevant intracranial hemorrhage in elderly patients taking Coumadin, most data suggest that normal GCS and physical examination cannot reliably exclude significant intracranial pathology in the elderly trauma patients who has even minor head trauma [50]. All patients older than 65 years who have closed head injury are at high risk for neurosurgical intervention (Canadian CT Head Rule [CCHR] and New Orleans Criteria [NOC]) [51,52]. Most studies support the liberal use of CT in the evaluation of elderly trauma patients who have closed head injuries as cost effective and clinically appropriate [53].

There is some debate in the literature concerning the evaluation of mild or minor head trauma in the elderly patient. Currently, there are no validated clinical pathways for identifying elderly TBI patients who can be safely managed without cranial CT. The two largest studies examining cranial CT in minor head injuries, the NOC and CCHR, categorized elderly patients as high risk and therefore excluded them from the algorithm. Other studies confirm the relationship between age and increased rates of TBI.

Gittleman and colleagues [54] reported that adult patients who had head trauma and a GCS of less than 15 were 42 times more likely to have abnormal cranial CT than younger patients. Similarly, Stein and Ross reported a 40% abnormal CT rate in adult patients who had closed head injury and GCS less than 13. In one recent study of geriatric patients who had mild head injury, 14% of patients had evidence of injury on cranial CT and one fifth of these required neurosurgical intervention [50].

Management

The elderly have increased mortality across all categories of the trimodal death curve: immediate (ie, at the scene), early (ie, within the first 24–48 hours), and delayed (ie, after 48–72 hours). Aggressive resuscitation, liberal radiographic examination, and early intensive monitoring or operative intervention are essential for reducing early mortality in the elderly trauma patient. Preventing delayed complications of trauma, such as cardiovascular compromise, sepsis, pneumonia, and multiorgan failure, is critical. Elderly trauma patients have reported in-hospital complication rates of 33%, compared with 19% for younger patients [10]. Cardiovascular events (23%) and pneumonia (22%) are the most common and most clinically significant. Prevention of these delayed complications begins in the emergency department.

Resuscitation

Elderly trauma patients have increased mortality for given ISS, RTS, and GCS than younger cohorts. Shock and occult hypoperfusion (OH) reliably predict mortality in the elderly trauma patient [10,55]. Two retrospective studies showed that in elderly blunt trauma a systolic blood pressure less than 90 mm Hg was associated with mortality rates of 82% to 100% [10,11]. Unfortunately, preexisting conditions can obscure the diagnosis of these entities and complicate resuscitation efforts. Congestive heart failure, coronary artery disease (CAD), and renal insufficiency commonly result in baseline fluid overload, further complicating the clinical picture.

Patients in florid shock should undergo aggressive resuscitation with IV fluid or blood and the cause of the shock should be identified. Crystalloid is the suggested initial resuscitation fluid for volume repletion in traumatic shock [56]. No convincing evidence exists to recommend either normal saline (NS) or lactated ringers (LR) as superior to the other. In large volume resuscitation, especially in patients who have impaired renal function, NS can theoretically result in hyperchloremic metabolic acidosis, worsening the shock state. Conversely, the calcium in LR may overwhelm the citrate in stored packed red blood cells (PRBC) and result in clotting during transfusion. A recent meta-analysis demonstrated that colloids do not have a significant beneficial effect in trauma resuscitation but do present a major additional cost. Most authors recommend 1 to 2 L of crystalloid be administered initially. A reasonable strategy is to administer boluses of 500 mL (based on clinical status) with continuous reassessment of patient response.

Blood transfusion is an independent predictor of mortality in blunt trauma [57]. Although selection bias certainly accounts for some of this increased mortality, the immunomodulatory effects of PRBC may play a role in subsequent multiorgan failure, sepsis, and death [58]. Despite these recent studies, hemorrhage shock is undoubtedly associated with elevated mortality. Early blood transfusion in the unstable elderly trauma patient should be strongly considered.

Age affects traditional measures of response to resuscitation. The physician must use a combination of clinical and laboratory parameters to judge the effectiveness of the resuscitation. Foley catheters should be placed in all major trauma patients who lack contraindication. Urine output, although not a reliable marker of fluid status in the elderly, can still provide clinically relevant information and should be monitored in the emergency department. Initial arterial blood gas and venous lactate are recommended. Base deficit (BD) and serum lactate provide important information in the triage and resuscitation of the elderly trauma patient. Lactate and BD levels correlate with systemic hypoperfusion and shock. Admission levels of these markers correlate with ICU length of stay (LOS), hospital LOS, ISS, and mortality. In the elderly patient who has clear signs of shock, normalizing lactate and BD levels are useful markers of adequate resuscitation. The concept of "lac time" or clearance of BD has been shown to correlate with successful resuscitation and mortality [59,60]. Any trauma patient who remains in the emergency department for more than 45 minutes should have serial lactate levels drawn. Although an abnormal base deficit clearly suggests significant pathology, a normal BD does not rule out disease. In a study by Davis and colleagues [61] elderly patients who had a normal BD had mortality rates of 24%. The use of lactate and BD in the emergency department is to quickly identify OH and guide early aggressive resuscitation. In an apparently hemodynamically stable patient, admission BD of −6 or less or lactate of 2.4 mmol or greater suggests occult hypoperfusion and should prompt further clinical investigation and aggressive resuscitation.

Invasive monitoring with pulmonary artery catheters (PAC) seems superior to central venous catheters and central venous pressure measurement for guiding the resuscitation of elderly trauma patients. In a study of 67 elderly patients who had hip fractures, Schultz and colleagues [62] showed that use of a PAC to guide resuscitation decreased mortality from 29% to 2.9% [63]. Scalea and colleagues [64], in a study of pedestrian motor vehicle trauma, found that elderly patients who had systolic blood pressure 130 to 150 mm Hg had high rates of occult hypoperfusion. In these patients, PAC-guided resuscitation to cardiac index of at least 4 L/min/m^2 and an oxygen consumption of 170 mL/min/m^2 improved mortality. These resuscitation endpoints are used in several trauma centers around the country.

Recently, Brown and colleagues [65] demonstrated in a retrospective analysis that noninvasive monitoring with bioelectrical impedance devices was comparable to PAC thermodilution techniques for estimating cardiac index in the geriatric trauma patient. Future prospective trails may show this promising technique to be easier, safer, and as effective as the PAC.

Summary

1. Any elderly patient who has physiologic compromise, significant injury (TS < 14), high risk mechanism, or preexisting medical condition with altered cardiovascular function, should be monitored with pulmonary artery catheter.
2. Reasonable resuscitation endpoints are cardiac index of 4 $L/min/m^2$ or O_2 consumption index of 170 $mL/min/m^2$.
3. BD and lactate clearance provide guidance as to the status of hemodynamic resuscitation.
4. Aggressive intravenous fluid, blood, and maximizing cardiac index with inotropes improves survival.

Solid organ injuries

The management of blunt abdominal trauma and solid organ injury in elderly patients continues to evolve. In the emergency department, fluid resuscitation, aggressive hemodynamic monitoring, and early diagnosis of injuries are fundamental. Historically, surgeons have considered advanced age as a prohibitive risk for consideration of NOM of blunt solid organ injury [66]. Early studies suggested a 60% to 90% failure rate for NOM of blunt splenic trauma in patients greater than 55 years old [57]. More recent studies indicate that in properly selected elderly blunt trauma patients, NOM has success rates of 62% to 85% [67–69]. Some 90% of hepatic trauma is managed nonoperatively with failure rate ranging from 5% to 15% across all age groups [70,71]. The Eastern Association for the Surgery of Trauma reported that hemodynamic stability, grade of injury, and the GCS score predicted the success of NOM of blunt splenic injuries in adults. Other studies show that successful NOM rates are equivalent between elderly and younger cohort. Accordingly, patients of advanced age who have solid organ injury can be managed nonoperatively.

Complications of NOM occur in approximately 3% to 11% of adult patients. Operative reports suggest a 1% to 3% rate of missed bowel injuries, delayed hemorrhage, delayed infections, bilomas, and hemobilia [72]. Higher ISS, increased hemoperitoneum, continued contrast blush or extravasation, and hemodynamic instability predict the need for surgery. Most elderly patients who fail NOM do so within the first 48 to 72 hours after injury [73]. Elderly patients who fail NOM seem to have worse clinical outcomes than younger patients [39]. Consideration of operative intervention should occur with unstable hematocrit, increasing abdominal pain, persistent unexplained tachycardia, or hemodynamic decompensation or instability. Markers of occult hypoperfusion, such as lactate and base excess, may play an important role in identifying the elderly trauma patient who has a solid organ injury and impending hemodynamic collapse.

Angiographic embolization (AE) is playing an increasingly important role in the NOM of solid organ injuries in the elderly. No reports specifically address the use of angiographic embolization in the elderly population. Several conclusions may be extrapolated from the adult trauma literature, however. Two techniques exist for splenic embolization: proximal (ie, main splenic artery) and distal (ie, selective embolization). In a series of 150 adult patients, Sclafani and colleagues [74] demonstrated a 98.5% salvage rate with splenic AE on hemodynamically stable trauma patients. Other studies report failure rates closer to 10% to 13.5% with a 20% complication rate (eg, recurrent hemorrhage, missed injuries, or infection) [75]. Success and complication rates are likely somewhat institution dependent [76]. Angiography is a reasonable option for the elderly trauma patient who has solid organ injury and demonstrable blush or extravasation on CT regardless of hemodynamic stability [72]. The physician should ensure that the hemodynamic collapse is not attributable to other injuries before transferring the patient to the angiography suite.

Pelvic fractures

Pelvic fractures in the elderly are a distinct clinical entity. In general, pelvic fractures require a significant transfer of kinetic energy and are associated with a high incidence of polytrauma. In the elderly, however, low-energy trauma (eg, fall from standing) is the most common mechanism of injury, followed closely by motor vehicle crash (MVC). Despite this fact, polytrauma is as common as with younger patients and the incidence of associated thoracic trauma in the elderly is significantly increased [77].

Age is an independent predictor of mortality in trauma patients who have pelvic fractures. Overall mortality from either acute or delayed complications (hemorrhage, multiorgan failure, sepsis) is 9% to 30% The disparity is most pronounced in the moderate severity patients (ie, ISS of 16–25) in whom elder mortality is 21% compared with 6% in the younger cohort [78]. The elderly do particularly poorly with open pelvic fractures; one study demonstrated mortality up to 81% [78].

Fracture patterns are similar between elderly and younger trauma patients. The pubic rami is most commonly fractured (56%), followed by the acetabulum (19%) and ischium (11%). More than 50% of patients suffer multiple fractures. The mechanisms and clinical sequelae differ significantly in the elderly, however. The elderly are less likely to have "severe" pelvic fractures as defined by the American Orthopedic Association, yet suffer far higher mortality. Lateral compression (LC) fractures are nearly five times more common that anteroposterior (AP) fractures [78]. In contrast to younger patients in whom LC fractures are associated with lower transfusion rates and increased survival, these fractures in the elderly trauma patient result in significantly higher rates of hemorrhage, transfusion, angiographic embolization, and admission to the ICU.

Emergent treatment of the elderly patient who has a pelvic fracture focuses on control of hemorrhage, stabilization of the fracture, pain control, and resuscitation. The elderly have higher rates of hemorrhage despite lower fracture severity perhaps secondary to atherosclerotic changes that retard vasospasm and "loose" periosteum that limits tamponade. Blackmore and colleagues [79] proposed a clinical decision rule for predicting major hemorrhage after pelvic fractures. In this study, heart rate greater than 130 bpm, hematocrit less than 30, obturator ring fractures greater than 1 cm, and greater than 1-cm disruption of the pubic symphysis diastasis were associated with major pelvic fracture–related hemorrhage. The NPV of this decision rule is limited in the elderly given higher rates of lateral compression fractures and blunted ability to mount a tachycardic response to hypovolemia.

All elderly trauma patients who have suspected pelvic fractures should be typed and crossed for four to six units of blood. Attaining hemostasis is a priority in the trauma bay. Disruption of the posterior pelvic ring is associated with increased hemorrhage and subsequent hypotension. External fixation is useful for reducing pelvic volume in patients who have AP-type pelvic fractures. External fixation is not useful in the patient who has an LC fracture, the major clinically significant pelvic fracture seen in elderly blunt trauma patient.

Retroperitoneal hemorrhage is common after geriatric pelvic trauma and is not amenable to surgical repair; thus AE is an important treatment modality for elderly patients who have pelvic fractures. Timing of embolization is debated in the literature. Some studies suggest AE after a transfusion threshold of six units; these studies have reported mortality rates of approximately 30% [80]. Alternatively, it can be offered early in the clinical course based on fracture patterns, pelvic hematoma on CT, tachycardia, and declining hematocrit. Liberal arterial embolization seems to increase the effectiveness of hemostasis but with the expected increase in rates of unnecessary procedures. Age greater than 55 years is a powerful indication for angiographic embolization in the patient who has a pelvic fracture given the eightfold increase in risk for major hemorrhage [81]. Age greater than 60 is associated with an even higher rate of retroperitoneal bleed and need for embolization (PPV 94%). In these patients, embolization decreases mortality despite admission hemodynamic status.

Given the low rates of complication from AE (3%–4% commonly reported) and the high mortality from ongoing hemorrhage, early AE should be considered in elderly patients who have pelvic fracture, any suggestion of hemodynamic compromise, evidence of pelvic hematoma on CT, or transfusion requirements of greater than four units. Most pelvic fractures in the elderly require admission to the hospital. Any signs of continued hemorrhage or instability warrant admission to the ICU.

Traumatic brain injury

TBI and intracranial hemorrhage (ICH) are common injuries in the elderly trauma patient, accounting for approximately 80,000 emergency department visits annually [82]. Seventy five percent of these patients require admission with an age-adjusted hospitalization rate of 156 per 100,000 population, twice that of trauma patients less than 65 years of age [83,84]. Age is an independent predictor of mortality and disability in patients who have moderate to severe head trauma [85]. Compared with younger patients, even with equivalent or lower trauma triage scores (ISS, RTS, and GCS), the elderly have longer hospital stays, increased ICU usage, lower rates of functional recovery, and significantly higher mortality [86]. Patients older than 65 years have mortality rates two to five times those of younger patients with matched GCS and intracranial pathology [87]. Overall mortality rates in elderly patients who have TBI with ICH range from 30% to 85% [84,88].

Multiple factors contribute to the increased morbidity and mortality observed in elderly patients who have TBI. Brain weight decreases 10% between ages 30 to 70 years [89]. This age-related cerebral atrophy increases the distance traversed by bridging veins resulting in a loss of venous tortuosity. The veins remain firmly adhered to brain and dura and are more susceptible to traumatic tears with subsequent subdural hematomas. Cerebral atrophy also increases intracranial free space, potentially masking ongoing bleeds, resulting in subtle presentations and delaying the diagnosis. In addition to these anatomic changes, elderly trauma patients have significantly higher rates of comorbidities (eg, COPD, CAD, hypothyroidism, and so forth) that can exacerbate the dangerous triad of hypotension, hypoxia, and hypocoagulability. Dementia and cognitive deterioration are frequently encountered in the elderly trauma patient. In addition to being an independent risk factor for falls and TBI, cognitive impairment may complicate the emergency assessment of the elderly trauma patient and delay diagnosis and treatment. Finally, the use of medications, such as Coumadin, aspirin, and clopidogrel bisulfate (Plavix), dramatically increases the morbidity associated with elderly TBI [84,90,91].

Currently, physicians prescribe warfarin to more than 1 million Americans and in elderly trauma patients who have TBI, nearly 9% are on Coumadin [92]. Coumadin, aspirin, Plavix and Lovenox are critical medications responsible for the improved survivability from strokes, acute myocardial infarction, thromboembolic events, and atrial fibrillation. The incidence of adverse thromboembolic events in subtherapeutically anticoagulated patients who have mechanical heart valves or atrial fibrillation is 2% to 12%

per year depending on age, coexisting risk factors, and prior ischemic events [93]. The use of Coumadin decreases these adverse events by 50% to 75% [94]. These agents also dramatically increase the morbidity and mortality from traumatic intracerebral hemorrhage, however [87]. Recent reports indicate that spontaneous ICH rates in anticoagulated patients range from 0.3% to 5.4% per year [95]. In anticoagulated patients who have blunt head trauma and minimal or no symptoms, the rate of significant intracranial hemorrhage approaches 7% to 14% [96].

The elderly patient who has TBI and is on anticoagulation, specifically Coumadin, poses a significant diagnostic and management challenge. Most studies show that Coumadin is an independent predictor of mortality in traumatic brain injuries resulting in a 3- to 10-fold increase in mortality from TBI in the elderly [91,97–99]. Several studies also indicate that the elderly are significantly more likely to present with supratherapeutic international normalized ratio (INR). Increased rates of hepatic disease, poor nutrition, and variable medical compliance likely contribute to this dangerous trend.

The physician should order an INR and cranial CT on all elderly trauma patients who have suspected TBI. Clinical demise, evidence of intracranial hemorrhage, or supratherapeutic INR are all indications for pharmacologic reversal of anticoagulation [97,100,101]. In these situations, the risk for immediate mortality far outweighs the risk for adverse embolic events from the preexisting condition. Several studies have demonstrated that temporary discontinuation of warfarin, aspirin, or Plavix in the setting of ICH does not increase the risk for thrombotic or ischemic events [92,102–104].

Multiple reversal strategies exist. Volume of blood from the ruptured vessel and hematoma expansion are the most important determinants of morbidity and mortality in intracerebral hemorrhage [105]. All efforts should be made to limit continued bleeding. Ivascu and colleagues [97] found that implementation of a reversal protocol using early cranial CT from triage, immediate transfusion of two units of unmatched fresh frozen plasma (FFP) followed by two units of matched FFP decreased the time to reversal from 4.3 to 1.9 hours. In this study, progression of ICH dropped from 40% to 11% and subsequent mortality improved from 50% to 10%. The volume of FFP required to reverse fully the anticoagulation may range from 2 to 4 L, creating potential limitations in the elderly trauma patient who has concomitant fluid overload [101]. In these instances, alternative protocols may be useful.

Cryoprecipitate, vitamin K, prothrombin complex concentrates (PCC), and recombinant activated factor VIIa (rfVIIa) are also viable options in the treatment of anticoagulated patients who have TBI. In multiple studies of nontraumatic intracranial hemorrhage, immediate administration of PCC was associated with more rapid reversal of INR and subsequent decreased hematoma growth than vitamin K and FFP [106,107]. Typical PCC dosages are 25 to 50 IU/kg based on body weight, degree of anticoagulation, and desired level of correction [108]. Several studies of atraumatic cerebral hemorrhage suggest that administration of rFVIIa within 4 hours after the onset of insult limits the growth of the hematoma, reduces mortality, and improves functional outcomes at 90 days [109]. Future studies will delineate the role of rFVIIa in the management of acute traumatic intracerebral hemorrhage in the anticoagulated patient. Reasonable strategies include vitamin K (10 mg IV or 5 to 10 mg subcutaneously) coupled with a faster acting reversal agent, such as FFP, PCC, or rFVIIa.

Antiplatelet agents, such as aspirin and clopidogrel, are also becoming increasingly common in the elderly population. As with Coumadin, aspirin and clopidogrel have untoward effects on the elderly trauma patient who has TBI. The cardiology literature suggests that clopidogrel is a more effective antiplatelet agent than aspirin; many patients are on dual therapy. In small studies of TBI in elderly patients on single-medication regimens, aspirin and clopidogrel seem to have similar mortality. There also seems to be no significant difference in mortality for patients on combination antiplatelet therapy versus single-agent regimens [90]. Reversal strategies for these patients are based on bench science, in vitro studies, and theoretic physiologic principles. Platelet transfusions may offset some of the bleeding consequences of aspirin and Plavix. Although no data exist in the trauma literature, some cardiothoracic surgery literature suggests that Desmopressin at doses of 15 μg/L may also slow hemorrhage in patients taking aspirin [110]. One recent study successfully used recombinant factor VIIa to reverse the inhibitory effects of aspirin or aspirin and clopidogrel on in vitro thrombin formation [111].

Any elderly trauma patient who has TBI on anticoagulation or with documented intracranial pathology on head CT should be admitted to the neurosurgical service. These patients are particularly susceptible to rapid clinical deterioration and aggressive hemodynamic monitoring is advisable. A recent study by Cohen and colleagues [112] of anticoagulated patients who had head trauma demonstrated two disturbing points. First, most of their patients were supratherapeutic with INR greater than 5.0 in 50% of patients who had severe head injuries and greater than 3.0 in 47% of patients who had minor head injuries. Second, of 77 patients who had GCS 13 to 15 who were either initially discharged or admitted for observation, 56 deteriorated clinically with a mortality rate for these patients who had minor head injury of greater than 80%. Although this mortality is likely multifactorial and related to the high rate of supratherapeutic anticoagulation, the point is clear: anticoagulated elderly patients who have traumatic brain injuries are extremely high risk [88]. Elderly patients who have isolated head trauma, normal cranial CT, and elevated INR do not require pharmaceutical reversal but should be observed in the hospital for 12 to 24 hours [113]. Elderly patients who have normal head CT, normal INR, and no other associated injuries may be discharged if they have a responsible care provider and have reliable follow up.

Rib fractures

Blunt thoracic trauma is responsible for 25% of all trauma deaths in the United States. Two thirds of these patients have rib fractures and up to 35% are affected by pulmonary complications [31]. The elderly are more susceptible to rib fracture from relatively minor trauma. In the study by Bergeron and colleagues [114], falls from standing accounted for greater than 50% of elderly patients who had blunt trauma admitted with rib fractures followed closely by MVCs. In MVCs, the elderly are more susceptible to rib fractures from seat belts in low-speed and medium-speed accidents [115].

Despite lower indices of injury severity, elderly patients have twice the mortality and thoracic morbidity of younger patients (22% versus 10%) [114,116]. In Bulger and colleagues' [21] study of 277 patients older than 65 years of age who had rib fractures, mortality increased 19% and the risk for pneumonia increased 27% for each rib fracture. Further, the presence of rib fractures in thoracic trauma patients correlated with a 1.7-time increase in hepatic injury and 1.4-time increase in splenic injury. This finding is of added significance in the elderly trauma patient in whom baseline hepatic dysfunction significantly increases trauma-related mortality.

The elderly patient who has rib fractures is more likely to present with hypotension and has a significantly higher risk for sternal fracture [21]. Aggressive pain management and hemodynamic monitoring are particularly important. Control of fracture-associated pain decreases splinting, reduces atelectasis, and may limit subsequent pulmonary sequelae. Multiple strategies exist for pain management in the elderly. IV narcotic analgesia and patient-controlled analgesia are often effective but may be limited by central nervous system effects and further depression of respiratory drive [117]. The use of epidural analgesia with agents such as bupivacaine and fentanyl reportedly provides superior pain control without the sedating effect of parenteral opioids [114,118].

Scant prospective data exist concerning the use of epidurals in elderly trauma patients who have rib fractures and retrospective mortality data are mixed. Some studies suggest that the use of epidural analgesia correlates with increased length of stay and pulmonary complications [117]. This finding may represent selection bias toward using this procedure with more severely injured patients. Other reports indicate that epidural analgesia is associated with a decrease in the rate of nosocomial pneumonia and a shorter duration of mechanical ventilation after rib fractures [21]. In one large study, epidural use demonstrated a significant reduction in mortality from 16% to 10% at 48 hours postinjury [119]. The use of epidural analgesia may be limited in the elderly trauma population because of numerous exclusion criteria (eg, thoracic vertebral body fractures, spinal cord injuries, ongoing coagulopathy, bacteremia, and severe head injury) [21]. In appropriate patients, however, it seems to decrease mortality and should be considered early in the course of treatment of multiple rib fractures in selected elderly trauma patients.

Age and ISS predict mortality in patients who have rib fractures and multisystem injury [120]. Elderly trauma patients who have greater than two isolated rib fractures should be admitted to the hospital for observation. With greater than six rib fractures, morbidity and mortality are high; the patient should be admitted to an intensive care unit [117]. Aggressive pulmonary toilet, airway monitoring, and pain control should be initiated early in the emergency department.

Summary

Elderly trauma patients present unique challenges and face more significant obstacles to recovery than younger patients. Despite overall higher mortality, longer LOS, increased resource use, and higher rates of discharge to rehabilitation, most elderly trauma patients return to independent or preinjury functional status. Critical to improving these outcomes is an understanding that although similar trauma principles apply to the elderly, they require more aggressive evaluation and resuscitation.

References

[1] U.S. Bureau of the Census. Jennifer Cheeseman day, population projections of the United States, by age, sex, race, and Hispanic origin: 1993 to 2050, current population reports, P25–1104. Washington, DC: U.S. Government Printing Office; 1993.

[2] Broos P. Multiple trauma in elderly patients: factors influencing outcome. Injury 1993; 24(6):365–8.

[3] Champion HR, Copes SW, Buyer D, et al. Major trauma in geriatric patients. Am J Public Health 1989;79(9):1278–82.

[4] Osler T, Hales K, Baack B, et al. Trauma in the elderly. Am J Surg 1988;156(6):537–43.

[5] Jacobs DG, Plaisier BR, Barie PS, et al. Practice management guidelines for geriatric trauma: the EAST practice management guidelines work group. J Trauma 2003;54: 391–416.

[6] Ma MH, MacKenzie EJ, Alcorta R, et al. Compliance with prehospital triage protocols for major trauma patients. J Trauma 1999;46:168–75.

[7] Phillips S, Rond PC, Kelly SM, et al. The failure of triage criteria to identify geriatric patients with trauma: results from the Florida trauma triage study. J Trauma 1996;40:278–83.

[8] Mandavia D, Newton K. Geriatric trauma. Emerg Clin North Am 1998;16:257–74.

[9] Sterling DA, O'Connor JA, Bonadies J. Geriatric falls: injury severity is high and disproportionate to mechanism. J Trauma 2001;50(1):116–9.

[10] Knudson MM, Lieberman J, Morris J, et al. Mortality factors in geriatric blunt trauma patients. Arch Surg 1994;129(4):448–53.

[11] Horst HM, Obeid FN, Sorensen VJ, et al. Factors influencing survival of elderly trauma patients. Crit Care Med 1986;14(8):681–4.

[12] Tornetta P, Mostafavi M, Riina J, et al. Morbidity and mortality in elderly trauma patients. J Trauma 1999;46(4):702–6.

[13] Demaria EJ, Kenney PR, Merriam MA, et al. Survival after trauma in geriatric patients. Ann Surg 1987;206(6):738–43.

[14] American College of Surgeons. Advanced trauma life support for doctors. American College of Surgeons Committee on Trauma. 7th edition. Chicago (IL): American College of Surgeons; 2004.

[15] Demetriades D, Sava J, Alo K, et al. Old age as a criterion for trauma team activation. J Trauma 2001;51:754–6.
[16] Demaria EJ, Kenney PR, Merriam MA, et al. Aggressive trauma care benefits the elderly. J Trauma 1987;27(11):1200–6.
[17] Trauma. 3rd edition. 1996. In: Felician DV, Moore EE, Mattox KL. editors. McGraw-Hill; 2003.
[18] Aziz L, Jahangir SM, Choudhury SN, et al. The effect of priming with vecuronium and rocuronium on young and elderly patients. Anesth Analg 1997;85(3):663–6.
[19] Narang AT, Sikka R. Resuscitation of the elderly. Emerg Med Clin North Am 2006;24(2): 261–72, v.
[20] Allolio B, Dorr H, Stuttmann R, et al. Effect of a single bolus of etomidate upon eight major corticosteroid hormones and plasma ACTH. Clin Endocrinol (Oxf) 1985;22(3): 281–6.
[21] Bulger EM, Arneson MA, Mock CN, et al. Rib fractures in the elderly. J Trauma 2000; 48(6):1040–7.
[22] Rozycki GS, Ballard RB, Feliciano DV, et al. Surgeon-performed ultrasound for the assessment of truncal injuries: lessons learned from 1540 patients. Ann Surg 1998;228(4): 557–67.
[23] McGahan JP, Richards J, Fogata ML. Emergency ultrasound in trauma patients. Radiol Clin North Am 2004;42(2):417–25, [review].
[24] Richards JR, McGahan JP, Pali MJ, et al. Sonographic detection of blunt hepatic trauma: hemoperitoneum and parenchymal patterns of injury. J Trauma 1999;47(6):1092–7.
[25] Lee BC, Ormsby EL, McGahan JP, et al. The utility of sonography for the triage of blunt abdominal trauma patients to exploratory laparotomy. AJR Am J Roentgenol 2007;188(2):415–21.
[26] Blackbourne LH, Soffer D, McKenney M, et al. Secondary ultrasound examination increases the sensitivity of the FAST exam in blunt trauma. J Trauma 2004;57(5):934–8.
[27] Baumgarten M, Margolis DJ, Localio AR, et al. Pressure ulcers among elderly patients early in the hospital stay. J Gerontol A Biol Sci Med Sci 2006;61(7):749–54.
[28] Morris JA, MacKenzie EJ, Edelstein SL. The effect of preexisting conditions on mortality in trauma patients. JAMA 1990;263(14):1942–6.
[29] Rozzelle CJ, Wofford JL, Branch CL. Predictors of hospital mortality in older patients with subdural hematoma. J Am Geriatr Soc 1995;43:240–4.
[30] Reuter F. Traumatic intracranial hemorrhages in elderly people. Advances in Neurosurgery 1989;17:43–8.
[31] Ziegler DW, Agarwal NN. The morbidity and mortality of rib fractures. J Trauma 1994;37: 975–9.
[32] Palvanen M, Kannus P, Niemi S, et al. Hospital-treated minimal-trauma rib fractures in elderly Finns: long-term trends and projections for the future. Osteoperosis International 2004;15(8):649–53.
[33] Obaid AK, Barleben A, Porral D, et al. Utility of plain film pelvic radiographs in blunt trauma patients in the emergency department. Am Surg 2006;72(10):951–4.
[34] Gross EA, Niedens BA. Validation of a decision instrument to limit pelvic radiography in blunt trauma. J Emerg Med 2005;28(3):263–6.
[35] Pehle B, Nast-Kolb D, Oberbeck R, et al. [Significance of physical examination and radiography of the pelvis during treatment in the shock emergency room]. Unfallchirurg 2003;106(8):642–8.
[36] Gonazalez RP, Fried PQ, Bukahlo M. The utility of clinical examination in screening for pelvic fractures in blunt trauma. J Am Coll Surg 2002;194(2):121–5.
[37] Stuhlfaut JW, Soto JA, Lucey BC, et al. Blunt abdominal trauma: performance of CT without oral contrast material. Radiology 2004;233(3):689–94, [E-pub 2004 Oct 29].
[38] Tsugawa K, Koyanagi N, Hashizume M, et al. New insight for management of blunt splenic trauma: significant differences between young and elderly. Hepatogastroenterology 2002; 49(46):1144–9.

[39] Harbrecht BG, Peitzman AB, Rivera L, et al. Contribution of age and gender to outcome of blunt splenic injury in adults: multicenter study of the Eastern Association for the Surgery of Trauma. J Trauma 2001;51(5):887–95.
[40] Willmann JK, Roos JE, Platz A, et al. Multidetector CT: detection of active hemorrhage in patients with blunt abdominal trauma. AJR Am J Roentgenol 2002;179(2):437–44.
[41] Anderson SW, Varghese JC, Lucey BC, et al. Blunt splenic trauma: delayed-phase CT for differentiation of active hemorrhage from contained vascular injury in patients. Radiology 2007 [E-pub ahead of print].
[42] Weisbord SD, Palevsky PM. Radiocontrast-induced acute renal failure. J Intensive Care Med 2005;20:63–75.
[43] Barrett BJ, Parfrey PS. Preventing nephropathy induced by contrast medium. N Engl J Med 2006;354:379–86.
[44] Toprak O, Cirit M. Risk factors and therapy strategies for contrast-induced nephropathy. Ren Fail 2006;28(5):365–81, [review].
[45] Papaioannou A, Watts NB, Kendler DL, et al. Diagnosis and management of vertebral fractures in elderly adults. Am J Med 2002;113(3):220–8, [review].
[46] Berry GE, Adams S, Harris MB, et al. Are plain radiographs of the spine necessary during evaluation after blunt trauma? Accuracy of screening torso computed tomography in thoracic/lumbar spine fracture diagnosis. J Trauma 2005;59(6):1410–3, [discussion: 1413].
[47] Brown CV, Antevil JL, Sise MJ, et al. Spiral computed tomography for the diagnosis of cervical, thoracic, and lumbar spine fractures: its time has come. J Trauma 2005;58(5):890–5, [discussion: 895–6].
[48] Mosenthal AC, Livingston DH, Elcavage J, et al. Falls: epidemiology and strategies for prevention. J Trauma 1995;38:753–6.
[49] Ibanez J, Arikan F, Pedraza S, et al. Reliability of clinical guidelines in the detection of patients at risk following mild head injury: results of a prospective study. J Neurosurg 2004;100(5):825–34.
[50] Mack LR, Chan SB, Silva JC, et al. The use of head computed tomography in elderly patients sustaining minor head trauma. J Emerg Med 2003;24(2):157–62.
[51] Clement CM, Stiell IG, Schull MJ, et al. CCC Study Group. Clinical features of head injury patients presenting with a Glasgow Coma Scale score of 15 and who require neurosurgical intervention. Ann Emerg Med 2006;48(3):245–51.
[52] Haydel MJ, Preston CA, Mills TJ, et al. Indications for computed tomography in patients with minor head injury. N Engl J Med 2000;343(2):100–5.
[53] Stein SC, Burnett MG, Glick HA. Indications for CT scanning in mild traumatic brain injury: a cost-effective study. J Trauma 2006;61:558–66.
[54] Gittleman AM, Ortiz AO, Keating DP, et al. Indications for CT in patients receiving anticoagulation after head trauma. Am J Neuroradiol 2005;26:603–6.
[55] van Aalst JA, Morris JA Jr, Yates HK, et al. Severely injured geriatric patients return to independent living: a study of factors influencing function and independence. J Trauma 1991;31(8):1096–101; [discussion 110–12].
[56] Roberts I, Alderson P, Bunn F, et al. Colloids versus crystalloids for fluid resuscitation in critically ill patients. Cochrane Database Syst Rev 2004;18(4):CD000567, [review].
[57] Charles A, Shaikh AA, Walters M, et al. Blood transfusion is an independent predictor of mortality after blunt trauma. Am Surg 2007;73(1):1–5.
[58] Claridge JA, Sawyer RG, Schulman AM, et al. Blood transfusions correlate with infections in trauma patients in a dose-dependent manner. Am Surg 2002;68:566–72.
[59] McNelis J, Marini CP, Jurkiewicz A, et al. Prolonged lactate clearance is associated with increased mortality in the surgical intensive care unit. Am J Surg 2001;182(5):481–5.
[60] Husain FA, Martin MJ, Mullenix PS, et al. Serum lactate and base deficit as predictors of mortality and morbidity. Am J Surg 2003;185(5):485–91.
[61] Davis JW, Kaups KL. Base deficit in the elderly: a marker of severe injury and death. J Trauma 1998;45:873–7.

[62] Schultz RJ, Whitfield GF, LaMurra JJ, et al. The role of physiologic monitoring in patients with fractures of the hip. J Trauma 1985;45:309–16.
[63] Victorino GP, Chong TJ, Pal JD. Trauma in the elderly patient. Arch Surg 2003;138: 1093–8.
[64] Scalea TM, Simon HM, Duncan AO, et al. Geriatric blunt multiple trauma: improved survival with early invasive monitoring. J Trauma 1990;30(2):129–34, [discussion 134–6].
[65] Brown CV, Shoemaker WC, Wo CC, et al. Is noninvasive hemodynamic monitoring appropriate for the elderly critically injured patient? J Trauma 2005;58:102–7.
[66] Godley CD, Warren RL, Sheridan RL, et al. Nonoperative management of blunt splenic injury in adults: age over 55 years as a powerful indicator for failure. J Am Coll Surg 1996;183(2):133–9.
[67] Barone JE, Burns G, Svehlak SA, et al. Management of blunt splenic trauma in patients older than 55 years. Southern Connecticut Regional Trauma Quality Assurance Committee. J Trauma 1999;46(1):87–90.
[68] Falimirski ME, Provost D. Nonsurgical management of solid abdominal organ injury in patients over 55 years of age. Am Surg 2000;66(7):631–5.
[69] Albrecht RM, Schermer CR, Morris A. Nonoperative management of blunt splenic injuries: factors influencing success in age > 55 years. Am Surg 2002;68(3):227–30, [discussion: 230–1].
[70] Hurtuk M, Reed RL 2nd, Esposito TJ, et al. Trauma surgeons practice what they preach: the NTDB story on solid organ injury management. J Trauma 2006;61(2):243–54, [discussion: 254–5].
[71] Richardson JD. Changes in the management of injuries to the liver and spleen. J Am Coll Surg 2005;200(5):648–69, [review].
[72] Schurr MJ, Fabian TC, Gavant M, et al. Management of blunt splenic trauma: computed tomographic contrast blush predicts failure of nonoperative management. J Trauma 1995; 39(3):507–12, [discussion: 512–3].
[73] Cocanour CS, Moore FA, Ware DN, et al. Delayed complications of nonoperative management of blunt adult splenic trauma. Arch Surg 1998;133:619–24.
[74] Sclafani SJ, Shaftan GW, Scalea TM, et al. Nonoperative salvage of computed tomography-diagnosed splenic injuries: utilization of angiography for triage and embolization for hemostasis. J Trauma 1995;39(5):818–25, [discussion: 826–7].
[75] Haan JM, Bochicchio GV, Kramer N, et al. Nonoperative management of blunt splenic injury: a 5-year experience. J Trauma 2005;58(3):492–8.
[76] Dent D, Alsabrook G, Erickson BA, et al. Blunt splenic injuries: high nonoperative management rate can be achieved with selective embolization. J Trauma 2004;56(5): 1063–7.
[77] O'Brien DP, Luchette FA, Pereira SJ, et al. Pelvic fracture in the elderly is associated with increased mortality. Surgery 2002;132:710–4.
[78] Martin RE, Teberian G. Multiple trauma and the elderly patient. Emerg Med Clin North Am 1990;8(2):411–20.
[79] Blackmore CC, Cummings P, Jurkovich GJ, et al. Predicting major hemorrhage in patients with pelvic fracture. J Trauma 2006;61(2):346–52.
[80] Kimbrell BJ, Velmahos GC, Chan LS, et al. Angiographic embolization for pelvic fractures in older patients. Arch Surg 2004;139(7):728–32, [discussion: 732–3].
[81] Velmahos GC, Toutouzas KG, Vassiliu P, et al. A prospective study on the safety and efficacy of angiographic embolization for pelvic and visceral injuries. J Trauma 2002;53(2): 303–8, [discussion: 308].
[82] Thompson HJ, McCormick WC, Kagan SH. Traumatic brain injury in older adults: epidemiology, outcomes, and future implications. J Am Geriatr Soc 2006;54:1590–5.
[83] Coronado VG, Thomas KE, Sattin RW, et al. The CDC traumatic brain injury surveillance system: characteristics of persons aged 65 years and older hospitalized with a TBI. J Head Trauma Rehabil 2005;20:215–28.

[84] Lavoie A, Ratte S, Clas D, et al. Preinjury warfarin use among elderly patients with closed head injuries in a trauma center. J Trauma 2004;56:802–7.
[85] Masson F, Thicoipe M, Mokni T, et al. Aquitaine group for severe brain injury study. Epidemiology of traumatic comas: a prospective population-based study. Brain Inj 2003; 17(4):279–93.
[86] Susman M, DiRusso SM, Sullivan T, et al. Traumatic brain injury in the elderly: increased mortality and worse functional outcome at discharge despite lower injury severity. J Trauma 2002;53:219–24.
[87] Cohen DB, Rinker C, Wilberger JE. Traumatic brain injury in anticoagulated patients. J Trauma 2006;60:553–7.
[88] Amacher AL, Bybee DE. Toleration of head injury by the elderly. Neurosurgery 1987;20:954–8.
[89] Ellis GL. Subdural hematoma in the elderly. Emerg Med Clin North Am 1990;8(2):281–94.
[90] Ohm C, Mina A, Howells G, et al. Effects of antiplatelet agents on outcomes for elderly patients with traumatic intracranial hemorrhage. J Trauma 2005;58:518–22.
[91] Franko J, Kish KJ, O'Connell BG, et al. Advanced age and preinjury warfarin anticoagulation increase the risk of mortality after head trauma. J Trauma 2006;61:107–10.
[92] Kirsch MJ, Vrabec GA, Marley RA, et al. Preinjury warfarin and geriatric orthopedic trauma patients: a case-matched study. J Trauma 2004;57:1230–3.
[93] Cannegieter SC, Rosendaal FR, Wintzen AR, et al. Optimal oral anticoagulant therapy in patients with mechanical heart valves. N Engl J Med 1995;333(1):11–7.
[94] Wijdicks EF, Schievink WI, Brown RD, et al. The dilaemma of discontinuation of anticoagulation therapy for patients with intracranial hemorrhage and mechanical heart valves. Neurosurgery 1998;42(4):769–73.
[95] Shireman TI, Mahnken JD, Howard PA, et al. Development of a contemporary bleeding risk model for elderly warfarin recipients. Chest 2006;130:1390–6.
[96] Li J, Brown J, Levine M. Mild head injury, anticoagulants, and risk of intracranial injury. Lancet 2001;357:771–2.
[97] Ivascu FA, Janczyk RI, Junn FS, et al. Treatment of trauma patients with intracranial hemorrhage on preinjury warfarin. J Trauma 2006;61:318–21.
[98] Ivascu FA, Howells GA, Junn FS, et al. Rapid warfarin reversal in anticoagulated patients with traumatic intracranial hemorrhage reduces hemorrhage progression and mortality. J Trauma 2005;59:1131–9.
[99] Karni A, Holtzman R, Bass T, et al. Traumatic head injury in the anticoagulated elderly patient: a lethal combination. Am Surg 2001;67(11):1098–100.
[100] Rathlev N, Medzon R, Lowery D, et al. Intracranial pathology in the elderly with minor head injury. Acad Emerg Med 2006;13(3):302–7.
[101] Aguilar MI, Hart RG, Kase CS, et al. Treatment of warfarin-associated intracerebral hemorrhage: literature review and expert opinion. Mayo Clin Proc 2007;82(1):82–92, [review. erratum in: Mayo Clin Proc. Mar 2007;82(3):387].
[102] Phan TG, Koh M, Wijdicks EF. Safety of discontinuation of anticoagulation in patients with intracerebral hemorrhage at high thromboembolic risk. Arch Neurol 2000; 57:1710–3.
[103] Babikian VL, Kase CS, Pressin MS, et al. Resumption of anticoagulation after intracranial bleeding in patients with prosthetic heart valves. Stroke 1988;19:407–8.
[104] Kawamata T, Takeshita M, Kubo O, et al. Management of intracranial hemorrhage associate with anticoagulation therapy. Surg Neurol 1995;44:438–42.
[105] Goldstein JN, Thomas SH, Frontiero V, et al. Timing of fresh frozen plasma administration and rapid correction of coagulopathy in warfarin-related intracerebral hemorrhage. Stroke 2006;37:151–5.
[106] Cartmill M, Dolan G, Byrne JL, et al. Prothrombin complex concentrate for oral anticoagulant reversal in neurosurgical emergencies. Br J Neurosurg 2000;14(5):458–61.
[107] Huttner HB, Schellinger PD, Hartmann M, et al. Hematoma growth and outcome in treated neurocritical care patients with intracerebral hemorrhage related to oral

anticoagulant therapy: comparison of acute treatment strategies using vitamin K, fresh frozen plasma, and prothrombin complex concentrates. Stroke 2006;37(6):1465–70, [E-pub 2006 May 4].

[108] Preston FE, Laidlaw ST, Sampson B, et al. Rapid reversal of oral anticoagulation with warfarin by a prothrombin complex concentrate (Beriplex): efficacy and safety in 42 patients. Br J Haematol 2002;116:619–24.

[109] Mayer SA, Brun NC, Begtrup K, et al. Recombinant activated factor VII intracerebral hemorrhage trial investigators. Recombinant activated factor VII for acute intracerebral hemorrhage. N Engl J Med 2005;352(8):777–85.

[110] Aschkenasy MT, Rothenhaus TC. Trauma and falls in the elderly. Emerg Med Clin N Am 2006;24:413–32.

[111] Altman R, Scazziota A, DE Lourdes Hererra M, et al. Recombinant factor VIIa reverses the inhibitory effect of aspirin or aspirin plus clopidogrel on in vitro thrombin generation. J Thromb Haemost 2006;4(9):2022–7.

[112] Cohen DB, Rinker C, Wilberger JE. Traumatic brain injury in anticoagulated patients. J Trauma 2006;60(3):553–7.

[113] Itshayek E, Rosenthal G, Fraifield S, et al. Delayed posttraumatic acute subdural hematoma in elderly patients on anticoagulation. Neurosurg 2006;58(5):E851–6.

[114] Bergeron E, Lavoie A, Clas D, et al. Elderly patients with rib fractures are at greater risk of death and pneumonia. J Trauma 2003;54:478–85.

[115] Shimamura M, Ohhashi H, Yamazaki M. The effects of occupant age on patterns of rib fractures to belt-restrained drivers and front passengers in frontal crashes in Japan. Stapp Car Crash J 2003;47:349–65.

[116] Sirmali M, Turut H, Topcu S, et al. A comprehensive analysis of traumatic rib fractures: morbidity, mortality and management. Eur J Cardiothorac Surg 2003;24(1):133–8.

[117] Keininger AN, Bair HA, Bendick PJ, et al. Epidural versus intravenous pain control in elderly patients with rib fractures. Am J Surg 2005;180:327–30.

[118] Wu CL, Jani ND, Perkins FM, et al. Thoracic epidural analgesia versus intravenous patient-controlled analgesia for treatment of rib fracture pain after motor vehicle crash. J Trauma 1999;47(3):564–7.

[119] Bakhos C, O'Connor J, Kyriadides T, et al. Vital capacity as a predictor of outcome in elderly patients with rib fractures. J Trauma 2006;61:131–4.

[120] Brasel KJ, Guse CE, Layde P, et al. Rib fractures: relationship with pneumonia and mortality. Crit Care Med 2006;34(6):1642–6.

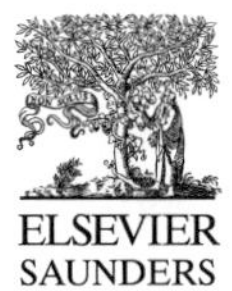

ELSEVIER
SAUNDERS

Emerg Med Clin N Am 25 (2007) 861–872

EMERGENCY
MEDICINE
CLINICS OF
NORTH AMERICA

Trauma in Pregnancy

Seric S. Cusick, MD[a], Carrie D. Tibbles, MD[b,*]

[a]*Department of Emergency Medicine, UC Davis School of Medicine, PSSB, 4150 V Street, #2100, Sacramento, CA 95817, USA*

[b]*Department of Emergency Medicine, Harvard Affiliated Emergency Medicine Residency, Beth Israel Deaconess Medical Center, One Deaconess Road, West Campus Clinical Center CC2, Boston, MA 02215, USA*

The care of the pregnant trauma patient provides unique challenges and holds profound implications for both fetal and maternal outcomes. The incidence of trauma in pregnant patients is low, approximately 5% [1], but it is the leading cause of nonobstetric mortality, and the associated fetal morbidity and mortality increases with the severity of the maternal injuries.

The management of these patients is influenced by unique anatomic and physiologic changes, increased concern for deleterious radiation and medication exposures, and the need for multidisciplinary care. This article reviews the critical features necessary in the assessment, diagnosis, treatment, and disposition of pregnant trauma patients with a focus on recent developments reported in the literature pertinent to emergency management.

Incidence

As described previously, trauma represents a significant cause of maternal death despite its relatively low absolute incidence. In a review of 95 maternal deaths, Fildes and colleagues [2] reported 46.3% to be of traumatic etiology. This rate increases in younger women and those of certain ethnic and socioeconomic groups. The nature of these traumatic insults has been reported as 55% motor vehicle collisions, 22% falls, 22% assaults, and 1% burns [3]. Although sampling of certain patient populations yields higher rates of penetrating trauma and mortality associated with violent crimes [2], Weiss and colleagues [4] identified motor vehicle collisions as the leading traumatic cause of fetal death (82%). This study also notes

* Corresponding author.
E-mail address: ctibbles@bidmc.harvard.edu (C.D. Tibbles).

doi:10.1016/j.emc.2007.06.010

that the causes of maternal and fetal mortality differ, with 11% of all fetal deaths being independent of maternal death.

Even minor maternal trauma may have immediate and long-term impacts on fetal well-being, highlighting the need for prevention, appropriate recognition, and multidisciplinary care.

General considerations

Typical prehospital and Advanced Trauma Life Support protocols must be modified in assessing the pregnant trauma patient because of alterations in anatomy and physiology. Additionally, the providers must consider the assessment and well being of the second patient—the fetus. These factors demand attention most immediately during the initial assessment and hold implications in the effective resuscitation, diagnosis, and treatment.

The uterus first becomes an intra-abdominal organ at 12 weeks, and as it enlarges it displaces abdominal contents upwards, reaching the costal margin between 34 and 38 weeks. The diaphragm may be elevated as much as 4 cm, with accompanying displacement of associated thoracoabdominal organs, altering interpretation of physical examination and radiographic findings. In a supine patient, the enlarged uterus compresses the inferior vena cava, decreasing venous return and potentially causing supine hypotension syndrome.

The maternal cardiopulmonary system displays significant alterations. By the second trimester, a mild increase in resting heart rate and decrease in systolic blood pressure are accompanied by moderate hypocapnia caused by increased minute ventilation. Multiple factors affect maternal hemodynamics. Increases in maternal blood volume (by 50%) and relatively smaller increases in red blood cell volume (by 30%) create a physiologic anemia of pregnancy with expected hematocrit values between 30% and 35% in the final trimester. These factors result in increased cardiac output, an increasing portion of which is shunted to the developing fetus and uterus.

Prehospital considerations

In the prehospital setting, information regarding the status of the pregnancy and the clinical condition of the patient should be obtained. In general, most pregnant patients following major trauma should be transported to a Level 1 trauma center with obstetric capabilities, particularly if there is hemodynamic compromise, loss of consciousness, or a third-trimester gestation [5]. Appropriate spine precautions should be observed, and a left lateral tilt position or manual displacement of the uterus may be used to avoid the supine hypotension syndrome. In late third-trimester patients, a supine position may be intolerable because of the associated respiratory distress, and the prehospital team may use up to 30° of reverse Trendelenberg positioning as allowed by hemodynamic parameters [6].

Appropriate emergency department management can proceed only if the patient is identified as pregnant. Emergency medical service personnel, family or friends, physical examination, and serum or urine pregnancy testing may provide this information, but not without the potential for delay or misinformation. In 2002 Bochicchio and colleagues [7] recommended that all female trauma patients of reproductive age receive a Focused Assessment with Sonography in Trauma with the secondary intent to screen for pregnancy. On retrospective review, these ultrasound examinations revealed a small number of newly diagnosed pregnancies with subsequent modification to the diagnostic evaluation of these patients. Once pregnancy is identified, the evaluation of a pregnant trauma patient should be multidisciplinary, including a combination of emergency physicians, trauma surgeons, and obstetricians.

Initial evaluation of the pregnant trauma patient

The primary survey is performed according to standard Advanced Trauma Life Support protocols, but special consideration must be paid to the cardiopulmonary alterations described earlier. Rapid-sequence induction is accepted as safe and is the preferred method for intubation. Appropriate techniques, such as Sellick's maneuver and adequate preoxygenation, are necessary to avoid complications, because pregnant patients are prone to aspiration and desaturation. Disturbances of respiration (eg, pneumothorax) may be more challenging to detect and may be associated with an accelerated decompensation because of alterations in respiratory mechanics. If tube thoracostomy is performed, a higher intercostal space should be used to avoid the elevated diaphragm. When evaluating the patient's circulatory status, the physiologic changes present in later pregnancy must be taken into account. The 50% increase in maternal blood volume and increased cardiac output may mask significant blood loss; fetal distress may be the earliest indicator of impending hemodynamic instability. Resuscitation with crystalloid should be initiated as appropriate, and, if needed before the availability of type-specific blood, O negative packed red blood cells should be used. Because of the susceptibility of the uterine blood supply, the use of vasopressors should be avoided.

After the primary survey is completed, a secondary survey should be performed with several important modifications. As early as possible in the resuscitation, fetal monitoring should be initiated for all viable gestations (> 23 weeks) and continued for at least 4 to 6 hours [8]. The decision to cease fetal monitoring should be made by the consulting obstetrician and should take into account documented uterine contractions, fetal well-being, and any plans for operative intervention. A vaginal examination should be completed to assess for the presence of blood or amniotic fluid and cervical effacement and dilation. Vaginal fluid may be examined for the presence of ferning and an elevated pH near 7, which would be consistent with traumatic rupture of membranes.

The standard Focused Abdominal Sonography for Trauma examination should be performed during the secondary survey, providing a screening examination for intraperitoneal hemorrhage with sensitivities of 80% to 83% and specificities of 98% to 100% for intraperitoneal fluid [9–11]. Bedside ultrasound also can be used to assess the fetal heart rate rapidly. With the advent of bedside ultrasound and rapid CT scans, diagnostic peritoneal lavage (DPL) has largely fallen out of routine use in the evaluation of trauma patients. The limited data on DPL in pregnancy report that it is accurate in pregnant patients and can be performed safely with no increases in fetal loss [12,13]. If performed during pregnancy, a DPL should be done by the supraumbilical approach using an open technique.

Diagnostic evaluation

Many trauma centers evaluate patients with a standardized laboratory panel. Alterations in pregnancy that should be considered in interpreting laboratory results include a physiologic anemia, slight elevation of the white blood cell count, mildly decreased serum bicarbonate, and an increased fibrinogen. Arterial blood gas analysis may reveal a slightly elevated pH and mild hyperventilation with pCO_2s near 30 mm Hg.

Kleihauer-Betke (KB) testing identifies fetal red blood cells within a maternal blood sample, indicating fetomaternal hemorrhage of at least 5 mL using current methods, although the development of flow cytometry techniques may lower this threshold [14]. The Rh-positive fetus possesses this antigen after 6 weeks' gestation, and transplacental hemorrhage of as little as 0.0001 mL of fetal blood can cause maternal sensitization. Consequently, the American College of Emergency Physicians recommends administration of immune globulin after even minor trauma [15]. Similarly, the American College of Obstetrics and Gynecology recommends administering Rh immune globulin to all Rh-negative trauma patients who have a positive KB test [16]. Further dosing to account for larger transplacental hemorrhage may be administered according to the dosing schedule of 300 μg of immune globulin per 30 cm^3 of estimated fetomaternal hemorrhage.

In 2004 Muench and colleagues [17] recommended routine KB testing in all cases of maternal trauma, regardless of maternal Rh status. In a retrospective review of 71 trauma patients, they report a positive KB test holding a sensitivity of 100% in the prediction of uterine contractions and labor with a specificity of 96% and 54% for the prediction of contractions and preterm labor, respectively. Dhanraj and Lambers [18], however, comparing low-risk third-trimester volunteers with pregnant trauma historical controls, revealed no significant difference in the incidence of a positive KB test. The authors concluded that an isolated positive result therefore is not indicative of pathologic transplacental hemorrhage. Although this retrospective review has obvious limitations, it questions the potential utility of the negative predictive value of the KB test.

Diagnostic imaging in pregnancy

As mentioned previously, ultrasound is an ideal tool for imaging the pregnant trauma patient, because it provides valuable information about both the fetus and mother and has no associated radiation exposure. Often, however, additional diagnostic imaging is required. In general, clinically necessary imaging studies should not be deferred because of concern about radiation, and the uterus should be shielded as much as feasible given the intended study [19]. The cumulative radiation dose associated with an increased risk of fetal malformation is 5 to 10 rads, significantly higher than many studies commonly used in trauma patients [20]. A pelvic CT alone (with mandated absence of shielding) will administer between 3 to 9 rads to the fetus and should be be undertaken only in critical patients, as the clinical situation requires [19,21]. Although the literature suggests radiographic studies should not be deferred in the pregnant trauma patient, the increased use of CT in blunt trauma patients results in radiation doses that often exceed previously described thresholds [22]. Clinicians are encouraged to consider these factors in the choosing appropriate imaging studies [23].

Injury severity scores and outcome in pregnant trauma patients

Much literature has been devoted to the description of factors associated with adverse maternal and fetal outcomes in trauma [2,4,13,24–32]. As described previously, trauma is one of the leading causes of maternal death and accounts for at least 5% of fetal deaths [2,4]. Pregnancy, however, does not influence morbidity or mortality independently from trauma; overall rates are similar to those in nonpregnant patients and are consistent with markers of injury severity [33,34]. Shah and colleagues [33] reported a mortality rate of 3.5% in a retrospective case-control analysis of 114 patients, which did not differ significantly from controls. The authors, however, did identify a trend in the pattern of injury toward more severe abdominal injuries and less severe head injuries.

Several factors have been investigated to identify predictors of fetal injury and loss. It is well documented that the maternal Injury Severity Score (ISS) correlates well with adverse fetal outcomes [13,26,29–31,33–35]. Rogers and colleagues [35] reported a 50% fetal mortality rate with an ISS greater than 25, whereas Kissinger and colleagues [30] identified a significant difference in mean ISS when comparing trauma with (ISS 21.6) and without (ISS 6.2) associated fetal mortality. This scoring system provides little assistance in the acute management of these patients, however, and may not be useful in prospectively identifying those at risk for adverse fetal outcomes [31]. The assessment of a Revised Trauma Score in the initial resuscitation has been investigated as a potential marker of clinical course. A small retrospective analysis failed to identify a predictive value in assigning a Revised Trauma Score when examining for untoward outcomes or the need for prolonged monitoring [27]. In a retrospective analysis of 20 patients who had an ISS higher than 12, Ali and colleagues [26] identified the presence of disseminated intravascular coagulation (DIC) as a major predictor of fetal mortality. DIC was identified with equal incidence in patients with and without evidence of placental abruption but was present only in the group with associated fetal mortality. Laboratory values consistent with DIC were found in 61.5% of these patients. Despite a small study size and previous reports with contradictory data [36], the authors recommend that patients who have DIC be considered for imminent delivery of a fetus of viable gestational age. Additional criteria that have been associated with fetal mortality include decreased Glascow Coma Scale, maternal acidosis, decreased serum bicarbonate, maternal hypoxia, and a single documented fetal heart rate below 110 beats per minute [13,29,30,33,35]. Although various analyses differ in the statistical significance of each of these features, markers of maternal malperfusion and hypoxia, direct uteroplacental injury, and severe maternal head injury are associated consistently with adverse fetal outcome. Sperry and colleagues [32] noted that even women discharged after minor traumatic injury with a viable pregnancy have increased risk of a preterm delivery and a low birth weight infant and identified trauma as an independent risk factor for these outcomes.

Perimortem cesarean section

A perimortem cesarean section should be performed in the pregnant patient in traumatic arrest if the fetus is potentially viable. This procedure originally was proposed by Katz and colleagues [37] in 1986 in light of data suggesting the inefficacy of cardiopulmonary resuscitation in the third trimester. Emptying the uterus relieves uterocaval compression and improves venous return and, consequently, cardiac output. The initial recommendation was to perform the procedure within 4 minutes of maternal arrest to minimize the potential for adverse maternal neurologic outcome in reversible causes of cardiac arrest. Subsequent studies have reported fetal and maternal survival rates of 45% and 72%, respectively [38]. Recently, a review of 38 case reports provided tentative evidence that maternal and fetal outcomes are improved by initiation of perimortem cesarean section within 4 minutes of maternal cardiac arrest. Eight of these cases were traumatic, although no subgroup analysis was provided. Both return of spontaneous circulation and delivery of normal infants was reported in several cases despite delay of the procedure for more than 15 minutes after arrest. Despite an acknowledged reporting bias affecting the review, the authors recommend a caesarean delivery be performed if pulses cannot be obtained in the case of maternal arrest [39].

Injuries unique to the pregnant trauma patient

Placental abruption

Placental abruption can occur even after minor abdominal trauma. It is the second most common cause of fetal mortality in this patient population [40]; the incidence ranges between 1% and 60% [5,24,41]. In minor trauma the rate of placental abruption is between 1% and 5% with significant mechanisms associated with rates of 20% to 60% [5,33,36].

Placental abruption results from the placenta shearing away from the uterus with bleeding into this space and clot formation. The elasticity of the uterus, matched against the relative stiffness of the placenta, creates a vulnerable interface. A placental abruption can result in the patient experiencing abdominal pain, cramping, and vaginal bleeding. The clinician may detect uterine tenderness on physical examination. Unfortunately, the absence of these features does not exclude the diagnosis of placental abruption reliably.

Several diagnostic modalities may be used in the evaluation of placental abruption. Ultrasound may detect a placental abruption, has the benefit of the absence of ionizing radiation, and provides additional information about fetal well-being. Its sensitivity for placental abruption, however, is poor—around 50%—so a negative ultrasound does not rule out a placental abruption [36,42]. Use of the KB test as an indicator of the fetomaternal hemorrhage likely to accompany abruption is not of great clinical utility because of its low specificity, particularly in light of the data presented earlier from Dhanraj and Lambers [18], and currently is not recommended for this application by the American College of Obstetrics and Gynecology [16]. Continuous fetal monitoring is the preferred test and should be initiated as early in the evaluation as possible. In the absence of symptoms consistent with placental abruption, an observation period of 4 to 6 hours is adequate [24,42]. Because of the potential for delayed manifestation (24–48 hours) of significant placental abruption, the Eastern Association for the Surgery of Trauma recommends continuation of fetal monitoring in the presence of uterine contractions, a nonreassuring fetal heart rate pattern, vaginal bleeding, significant uterine tenderness or irritability, or serious maternal injury [8]. This recommendation applies to even minor trauma, because these patients are particularly prone to delayed recognition of placental abruption.

Uterine rupture

Uterine rupture is a rare consequence of maternal trauma, one that carries a grave outcome for the fetus. This diagnosis is present in less than 1% of blunt trauma and is found typically in patients who have had a previous cesarean section. Associated fetal mortality is nearly universal, with an associated 10% maternal mortality rate [42]. Presenting features may include uterine tenderness and variable shape, hemodynamic instability, and the ability to palpate fetal parts on abdominal examination. In patients without a previous cesarean section, the uterus is more likely to rupture posteriorly, making detection of these physical examination findings more difficult [43].

Pelvic fracture

As expected from proximity alone, injuries to the bony pelvis are complicated to manage in pregnancy. Leggon and colleagues [44] described maternal and fetal mortality rates of 9% and 35%, respectively, in a retrospective review of 101 pelvic and acetabular fractures sustained during pregnancy. The major causes of fetal deaths were direct injury to the uterus, placenta, or fetus (52%) and maternal hemorrhage (36%). Fatal insults to the fetus were identified in all three trimesters, with no significant difference in the distribution of fetal mortality by gestational age. In subanalysis of this population according to injury severity, a fetal mortality rate of 10% was discovered in patients who had injuries of minor severity. These results are significantly higher than the generally accepted fetal mortality rates of 1% in this subset of pregnant trauma patients [5]. Although the research methodology has inherent limitations, this finding suggests that pelvic fractures may be an independent predictor of adverse fetal outcome.

The management of pelvic fractures in pregnant trauma patients has several critical modifications. Because of the increased risk of fetal morbidity and mortality, a thorough evaluation of the uterus and of fetal well-being must be undertaken. Recent reports, however, suggest that both percutaneous and open fixation may be performed with good fetal and maternal outcomes [45–47]. In addition to stabilization of unstable pelvic fractures, current management of hemodynamically unstable polytrauma victims often includes the use of angiography to coil or embolize bleeding pelvic or retroperitoneal vessels. The feasibility of this procedure in pregnant patients is not established.

In a large retrospective analysis of 3992 hospitalized pregnant patients who had fractures of any type, El Kady and colleagues [25] found lower extremity fractures were the most common, but pelvic fractures were associated with the highest risk of placental abruption and maternal and fetal death. Women who had pelvic fractures and who were discharged without delivering carried an increased risk of fetal, neonatal, and infant death, mostly attributed to abruption and low birth weight.

Injury prevention

Given the dramatic impact on fetal well-being and the prevalence of traumatic injuries in women of childbearing age, there are great potential benefits in the prevention of traumatic injuries in pregnant patients. Although there is discrepancy in the literature regarding the etiology, most authors identify motor vehicle collisions as the primary source of traumatic injuries. Even though the use of seatbelts is recommended, many pregnant patients do not use them. Approximately one third of pregnant patients do not use safety restraints properly, and a minority of women report physician counseling on this topic [48,49]. Previous literature suggests as few as 46% of pregnant women involved in motor vehicle collisions were properly restrained, with as few of half of all pregnant women reporting routine proper use of restraints [33,50–52]. Therefore a large emphasis has been placed on appropriate positioning of the lap and shoulder belts. Recently, the role of airbag deployment in obstetric complications has been investigated in case reports and series. Fusco and colleagues [53] reported the first case of uterine rupture associated with airbag deployment in 2001. Subsequently, a retrospective review by Metz and Abbott [54] of 30 cases involving airbag deployment failed to demonstrate a high rate of abruption or fetal compromise. Although preliminary experimental data suggest airbags may impart dangerous force to the uterus with improper use, the risk of airbags in late-trimester patients remains to be defined [55,56]. In 1997 the National Highway Traffic Safety Administration issued guidelines that describe the benefits of airbags as outweighing potential risks and recommended positioning the sternum and/or uterine fundus at least 10 inches away from the airbag cover [57]. At this time there remains great opportunity to impact pregnancy outcomes with both effective public health initiatives and patient education during interactions between pregnant patients and independent health care practitioners.

The prevalence of violence in pregnancy is estimated to be 10% to 15%, with some series identifying up to 31.5% of traumatic injuries as attributable to interpersonal violence [58–60]. Most of these assaults (70%–85%) are attributable to boyfriends or spouses [47]. The frequency and/or nature of abuse may escalate during pregnancy and is associated with late entry into prenatal care, prematurity, and low birth weight in addition to any immediate implications of the traumatic insult. In a large retrospective analysis of severely injured, hospitalized assault victims, El Kady and colleagues [28] identified increased rates of maternal mortality and uterine rupture. Furthermore, they reported adverse long-term effects on fetal outcome (eg, low birth weight) that persisted when controlling for socioeconomic factors previously viewed as confounding variables. The available structure of routine prenatal visits and the potential for increased use of emergency departments by this patient population may provide opportunities to detect patients subjected to domestic violence. Several methods for detection have been described, and guidelines for screening are available from the American College of Obstetrics and Gynecology [61–63].

Summary

Trauma in pregnancy presents unique challenges to the emergency physician. Knowledge of the anatomic and physiologic alterations in pregnancy, a thorough evaluation of both the mother and fetus, and careful consideration of conditions specific to pregnancy are essential to manage these cases expertly and ensure the best possible outcomes for both the mother and the fetus.

References

[1] Mattox KL, Goetzl L. Trauma in pregnancy. Crit Care Med 2005;33(10 Suppl):S385–9.
[2] Fildes J, Reed L, Jones N, et al. Trauma: the leading cause of maternal death. J Trauma 1992; 32(5):643–5.
[3] Connolly AM, Katz VL, Bash KL, et al. Trauma and pregnancy. Am J Perinatol 1997;14(6): 331–6.
[4] Weiss HB, Songer TJ, Fabio A. Fetal deaths related to maternal injury. JAMA 2001;286(15): 1863–8.
[5] Goodwin TM, Breen MT. Pregnancy outcome and fetomaternal hemorrhage after noncatastrophic trauma. Am J Obstet Gynecol 1990;162(3):665–71.
[6] Lavery JP, Staten-McCormick M. Management of moderate to severe trauma in pregnancy. Obstet Gynecol Clin North Am 1995;22(1):69–90.
[7] Bochicchio GV, Haan J, Scalea TM. Surgeon-performed focused assessment with sonography for trauma as an early screening tool for pregnancy after trauma. J Trauma 2002;52(6): 1125–8.
[8] The Eastern Association for the Surgery of Trauma. EAST Practice Management Guidelines Work Group. Diagnosis and management of inury in the pregnant patient. Available at: http://www.east.org/tpg/pregnancy.pdf. Accessed March 16, 2007.
[9] Ma OJ, Mateer JR, DeBehnke DJ. Use of ultrasonography for the evaluation of pregnant trauma patients. J Trauma 1996;40(4):665–8.
[10] Goodwin H, Holmes JF, Wisner DH. Abdominal ultrasound examination in pregnant blunt trauma patients. J Trauma 2001;50(4):689–93, [discussion: 694].
[11] Brown MA, Sirlin CB, Farahmand N, et al. Screening sonography in pregnant patients with blunt abdominal trauma. J Ultrasound Med 2005;24(2):175–81, [quiz: 183–4].
[12] Rothenberger DA, Quattlebaum FW, Zabel J, et al. Diagnostic peritoneal lavage for blunt trauma in pregnant women. Am J Obstet Gynecol 1977;129(5):479–81.
[13] Scorpio RJ, Esposito TJ, Smith LG, et al. Blunt trauma during pregnancy: factors affecting fetal outcome. J Trauma 1992;32(2):213–6.
[14] Davis BH, Olsen S, Bigelow NC, et al. Detection of fetal red cells in fetomaternal hemorrhage using a fetal hemoglobin monoclonal antibody by flow cytometry. Transfusion 1998;38(8):749–56.
[15] Clinical policy: critical issues in the initial evaluation and management of patients presenting to the emergency department in early pregnancy. Ann Emerg Med 2003;41(1):123–33.
[16] ACOG educational bulletin. Obstetric aspects of trauma management. Number 251, September 1998 (replaces Number 151, January 1991, and Number 161, November 1991). American College of Obstetrics and Gynecology. Int J Gynaecol Obstet 1999;64(1):87–94.
[17] Muench MV, Baschat AA, Reddy UM, et al. Kleihauer-Betke testing is important in all cases of maternal trauma. J Trauma 2004;57(5):1094–8.
[18] Dhanraj D, Lambers D. The incidences of positive Kleihauer-Betke test in low-risk pregnancies and maternal trauma patients. Am J Obstet Gynecol 2004;190(5):1461–3.

[19] Osei EK, Faulkner K. Fetal doses from radiological examinations. Br J Radiol 1999;72(860): 773–80.
[20] Lowe SA. Diagnostic radiography in pregnancy: risks and reality. Aust N Z J Obstet Gynaecol 2004;44(3):191–6.
[21] Damilakis J, Perisinakis K, Voloudaki A, et al. Estimation of fetal radiation dose from computed tomography scanning in late pregnancy: depth-dose data from routine examinations. Invest Radiol 2000;35(9):527–33.
[22] Bochicchio GV, Napolitano LM, Haan J, et al. Incidental pregnancy in trauma patients. J Am Coll Surg 2001;192(5):566–9.
[23] Goldman SM, Wagner LK. Radiologic management of abdominal trauma in pregnancy. AJR Am J Roentgenol 1996;166(4):763–7.
[24] Pearlman MD, Tintinallli JE, Lorenz RP. A prospective controlled study of outcome after trauma during pregnancy. Am J Obstet Gynecol 1990;162(6):1502–7, [discussion: 1507–10].
[25] El Kady D, Gilbert WM, Xing G, et al. Association of maternal fractures with adverse perinatal outcomes. Am J Obstet Gynecol 2006;195(3):711–6.
[26] Ali J, Yeo A, Gana TJ, et al. Predictors of fetal mortality in pregnant trauma patients. J Trauma 1997;42(5):782–5.
[27] Biester EM, Tomich PG, Esposito TJ, et al. Trauma in pregnancy: normal Revised Trauma Score in relation to other markers of maternofetal status–a preliminary study. Am J Obstet Gynecol 1997;176(6):1206–10, [discussion: 1210–2].
[28] El Kady D, Gilbert WM, Xing G, et al. Maternal and neonatal outcomes of assaults during pregnancy. Obstet Gynecol 2005;105(2):357–63.
[29] Hoff WS, D'Amelio LF, Tinkoff GH, et al. Maternal predictors of fetal demise in trauma during pregnancy. Surg Gynecol Obstet 1991;172(3):175–80.
[30] Kissinger DP, Rozycki GS, Morris JA Jr, et al. Trauma in pregnancy. Predicting pregnancy outcome. Arch Surg 1991;126(9):1079–86.
[31] Schiff MA, Holt VL. The injury severity score in pregnant trauma patients: predicting placental abruption and fetal death. J Trauma 2002;53(5):946–9.
[32] Sperry JL, Casey BM, McIntire DD, et al. Long-term fetal outcomes in pregnant trauma patients. Am J Surg 2006;192(6):715–21.
[33] Shah KH, Simons RK, Holbrook T, et al. Trauma in pregnancy: maternal and fetal outcomes. J Trauma 1998;45(1):83–6.
[34] Esposito TJ, Gens DR, Smith LG, et al. Trauma during pregnancy. A review of 79 cases. Arch Surg 1991;126(9):1073–8.
[35] Rogers FB, Rozycki GS, Osler TM, et al. A multi-institutional study of factors associated with fetal death in injured pregnant patients. Arch Surg 1999;134(11):1274–7.
[36] Dahmus MA, Sibai BM. Blunt abdominal trauma: are there any predictive factors for abruptio placentae or maternal-fetal distress? Am J Obstet Gynecol 1993;169(4):1054–9.
[37] Katz VL, Dotters DJ, Droegemueller W. Perimortem cesarean delivery. Obstet Gynecol 1986;68(4):571–6.
[38] Morris JA Jr, Rosenbower TJ, Jurkovich GJ, et al. Infant survival after cesarean section for trauma. Ann Surg 1996;223(5):481–8, [discussion: 488–91].
[39] Katz V, Balderston K, DeFreest M. Perimortem cesarean delivery: were our assumptions correct? Am J Obstet Gynecol 2005;192(6):1916–20, [discussion 1920–1].
[40] Tsuei BJ. Assessment of the pregnant trauma patient. Injury 2006;37(5):367–73.
[41] Baker DP. Trauma in the pregnant patient. Surg Clin North Am 1982;62(2):275–89.
[42] Pearlman MD, Tintinalli JE. Evaluation and treatment of the gravida and fetus following trauma during pregnancy. Obstet Gynecol Clin North Am 1991;18(2):371–81.
[43] Shah AJ, Kilcline BA. Trauma in pregnancy. Emerg Med Clin North Am 2003;21(3):615–29.
[44] Leggon RE, Wood GC, Indeck MC. Pelvic fractures in pregnancy: factors influencing maternal and fetal outcomes. J Trauma 2002;53(4):796–804.
[45] Dunlop DJ, McCahill JP, Blakemore ME. Internal fixation of an acetabular fracture during pregnancy. Injury 1997;28(7):481–2.

[46] Loegters T, Briem D, Gatzka C, et al. Treatment of unstable fractures of the pelvic ring in pregnancy. Arch Orthop Trauma Surg 2005;125(3):204–8.
[47] Parker B, McFarlane J, Soeken K. Abuse during pregnancy: effects on maternal complications and birth weight in adult and teenage women. Obstet Gynecol 1994;84(3):323–8.
[48] Pearlman MD, Phillips ME. Safety belt use during pregnancy. Obstet Gynecol 1996;88(6): 1026–9.
[49] McGwin G Jr, Russell SR, Rux RL, et al. Knowledge, beliefs, and practices concerning seat belt use during pregnancy. J Trauma 2004;56(3):670–5.
[50] Johnson HC, Pring DW. Car seatbelts in pregnancy: the practice and knowledge of pregnant women remain causes for concern. BJOG 2000;107(5):644–7.
[51] Schiff M, Kasnic T, Reiff K, et al. Seat belt use during pregnancy. West J Med 1992;156(6): 655–7.
[52] Tyroch AH, Kaups KL, Rohan J, et al. Pregnant women and car restraints: beliefs and practices. J Trauma 1999;46(2):241–5.
[53] Fusco A, Kelly K, Winslow J. Uterine rupture in a motor vehicle crash with airbag deployment. J Trauma 2001;51(6):1192–4.
[54] Metz TD, Abbott JT. Uterine trauma in pregnancy after motor vehicle crashes with airbag deployment: a 30-case series. J Trauma 2006;61(3):658–61.
[55] Pearlman MD, Viano D. Automobile crash simulation with the first pregnant crash test dummy. Am J Obstet Gynecol 1996;175(4 Pt 1):977–81.
[56] Moorcroft DM, Stitzel JD, Duma GG, et al. Computational model of the pregnant occupant: predicting the risk of injury in automobile crashes. Am J Obstet Gynecol 2003; 189(2):540–4.
[57] National conference on medical indications for air bag disconnection conducted by The Ronald Reagan Institute of Emergency Medicine and The National Crash Analysis Center, The George Washington University Medical Center. Washington DC, July 16–18, 1997.
[58] Guth AA, Pachter L. Domestic violence and the trauma surgeon. Am J Surg 2000;179(2): 134–40.
[59] Poole GV, Martin JN Jr, Perry KG Jr, et al. Trauma in pregnancy: the role of interpersonal violence. Am J Obstet Gynecol 1996;174(6):1873–7, [discussion 1877–8].
[60] Rudloff U. Trauma in pregnancy. Arch Gynecol Obstet 2007, in press.
[61] Dienemann J, Trautman D, Shahan JB, et al. Developing a domestic violence program in an inner-city academic health center emergency department: the first 3 years. J Emerg Nurs 1999;25(2):110–5.
[62] McFarlane J, Parker B, Soeken K, et al. Assessing for abuse during pregnancy. Severity and frequency of injuries and associated entry into prenatal care. JAMA 1992;267(23):3176–8.
[63] ACOG technical bulletin. Domestic violence. Number 209–August 1995 (replaces no. 124, January 1989). American College of Obstetrics and Gynecology. Int J Gynaecol Obstet 1995;51(2):161–70.

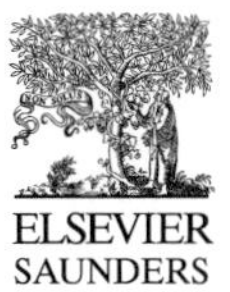

ELSEVIER
SAUNDERS

Emerg Med Clin N Am 25 (2007) 873–899

EMERGENCY
MEDICINE
CLINICS OF
NORTH AMERICA

Wound Management

Maria E. Moreira, MD[a,b,*], Vincent J. Markovchick, MD, FAAEM[c,d]

[a] *Denver Health Medical Center, Denver, CO, USA*
[b] *Division of Emergency Medicine, University of Colorado Health Sciences Center, 777 Bannock Street, Mailcode 0108, Denver, CO 80204, USA*
[c] *Emergency Medical Services, Denver Health, 777 Bannock Street, MC 0108, Denver, CO 80204, USA*
[d] *Division of Emergency Medicine, Department of Surgery, University of Colorado Health Sciences Center, 777 Bannock Street, Denver, CO 80204, USA*

Management of traumatic wounds is one of the most common procedures practiced in emergency medicine representing approximately 8% percent of emergency department (ED) presentations [1]. It is the most visible manifestation of emergency practice, in that the result of the physician's efforts is with the patient for their entire life. Wound care practices, however, have been based mostly on experience with a paucity of well-performed, randomized, controlled clinical trials to support these practices.

There has been controversy over different aspects of wound care including timing of wound closure, the best method of wound closure, the preparation of wounds, and antibiotic use in traumatic wounds. Studies relevant to these aspects of wound management are discussed further in this article. The article also discusses future innovative methods for wound management including the use of botulinum toxin, hyaluronidase injections, and porcine small intestinal submucosa (SIS). Emergency medicine physicians strive to provide patients with the best care in a timely fashion based on the current evidence. In wound management, this goal translates to providing painless, quick wound closure with an excellent cosmetic result and avoiding infection. New methods of wound closure that meet all these criteria are discussed.

* Corresponding author. Division of Emergency Medicine, University of Colorado Health Sciences Center, 777 Bannock Street, Mailcode 0108, Denver, CO 80204.

E-mail address: maria.moreira@dhha.org (M.E. Moreira).

doi:10.1016/j.emc.2007.06.008

Physiology

The goal in wound management is an ideal functional or cosmetic result without any complication. To achieve this goal, the clinician must have a basic understanding of wound physiology and factors that potentially can affect normal wound healing.

When wounding occurs, wound edges retract, and tissue contracts. Subsequently platelets aggregate on the exposed wound surface, the clotting cascade is activated, and a hemostatic coagulum is formed. The inflammatory response follows with granulocytes and lymphocytes migrating to the wound helping to control bacterial growth and suppress infection. Macrophages are the predominant cell present in the wound by day 5. These cells play a role in early fibroblast and collagen formation. As the inflammatory response evolves, epithelial cells form pseudopod-like structures and move over the wound surface. After laceration repair, initial epithelialization occurs within 24 to 48 hours. Peak synthesis of collagen occurs between days 5 and 7. Because of the balance between synthesis and lysis, however, there is a vulnerable period between days 7 and 10 after initial injury when wounds are prone to dehiscence. The wound will be at 5% of its ultimate tensile strength at 2 weeks and at about 35% at 1 month [2].

Clinical evaluation

History

A thorough history is paramount for discerning host factors affecting wound healing. Multiple patient conditions have been shown to increase the risk of infection. These conditions include extremes of age, diabetes mellitus, chronic renal failure, obesity, malnutrition, and inherited or acquired connective tissue disorders [3]. The use of certain medications is important also. Immunosuppressive medications such as corticosteroids have been shown to affect wound healing negatively and to increase the potential for infection [3].

Wound and environmental factors also contribute to wound healing. The clinician needs to ascertain if the wound was caused by a cut or by blunt trauma. Compressive forces as the mechanism of injury increase the risk for infection because of compromised circulation to the wound edges [4]. Retained foreign bodies increase the risk of an inflammatory response and subsequent infection and abscess formation. A "dirty" wound may or may not be a "contaminated" wound. Contaminated wounds are those in which there is a high degree of bacterial inoculation at the time of wounding. Mechanisms include mammalian bites, human bites, and wounds incurred in submerged bodies of water (eg, streams, lakes, ponds). Also "old" wounds should be considered contaminated because of the high level of bacteria 6 to 8 hours after wounding.

The time from injury to evaluation can affect the type of closure performed. The concept of the "golden period" stems from the assumption that bacterial proliferation within wounds is dependent on time from initial insult to repair. All wounds, including "clean" wounds, have bacteria introduced at the time of wounding. Although bacteria are in the wound at the time of presentation [5,6], however, most wounds have bacterial counts well below the infectious inoculum of 10^5 or more organisms per gram [6]. A period of 3 to 5 hours generally is required for proliferation of bacteria to produce infection [6], and after 8 hours the bacterial count rises exponentially.

A study undertaken in Jamaica suggested a 19-hour golden period for the repair of simple wounds in areas other than the head. Wounds sutured after 19 hours were less likely to heal. Healing of wounds involving the head was unaffected by the interval between injury and repair [7]. This study quotes time periods slightly longer than the standard period suggested for the interval before extremity wound closure. The accepted interval from injury to wound closure is up to 6 hours for wounds to the extremities and up to 24 hours for face and scalp wounds.

Some clinicians suggest that timing is not important if the wound is clean and not infected [8]. Each wound needs to be considered individually as to the time and mechanism of injury as well as wound and host characteristics affecting potential functional and cosmetic outcome. The clinician may decide to close a clean leg wound on a healthy patient after 10 hours and not to close a contaminated leg wound on a diabetic after 4 hours.

Other important aspects of the history include allergies to medications and tetanus immunization status. The incidence of tetanus has declined since tetanus toxoid vaccine was introduced in the 1940s. From 1998 to 2000, the average annual incidence of tetanus was 0.16 cases per million population. Most of the cases reported during that time occurred in people who had inadequate vaccination or unknown vaccination history and who sustained an acute injury [9].

If a patient has an inadequate immunization history or has never been immunized, tetanus immune globulin (250 IU) and tetanus toxoid (0.5 mL) are indicated. A primary series of tetanus toxoid induces protective levels of serum antitoxin persisting for 10 years or longer [10]. Booster for minor and uncontaminated wounds needs to be given only every 10 years. With other wounds, booster should be administered if the patient has not received tetanus toxoid within 5 years. Tetanus-diphtheria toxoid (0.5 mL) is preferred for patients 7 years of age and older, whereas diphtheria, pertussis, and tetanus (0.5 mL) should be used in patients under the age of 7 years. For the patient who has a tetanus-prone wound and unknown tetanus immunization or less than three tetanus toxoid doses, tetanus immune globulin as well as toxoid should be given. Tetanus immune globulin provides passive immunity. If the patient presents with a non–tetanus-prone wound, only toxoid is required. A wound is considered tetanus-prone if it has any of the following features: age of wound greater than 6 hours, stellate wound or avulsion, depth of wound greater than 1 cm, mechanism of injury is a missile, crush, burn, or frostbite, signs of infection are present, devitalized tissue is present, presence of contaminants (dirt, feces, soil, or saliva), or presence of denervated or ischemic tissue. If both tetanus immune globulin and toxoid are given, they need to be given in different syringes and at separate sites.

Physical examination

Proper physical examination and documentation of the wound includes location, length in centimeters, neurovascular examination, motor examination, exploration for tendon or joint involvement, and presence of foreign body. Some wound characteristics noted on physical examination portend a higher rate of infection. In a cross-sectional study of patients who had traumatic lacerations, wound characteristics associated with higher infection rates included jagged wound edges, stellate shape, injury deeper than the subcutaneous tissue, presence of a foreign body, and visible contaminants (ie, dirt and others) [11]. Infection was defined as the presence of a stitch abscess, purulent drainage, or cellulites more than 1 cm beyond the wound edges.

A thorough neurovascular examination needs to be performed before anesthetizing the wound. Two-point discrimination at the finger pads provides the best assessment of digital nerve function [12]. Any sensory deficits, problems with motor function, and the presence of pulses or capillary refill need to be documented. If there is a suspicion of a fracture, a radiograph should be obtained before moving a joint through full range of motion. The motor examination provides an evaluation of motor nerves, muscle groups, and tendons.

All wounds need to be explored to evaluate for tendon lacerations and foreign bodies. To obtain optimal examination of the wound, good lighting and a bloodless field are essential. Several methods are available to control bleeding from wounds. Direct external pressure almost always is successful in controlling bleeding. If the wound is in an extremity, and bleeding cannot be controlled with direct external pressure, the next option is to inflate a sphygmomanometer proximal to the site of bleeding. The cuff needs to be inflated to a pressure greater than the patient's systolic blood pressure. The clinician needs to keep track of the time of cuff inflation, which, in general, can be maintained for about 2 hours without producing injury to vessels or nerves. Digital tourniquets, on fingers or toes, should be used only for 20 to 30 minutes at a time.

Because the position of joints and tendons during injury can differ from the position during examination, once a bloodless field is obtained, the depth of the wound needs to be visualized while the extremity is taken through full range of motion. Remember that a tendon can be 90% lacerated and still maintain normal motor function. Avoid motor testing for tendon injury against resistance to prevent from converting a partial tendon laceration into a complete tendon laceration.

It also is important to detect and remove foreign bodies within the wound because the presence of a foreign body poses an increased risk of infection. Other reasons for removal of foreign bodies include impairment of mechanical function, potential for causing persistent pain, and potential for migration. When possible, all foreign bodies should be removed. For those that are minute or deep in tissue or muscle, the risks versus benefits of exploration and removal must be evaluated. If a foreign body does not meet an indication for removal and is not readily accessible, it should be left in place, and the patient must be informed of the risk/benefit assessment and the reason for leaving a retained foreign body in situ.

Careful consideration should be given to handling of tissues when exploring wounds. The clinician must avoid any further damage to the tissue while obtaining a clear visualization of the depth of the wound. Instead of using toothed forceps to grasp wound edges, a nontoothed forcep should be used or alternatively, the forcep should be used to push the edges apart. Skin hooks also can be used to lift wound edges apart. If skin hooks are not available, hooks can be created by bending the tips of a 20-gauge needle [12].

Diagnostic evaluation

The use of diagnostic adjuncts is unnecessary for most wounds. Physical examination and exploration after hemorrhage control usually provide a thorough evaluation of the wound. If the wound extends into muscle belly, and the mechanism is compatible with a foreign body (eg, broken glass), radiographs are indicated. Eighty percent to 90% of foreign bodies are detected by radiograph [13,14], but radiographs may not detect organic foreign bodies such as wood splinters and vegetable matter. In those instances, ultrasound may detect organic foreign bodies not visible on radiographs. CT is the modality of choice for the detection of foreign bodies when other techniques have failed.

Therapeutic intervention

Anesthesia

Proper wound evaluation, exploration, and closure are enhanced by good anesthesia. Modalities for administration of anesthesia include topical, direct wound infiltration, or regional nerve blocks. Certain patients may require procedural sedation as an adjunct to local anesthesia. In many cases more than one form of anesthesia is beneficial.

Although topical anesthetics decrease the pain of subsequent anesthetic injection, they require time to take effect. Investigators have shown that a topical anesthetic such as 4% lidocaine, 1:2000 epinephrine, and 0.5%

tetracaine can be applied effectively by nurses at triage [15]. This administration helps decrease the amount of time from presentation to repair. Table 1 provides a list of available topical anesthetics and their onset and duration of action.

There are two categories of local anesthetics: the amides and the esters. Allergy to one group is not associated with allergy to anesthetic from the other group. Most allergies are caused by preservatives used in the anesthetic. Therefore, a pure agent such as cardiac lidocaine can be used in patients who have allergies to anesthetics.

The maximum safe dose of an anesthetic must be considered when performing infiltration (Table 2). This maximum safe dose increases with the addition of epinephrine to the solution. Epinephrine should be avoided in areas with end arterioles and lack of collateral circulation. These sites include the fingers, toes, the tip of the nose, pinna, and penis.

The pain of local infiltration can be diminished by injecting subcutaneously through the open wound edge instead of directly into intact skin [16,17] with the smallest needle possible. Although 30-gauge needles can be used for direct infiltration, 25- or 27-gauge needles are better suited for regional nerve blocks to decrease the possibility of deflection of the needle [18]. Other available techniques to decrease pain of infiltration include buffering the anesthetic with sodium bicarbonate in a 1:10 solution, using warm solutions, using slow rates of infiltration, and pretreatment with topical anesthetic [19–21].

Regional anesthesia blocks the nerve supply to the area of the laceration. Regional anesthesia is preferred to local infiltration in three specific situations: (1) in wounds that otherwise would require large, toxic amounts of local anesthetic; (2) in wounds in which local tissue distortion needs to be avoided (eg, lips and digits); (3) in wounds where local infiltration is particularly painful (eg, plantar surface of the foot). In these cases the discomfort of percutaneous injection can be reduced using topical cryotherapy with an ice cube. A further description of regional nerve blocks can be found in any emergency medicine procedural textbook.

Procedural sedation and anesthesia may be required in cases of extensive wound repair, especially in children. The goal is to achieve a depressed level of consciousness while maintaining a patent airway. Procedural sedation can be performed safely and effectively by emergency physicians in both community- and university-based settings. Table 3 provides a partial list of drugs available for this type of anesthesia [22].

In the pediatric population there has been some emphasis on use of distraction techniques (ie, music, video games, or cartoon videos) to improve satisfaction with wound repair and decrease the stress of wound repair. With distraction, the child's attention is diverted away from the stressful stimulus and focused onto a more pleasant one. Sinha and colleagues [23] found these techniques to be effective in reducing situational anxiety in older children and also in lowering parental perception of pain distress in younger

Table 1
Topical anesthetics

Anesthetic Product	Methods	Onset/duration	Effectiveness	Complications
TAC	2–5 mL (1 mL/cm of laceration) applied to wound with cotton or gauze for 10–30 minutes	Onset: effective 10–30 minutes after application. Duration: not established.	May be as effective as lidocaine for lacerations on face and scalp	Rare severe toxicity, including seizures and sudden cardiac death
LET	1–3 mL applied directly to wound for 15–30 minutes	Onset: 20–30 minutes. Duration: not established.	Similar to TAC for face and scalp lacerations; less effective on extremities	No severe adverse effects reported
EMLA	Thick layer (1–2 g/10 cm^2) applied to intact skin with covering patch of transparent medical dressing	Onset: must be left on for 1–2 hours. Duration: 0.5–2 hours	Variable, depending on duration of application	Contact dermatitis, methemoglobinemia (very rare)

Abbreviations: EMLA, 2.5% lidocaine and 2.5% prilocaine; LET, 4% lidocaine, 1:2000 epinephrine, and 0.5% tetracaine; TAC, 0.5% tetracaine, 1:2000 epinephrine, and 11.8% cocaine.

Data from Kundu S, Achar S. Principles of office anesthesia: part II. Topical anesthesia. Am Fam Physician 2002;66:100.

Table 2
Local anesthetics

Agent	Class	Maximum allowable single dose	Onset of action	Duration of action
Lidocaine	Amide	4.5 mg/kg of 1%	Fast	1–2 h
Lidocaine with epinephrine	Amide	7 mg/kg of 1%	Fast	2–4 h
Bupivacaine	Amide	2 mg/kg of 0.25%	Intermediate	4–8 h
Bupivacaine with epinephrine	Amide	3 mg/kg of 0.25%	Intermediate	8–16 h
Procaine	Ester	7 mg/kg	Slow	15–45 min
Procaine with epinephrine	Ester	9 mg/kg	Slow	30–60 min

children. Distraction did not reduce self-reported pain intensity, however. The children enrolled in this study had uncomplicated lacerations less than 5 cm in length.

Wound preparation

Wound preparation is a crucial aspect of wound management that affects infection rate. Saline irrigation decreases the incidence of wound infection in proportion to the amount of irrigation used [12,24,25]. The pressure at which this irrigant is delivered is crucial in determining the efficacy of irrigation [26,27]. With high-pressure irrigation, there is a balance between achieving a reduction in bacterial wound counts and causing further tissue damage. The recommended irrigation pressure is 5 to 8 psi [18,26,28], which can be achieved by using a 30- to 60-mL syringe and a 19-gauge needle or splash shield. This pressure also can be obtained by using a saline bag inside a pressure cuff inflated to 400 mm Hg and connected to intravenous tubing with a 19-gauge angiocath [29] or by using a mechanical irrigator. The location of the wound also needs to be considered when determining the irrigation pressure. Although high-pressure irrigation is indicated for

Table 3
Agents for procedural sedation

Medication	Recommended dose	Route of administration
Fentanyl	1–3 μg/kg	Intravenous
Midazolam	0.02–0.1 mg/kg (adult)	Intravenous
	0.05–0.15 mg/kg (child)	
	0.05–0.15 mg/kg	Intramuscular
	0.5–0.75 mg/kg	Oral
Ketamine	1–2 mg/kg	Intravenous
	4–5 mg/kg	Intramuscular
Propofol	1 mg/kg	Intravenous
Etomidate	0.1–0.2 mg/kg	Intravenous

contaminated wounds in the extremities, it is not indicated in highly vascularized areas containing loose areolar tissue. High-pressure irrigation of chest wall lacerations may induce a hemo/pneumothorax.

Other considerations include the amount of irrigation and the temperature of the irrigant. In a study comparing different amounts of irrigation (250 cm^3, 500 cm^3, and 1000 cm^3), the incidence of infection was related inversely to the amount of irrigation; that is, the greater the irrigation, the lower was the incidence of infection [30]. A simple rule of thumb is to use 50 mL to 100 mL of irrigant per centimeter of laceration [31]. The more contaminated the wound, the greater the amount of irrigant required for proper wound preparation. Less irrigation may be acceptable with noncontaminated wounds in well-vascularized areas such as the face. Hollander and colleagues [32] found irrigation did not make a difference in clean, noncontaminated facial and scalp lacerations. When considering temperature of the irrigant, a single-blind, cross-over trial of irrigation of simple linear wounds demonstrated that warmed saline was more comfortable and soothing than room-temperature saline [33].

If saline is not available for irrigation, tap water may be a good alternative. Several studies have shown tap water to be an effective irrigant without increasing rates of infection or growth of unusual organisms [34–36]. On the other hand, detergents, hydrogen peroxide, and concentrated povidone-iodine should be avoided in wound irrigation because these agents are toxic to tissues [26,29]. If detergent must be used (eg, to remove grease), it should be followed by copious irrigation.

Débridement should be reserved for wounds in which nonviable tissue creates a nidus for infection [26,37]. Necrotic tissue also obstructs re-epithelialization and wound contraction [38]. Therefore, all crushed or devitalized tissue should be debrided.

Hair should not be shaved during wound preparation. Bacteria reside in hair follicles, and shaving has been noted to increase wound infection [26,39]. Instead, clippers or scissors should be used to reduce damage to hair follicles.

Caps and masks have not been shown to make a difference in infection rates. Recently a prospective, randomized, multicenter trial evaluating the use of sterile versus nonsterile gloves in laceration repair showed no difference in the two groups in the final outcome of rate of infection as reported by patients on a questionnaire at the time of suture removal. Another randomized study has reproduced these results [40]. Sterile gloves fit better than nonsterile gloves, however, and result in better control of instruments and sutures. Sterile gloves continue to be used in most laceration repair.

Types of wound closure

There are three types of wound closure: primary, secondary, and delayed. Primary closure is closure of the wound before formation of granulation tissue. All "clean" wounds can be closed primarily except puncture wounds that cannot be irrigated adequately. Contaminated wounds, noncosmetic animal bites, abscess cavities, and wounds presenting after a delay should be irrigated, hemorrhage controlled, and debrided. Delayed primary closure can be performed after 3 to 5 days to allow the patient's defense system to decrease the bacterial load. Bacterial load will be at its lowest approximately 96 hours after the time of initial impact (Fig. 1). Secondary closure is healing by granulation tissue. This type of closure is suited for partial-thickness avulsions (ie, fingertip injuries), contaminated small wounds (ie, puncture wounds, stab wounds), and infected wounds.

Techniques of wound closure

The balance between function and cosmesis is a major consideration in selecting the technique for wound closure. When the goal is to obtain the best function, the laceration should be closed in a single layer with the least amount of sutures. When cosmesis is most important, a multiple-layer closure should be used [41]. Intradermal sutures when placed in areas of high static and dynamic wound tension improve cosmesis by facilitating the placement of surface sutures. Singer and colleagues [42] evaluated determinants of poor outcome after laceration repair. In their evaluation the type of closure and the use of deep sutures had no effect on cosmesis or infection rates, but the wounds included in the study were small, with mean length

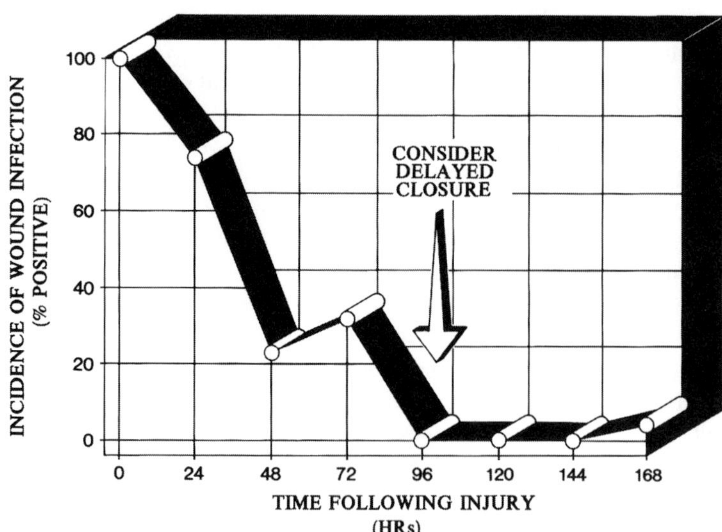

Fig. 1. This graph illustrates the best time for delayed wound closure from initial time of wounding. The incidence of infection is greatly reduced by 96 hours. (*From* Trott A. Decisions before closure–timing, debridement, consultation. In: Wounds and lacerations emergency care and closure. St. Louis (MO): Mosby; 1997. p. 119; with permission.)

of 2.2 ± 1.9 cm and mean width of 3.5 ± 3.8 mm. Table 4 lists the factors to consider when cosmesis is of utmost importance.

Stellate wounds that change directions or have multiple components are best closed with simple interrupted sutures. This type of suture would not be ideal for a wound with increased tension caused by swelling. For a wound under increased tension, such as over joints, horizontal mattress sutures can be used in a single-layer closure because they are naturally everting, hemostatic, and do not cut through skin edges if tension increases from movement or swelling. This type of closure is not used when the primary goal is cosmesis. Running sutures can be used in wounds under minimal tension or as the surface sutures in a layered closure.

Some lacerations need further manipulation by the clinician in preparation for closure. In gaping wounds, skin tension can be reduced by undermining the wound. Undermining is the procedure by which the dermis and superficial fascia are released from deeper attachments, allowing wound

Table 4
Factors contributing to scar visibility

Factors associated with scarring	Methods to minimize scarring
Direction of wound perpendicular to lines of static and dynamic tension	Layered closure; proper direction in elective incisions of wounds
Infection requiring removal of sutures and healing by secondary intention	Proper wound preparation; irrigation, and use of delayed closure in contaminated wounds
Wide scar secondary to tension	Layered closure, proper splinting, and elevation
Suture marks	Remove all percutaneous sutures within 7 days
Uneven wound edges	Careful, even approximation of wound superficial layer to prevent differential swelling of edges
Inversion of wound edges	Proper placement of simple sutures or use of horizontal mattress sutures
Tattooing secondary to retained dirt or foreign body	Proper wound preparation and débridement
Tissue necrosis	Use of corner sutures on flaps, splinting, and elevation of wounds with marginal circulation or venous return; excision of nonviable wound edges before closure
Compromised healing secondary to hematoma	Use of properly conforming dressing and splints
Hyperpigmentation of scar or abraded skin	Use of sun block with a sun protection factor ≥ 15 for 6 months
Superimposition of blood clots between healing wound edges	Proper hemostasis and closure; proper application of compressive dressings
Failure to align anatomic structures (eg, vermilion border) properly	Meticulous closure and alignment; use of regional blocks

Adapted from Markovchick V. Suture materials and mechanical after care. Emerg Med Clin North Am 1992;10:676.

edges to be brought together with less force. Undermining should be performed to a distance from the wound edge that approximates the extent of gaping of the wound edges [43].

Lacerations that are irregular in configuration and depth may require use of a mix of different techniques for closure. Triangular and circular lacerations can be converted into elliptical lacerations for better closure.

Materials

Various options are available for wound closure including sutures, staples, tissue adhesives, and adhesive tapes. Although each modality has its place in wound management, it is important to assess wound characteristics carefully to make the best choice in material.

Sutures

When selecting sutures the clinician must make two further decisions: absorbable versus nonabsorbable sutures and needle size. Absorbable sutures typically are used to close structures deeper than the epidermis. The synthetic absorbable sutures are less reactive and maintain greater tensile strength than the natural sources. The epidermis then is closed with nonabsorbable sutures such as nylon or polypropylene. The advantage of sutures over adhesives for this surface closure is that sutures can be used to ensure the opposed wound edges are even. These nonabsorbable sutures are relatively nonreactive and retain tensile strength for longer than 60 days [26,41].

Needle size depends on the location of the wound (Table 5). Typically, the epidermis is closed with 6.0 sutures on the face and 4.0 or 5.0 sutures on the extremities. Deep stitches typically are placed with 4.0 or 5.0 sutures.

Staples

Staples are a cosmetically acceptable alternative to sutures for the closure of scalp lacerations [44] and also are used for closure of linear perpendicular lacerations of the scalp, trunk, or extremities. Care must be taken to avoid uneven or overlapping wound edges when placing staples. Studies comparing staples and sutures have shown that staples provide more rapid wound repair [44–46] and have a lower rate of reactivity and infection [46]. The disadvantages of staples are the inability to provide a meticulous closure and the more painful process of removal [45].

Tissue adhesives

The cyanoacrylate adhesives were developed in 1945 to be applied topically to the epidermis, thus bridging the wound edges. Care must be taken to avoid getting any adhesive between cut wound edges. Although

Table 5
Guidelines for suture material dependent on body region

Body region	Suture material (skin)	Suture material (deep)	Special closure and dressing	Suture removal
Scalp	3-0 or 4-0 NA	4-0 SA	Interrupted in galea; single, tight layer for scalp	7–12 d
Pinna (ear)	6-0 NA	5-0 SA	Interrupted SA sutures for perichondrium; stint dressing	4–6 d
Eyebrow	6-0 NA	4-0 or 5-0 SA	Layered closure	4–5 d
Eyelid	6-0 NA	None	Single-layer horizontal mattress	4–5 d
Lip	6-0 NA	4-0 silk or SA (mucosa); 5-0 SA (subcutaneous, muscle)	Three-layered closure for through and through lacerations	4–6 d
Oral cavity	None	4-0 SA	Layered closure if muscularis of tongue involved	7–8 d or allow to dissolve
Face	6-0 NA	4-0 or 5-0 SA	Layered closure for full-thickness lacerations	4–6 d
Neck	5-0 NA	4-0 SA (subcutaneous)	Two-layered closure gives best cosmetic result	4–6 d
Trunk	4-0 or 5-0 NA	4-0 SA (subcutaneous, fat)	Single or layered closure	7–12 d
Extremity	4-0 or 5-0 NA	3-0 or 4-0 SA (subcutaneous, fat, muscle)	Splint if wound is over a joint	7–14 d
Hands and feet	4-0 or 5-0 NA	None	Only close skin; use horizontal mattress sutures if there is much tension on wound edges; splint if wound over joint	7–12 d
Nailbed	5-0 SA	None	Replace nail under cuticle	Allow to dissolve

Abbreviations: NA, nonabsorbable suture (eg, nylon, polypropylene); SA, synthetic absorbable suture.

Data from Markovchick V. Soft tissue injury and wound repair. In: Reisdorff EJ, Roberts MR, Wiegenstein JG, editors. Pediatric emergency medicine. Philadelphia: W.B. Saunders; 1993. p. 899–908; and Trott A. Special anatomic sites. In: Wounds and lacerations emergency care and closure. St. Louis (MO): Mosby; 1997. p. 179.

considered a relatively painless method of wound closure, the chemical reaction of polymerization when tissue adhesives are applied produces heat that can cause some discomfort [31]. Wound closure using this method is less painful and faster than closure with sutures. Tissue adhesive is an effective method of closing appropriately selected wounds. Use of tissue adhesives should be limited to linear lacerations less than 4 cm in length [47] in wounds devoid of significant tension or repetitive movement. If tissue adhesive is used to close the skin in an area of high tension, subcutaneous or subcuticular sutures are required to relieve this tension.

One of the largest studies comparing tissue adhesives with sutures was the manufacturer-sponsored study for the approval of 2-octylcyanoacrylate by the Food and Drug Administration. This study found that tissue adhesives had performance comparable to sutures in short-term infection rate, wound dehiscence, and 3-month cosmetic outcome [26,48]. Other studies have shown similar results [49,50]. When used for wound repair in athletes allowed to return to play immediately, tissue adhesive was found to retain its strength, durability, and skin apposition [51].

Wounds parallel to Langer's lines of skin tension tend to have a better outcome than those running against these physiologic lines (Fig. 2). Simon [52] evaluated facial lacerations closed with tissue adhesives or sutures, specifically studying laceration relationship to lines of skin tension. All wounds greater than 5 mm in length underwent placement of subcutaneous sutures.

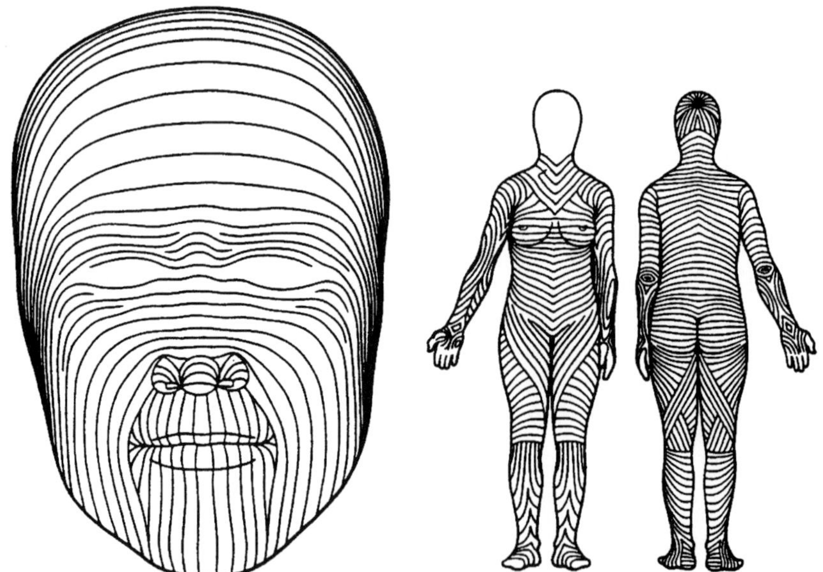

Fig. 2. Direction of lines of skin tension. (*From* Marx J, Hockberger R, Well R, et al, editors. Rosen's emergency medicine: concepts and clinical practice. 5th edition. Philadelphia: Mosby; 2002. p. 738–9; with permission.)

Then patients were assigned randomly to tissue adhesives or sutures for skin closure. He noted that cosmetic outcome of facial lacerations repaired by tissue adhesives was less affected by the initial orientation of the wound. The author's concluded that tissue adhesives can be used to close facial lacerations regardless of the orientation of the wound [52]. Several techniques are available for the removal of these tissue adhesives. Bathing accelerates removal, as does the application of antibiotic ointment or petroleum jelly. If more rapid removal is necessary, acetone can be used.

Adhesive tapes

Studies have shown adhesive tapes to be equal to staples in cosmesis and to pose less risk of infection than either staples or sutures [53]. Lacerations evaluated in this study were facial lacerations less than 2.5 cm in length and less than 12 hours old. Cosmetic outcomes were evaluated at 2 months, which may not correlate with long-term outcome.

Adhesive tapes can be applied in many different patterns, but a parallel, non-overlapping pattern with complete coating of the skin surface with Liquid adhesive has the highest degree of adherence [54]. At 10 days these wounds have tensile strength equal or superior to that of wounds closed with sutures [54].

Special situations in wound management

Scalp

A scalp wound requires palpation and exploration for the evaluation of a possible skull fracture. After proper exploration, the wound edges should be approximated tightly with sutures or staples to prevent hematoma formation. The double staple gun technique is a useful trick for use in pediatric lacerations requiring two staples. This technique involves two physicians holding a staple gun perpendicular to the laceration and firing the staple gun in unison. Placing the staples at the same time is less painful and decreases the emotional trauma for the patient [55].

Scalp lacerations 3 to 10 cm in length also can be closed using the patient's own hair. Hair strands need to be at least 3 cm in length. Strands from each side of the wound are twisted together to approximate the wound edges. The intertwined strands then are secured in place using a drop of tissue adhesive. This procedure is quick and cost effective as well as less painful for the patient [55].

Pinna

Anesthesia of the pinna is obtained with a field block. After repair, a pressure dressing must be applied to prevent formation of a hematoma between the skin and the perichondrium. A hematoma in this site is painful and may compromise the blood supply to the cartilage. The dressing is left in place for 24 to 48 hours.

The wound needs to be inspected for any cartilaginous involvement. These lacerations are closed by apposing the skin overlying the laceration in the cartilage. In a through-and-through laceration, the anterior and posterior portions of the wound are closed separately. If possible, one should avoid placing sutures through the cartilage. If the skin cannot be brought over the cartilage without tension, conservative débridement must be performed. No more than 5 mm of cartilage should be debrided. More than that will deform the cartilaginous skeleton [56].

Eyebrow

Excision of tissue is to be avoided. When débridement is necessary, it should be performed in a parallel direction of the hair follicle. Eyebrows should never be removed, because doing so can lead to abnormal growth. The eyebrow provides a useful guide for approximation of wound edges.

Eyelid

Eyelid lacerations require an examination for possible globe penetration. If the laceration is through the tarsal plate or involves the lacrimal apparatus, an ophthalmology consultation is advised. If simple sutures result in inversion or overlapping of wound edges, horizontal mattress sutures should be used.

Lip

Through-and-through lip lacerations require layered closure from the inside out. Suturing the oral mucosa first minimizes contamination of the wound from saliva. After the mucosa is closed with absorbable suture, the closure is checked by irrigating the wound and evaluating for leaks into the oral cavity. Subsequently the muscle layer is closed with 4.0 or 5.0 absorbable suture. Not closing the muscle layer can lead to a depression of the scar as the muscle fibers retract. In closing the outer aspect of the lip, priority is given to approximating the vermilion border with the first stitch or "stay" suture placed at this site. If part of the vermillion is missing with the laceration, a full-thickness wedge of lip tissue can be removed. This technique will produce a single linear scar with an intact vermilion, which is preferable to an irregular vermillion margin. Up to one third of the lip can be lost without appreciable distortion in the symmetry of the lip [57]. Because of the importance of the approximation of the vermilion border, regional anesthesia (infraorbital or mental nerve block) should be considered.

Oral cavity and mucous membranes

Lacerations of the buccal mucosa and gingiva generally heal without repair, but wounds that are longer than 2 cm, gaping, or continuing to bleed should be closed tightly with absorbable 4.0 or 5.0 suture. Likewise, the indications for repair of tongue lacerations are uncontrollable hemorrhage, airway compromise, the presence of a significant segment of severed tongue, or a gaping laceration. Tongue sutures should be placed wide and deep. These sutures should be tied loosely to allow room for swelling. Placing an instrument such as a closed hemostat between the suture and the tongue prevents overtying the knot [57]. All three layers (inferior mucosa, muscle, and superior mucosa) of a tongue laceration can be closed with one stitch or with two stitches including half of the thickness of the tongue in each stitch. If the wound involves the posterior pharynx, a lateral soft tissue radiograph may be of benefit in determining the extent of the wound. Air dissecting along fascial planes is indicative of deep space involvement.

Face

With cheek lacerations, there is potential for injury to the parotid gland and to the seventh cranial nerve. Discharge of clear fluid from the wound indicates parotid gland or Stensen's duct involvement. Involvement of these structures is an indication for consultation. Facial wounds should not undergo radical débridement. Because of the excellent blood supply to the head and neck, tissue can survive in this region on small pedicles [57].

Extremities

Lacerations over joints need to be evaluated for involvement of the joint capsule. Sterile saline can be injected into the joint to assess for a defect in the joint capsule. Extravasation is better appreciated by adding a few drops of methylene blue to the saline. Small defects in the capsule can be detected by the use of fluorescein. A drop of fluorescein is placed into 50 mL of saline and injected into the joint. The joint then is wrapped for 10 minutes. Once the wrap is removed, extravasation can be detected with a Wood's lamp [58].

Wounds over joints or under increased tension require suturing with interrupted horizontal mattress sutures and splinting for at least 1 to 2 weeks.

Hands

Conservative treatment with serial nonadherent dressings is advocated for pulp defects less than 1 cm^2 in adults and proportionately smaller in children with minimal or no bone exposure [59]. Lacerations less than 2 cm also may be treated conservatively without suturing. Quinn and colleagues [60] evaluated hand lacerations less than 2 cm long without associated tendon, joint, bone, or nerve injury. They randomly assigned patients to conservative management or suturing. Two independent physicians blinded to treatment assessed the end points. Cosmetic appearance at 3 months did not differ between the two groups. The mean time to treatment, however, was longer in the suture group than in the conservative group (19 minutes versus 5 minutes). Time to resume normal activities was reported as the same in both groups [60,61].

Many factors must be considered when deciding between replantation or amputation of a distal digit injury. In a study from Japan, replantation provided better functional outcomes, better appearance, and higher patient satisfaction with minimal pain. The other disadvantage of amputation is the potential for a painful stump. On the other hand, amputation provides a shorter recovery period and faster return to work [62].

Nail bed

The nail bed is damaged in 15% to 24% of fingertip injuries in children [59]. Simple lacerations through the sterile matrix are sutured with 6.0 or 7.0 absorbable suture [59]. If the nail plate has been removed, it should be replaced to maintain adequate space between the germinal matrix and the proximal nail fold. A small hole can be placed in the nail bed to allow for drainage. The nail plate then is secured with a 5.0 nylon suture through the hyponychium or with a horizontal mattress suture through the proximal nail fold. If a distal hyponychium suture is used, it can be left in place for 7 to 10 days. The nail plate also has been replaced using tissue adhesives [63,64] and chloramphenicol [65]. With chloramphenicol, a small amount of ointment is applied to the deep surface of the nail plate, and then the nail plate is slipped under the eponychial fold into position. The ointment forms an adhesive layer between the nail plate and the nail bed. The finger then is dressed, and the dressing is left in place for 1 week. The nail plate works itself loose on its own, usually when that occurs the nail bed is well healed and the new nail is growing from below. If the nail plate is not available, a piece of reinforced silicone sheeting or nonadherent gauze can be used instead.

For subungal hematomas there is no difference between nail bed removal with repair of the nail bed laceration and drainage of the hematoma without nail removal. The results of one study recommended conservative management of subungal hematoma regardless of size when the nail plate is still adherent to the bed and not displaced out of the nail folds. Roser and Gellman [66] compared nail trephinization and nail bed repair for subungal hematoma in children. Inclusion criteria for the study were an intact nail and nail margin with subungal hematoma and no previous nail abnormality. These authors found no difference in outcome for the two groups regardless of hematoma size, presence of fracture, age, or injury mechanism.

About 50% of nail bed injuries have an associated distal phalangeal fracture [66]. Although these injuries usually can be considered open fractures, antibiotics are not indicated for this type of wound.

Bites

Five percent of traumatic wounds evaluated in the ED result from mammalian bites, most commonly dog bites. Infection rates are highest for puncture wounds caused by cat bites, ranging from 29% to 50%

[67]. Chen and colleagues [68] studied primary closure of wounds caused by mammalian bites (dogs, cats, humans) and found the overall infection rate to be 6%. There was no difference between the incidence of infection in lacerations of the head and the upper extremities. This infection rate may be acceptable when closure is necessary and cosmesis is the main concern. Fig. 3 gives a suggested algorithm to be used for the care of bite wounds.

Gunshot wounds

The increased damage associated with high-velocity injuries is secondary to the dissipation of kinetic energy. Also, behind the bullet there is a sucking action that deposits clothing or dirt in the wound. Wounds caused by bullets should be debrided, irrigated, and left open to be repaired with delayed primary closure or by secondary closure.

Antibiotics in wound care

One of the continuing controversies in wound management is the use of prophylactic antibiotics. Studies looking at antibiotics in wound care have varied in definitions of infection and in protocols for outpatient wound surveillance. These studies also have been limited by the low number of subjects.

In 1961 Burke [69] looked at the effective period for preventive antibiotics in contaminated wounds. He noted this period to be from the time bacteria gained access to the wound to 2 to 3 hours after the initial inoculation. This finding suggests a golden period for administration of antibiotics of 3 hours to limit bacterial proliferation. When evaluating clinical studies, this estimate seems to be conservative.

Several studies have failed to show a benefit for prophylactic antibiotics in simple lacerations [4,26,70–72]. After performing a meta-analysis of randomized trials of prophylactic antibiotics for simple nonbite wounds,

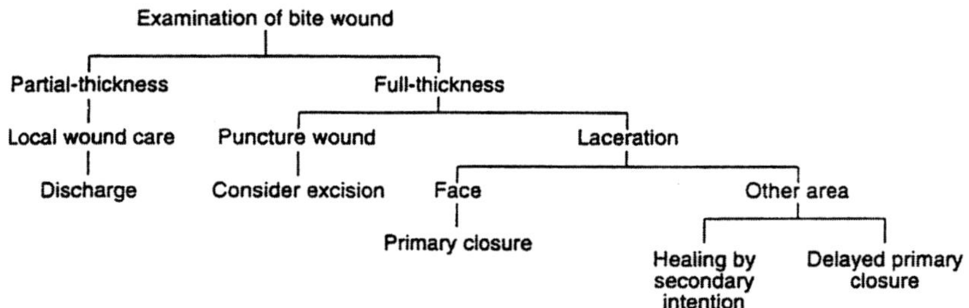

Fig. 3. Algorithm for the care of bite wounds. (*From* Markovchick V. Wound management. In: Markovchick V, Pons P, editors. Emergency medicine secrets. Philadelphia: Mosby Elsevier; 2006. p. 666; with permission.)

Cummings and Del Beccaro [73] concluded that there is no evidence that this practice offers protection against infection. Whittaker and colleagues [74] performed a prospective randomized, placebo-controlled, double-blinded study in adults looking at the use of antibiotics in clean, incised hand injuries including trauma to the skin, tendon, and nerve. Wound infection was defined as frank purulence, greater erythema than expected, or wound dehiscence. Infection also included a wound problem with a pathogenic bacterial growth on microbiologic swab results. Mild erythema or serous discharge without bacterial growth on swabs was described as a wound problem. Infection rates were 15% for placebo, 13% for intravenous flucloxacillin (a narrow-spectrum beta-lactam antibiotic), and 4% for the combination of intravenous antibiotic followed by an oral regimen. These differences were not statistically significant [74]. It is unclear, however, if antibiotics would benefit specific subgroups of patients who have characteristics placing them at a higher risk of infection (ie, diabetes mellitus). Antibiotics are indicated in patients prone to bacterial endocarditis, those who have an orthopedic prosthesis, and those who have lymphedema.

Because oral injuries are assumed to be contaminated with micro-organisms, it has been suggested that these wounds should be supported with prophylactic antibiotics. Clinical evidence for the use of antibiotics in this setting is lacking, however. The use of antibiotics for an oral wound may be warranted in heavily contaminated wounds where débridement is not optimal; wounds in which débridement is delayed for more than 24 hours; wounds associated with open reduction of jaw fractures; wounds in patients who have compromised defense systems; and wounds caused by human or animal bites [57].

Evidence supports the use of antibiotics in hand injuries involving fractures, contaminated wounds, crush injuries, animal bites, and human bites [74]. Zubowicz and Gravier [75] found mechanical wound care by itself to be insufficient therapy for human bites of the hand. In their study, oral and intravenous antibiotics were equivalent for prophylaxis.

Further evaluation of hand injuries involving fractures suggest that not all hand fractures associated with wounds warrant antibiotics. A study looking at the prophylactic use of flucloxacillin in the treatment of open fractures of the distal phalanx showed that the antibiotics did not confer any benefit over thorough wound preparation and careful soft tissue repair [76].

In dog bite wounds, débridement is more effective than prophylactic antibiotics in reducing infection. One study evaluating care of dog bites showed a 68% rate of infection in wounds without débridement, compared with an infection rate of 2% in the débridement group [77]. Wounds that could not be irrigated thoroughly, such as puncture wounds, had an infection rate twice that of wounds that could be irrigated thoroughly [77]. Therefore, high-risk wounds such as those on the hand or puncture wounds benefit from prophylactic antibiotics. Antibiotics are not required in low-risk wounds, such as deep wounds that can be adequately irrigated or in wounds of the face or scalp.

In conclusion, antibiotics are not beneficial in clean wounds even when these wounds involve the hand. In general, antibiotics are recommended for contaminated wounds or wounds that cannot be adequately debrided or irrigated. Also antibiotics need to be considered in patients who are more prone to infection including diabetics. Each wound needs to be considered individually, and the patient should have good follow-up, especially when the clinician decides not to provide antibiotics in potentially high-risk wounds.

Cosmesis

Although all wounds heal with a scar, the final appearance of this scar is influenced by patient factors, wound factors, and technical factors. Important patient factors include comorbid conditions, age, ethnicity, skin type, medications, and hereditary predisposition [78]. Wound factors include the nature of the wound (elective versus traumatic), location and orientation of the wound, vascularity of the tissues, elasticity and tension of soft tissues, and degree of contamination. Technical factors include the handling of tissues, débridement, sutures used, and method of wound repair. Avoiding rough tissue handling and the use of crushing instruments is important in preventing tissue ischemia, which leads to necrosis and poor scarring.

Wounds continue to remodel over 3 to 12 months. During that time period the scar may widen. Therefore, the long-term cosmetic outcome of the wound may not correlate with the short-term outcome [26].

Factors associated with patient-rated cosmesis scores may differ from those associated with doctor-rated cosmesis scores. Lowe and colleagues [79] found cosmetic outcome was the most important aspect of wound care for 33% of patients who had facial wounds and 17% of all patients who had lacerations. Patients in Lowe's study judged scar appearance using a 10-point numerical rating scale 14 days after repair and 3 months after repair. The site of laceration was the most significant factor related to satisfactory patient-rated cosmesis. Lacerations on the torso, leg, or foot received the lowest cosmesis scores. Another factor associated with poor cosmetic outcomes was increased time from injury to repair. Seniority of the practitioner performing the repair was not a significant factor in patient-rated cosmesis.

Aftercare instructions

If possible wounds should be covered with a nonadherent dressing for 24 to 48 hours. This period allows enough epithelialization to protect the wound from contamination [28]. Compression dressings should be applied to wounds with potential for hematoma formation. This dressing is left in place for 24 to 48 hours. After this time period, dressings should be removed, and wounds should be cleaned three to four times a day to minimize coagulum between wound edges. Thereafter, patients should be advised to administer a sun-blocking agent with a sun protective factor of 15 to the wound to prevent hyperpigmentation from exposure to sunlight. This process should be continued for 6 months.

Tissue adhesives do not require removal and will slough off over 5 to 10 days with wound epithelialization. Sutures and staples require removal on an average of 7 days after placement. Facial sutures can be removed in 3 to 5 days to avoid formation of sinus tracts. Sutures over joints or areas with a lot of movement should stay in for 10 to 14 days. Also lacerations overlying joint surfaces should be splinted in position of function for up to 10 days.

Future of wound care

Anesthesia with nitrous oxide

Bar-Meir and colleagues [80] evaluated the administration of nitrous oxide for repair of facial lacerations by plastic surgeons in the ED. The appealing aspects of this drug are its fast onset and rapid recovery characteristics, which make it an ideal drug for short procedures. It provides analgesia, anxiolysis, amnesia, and euphoria while having minimal cardiovascular and respiratory effects. The American Society of Anesthesiologists considers 50% nitrous oxide in oxygen as minimal sedation. Because administration of nitrous oxide requires a mask, there may be some limitations to its use. These investigators used a nasal mask for the administration of the drug, leaving the mouth uncovered. The mask could be removed immediately in case of emesis. The only lacerations covered by the mask were those on the nose. For nasal lacerations, the gas was administered first, followed by infiltration of local anesthetic while the patient was still under the influence of the gas. Also, because 50% nitrous oxide allows patients to maintain normal airway reflexes, fasting was not required before anesthesia. The authors of this study concluded that nitrous oxide could be safely administered in the ED [80].

Botulinum toxin

One group of investigators looked at the use of botulinum toxin in the repair of facial wounds. The study included 31 patients who had traumatic forehead lacerations or were undergoing elective excision of forehead masses. Patients were assigned randomly to injection of either botulinum toxin or placebo into the musculature in a diameter of approximately 1 to 3 cm around wound edges within 24 hours of wound closure. Immobilizing the wounds with the toxin enhanced healing and led to a superior cosmetic appearance at 6 months [81]. Further studies need to evaluate the use of chemoimmobilization in other types of lacerations in multiple different sites. Although this therapy may be a part of the future of wound management, its use in the ED may be limited by its cost.

Porcine small intestinal mucosa

Kragh and colleagues [82] reported better results in supination torque, appearance, and satisfaction when muscle was repaired with suture than with nonoperative management. Porcine SIS is a collagenous biomaterial that induces site-specific remodeling of various connective tissues. This product can act as a collagen scaffold allowing ingrowth of host tissue appropriate to the location of implantation. This product was tested on full-thickness muscle belly lacerations in rabbits. The study suggested that SIS, when added to a suture repair of muscle, may improve final outcomes and function [83]. The healed tissue after repair with SIS resembled normal muscle in morphology and function more closely than did nonsutured tissue, sutured tissue without use of SIS, or nonsutured tissue with use of SIS. At this time it is unclear if this product will be available for ED management of muscle wounds.

Hyaluronidase injections

Wounds from human bites typically are allowed to repair by secondary intention or undergo delayed closure. A new method described in the literature is the use of hyaluronidase injections around the wound site allowing immediate closure of wounds that otherwise might be considered for delayed closure. This product enzymatically breaks up the intercellular cement substance. When combined with external pressure in wounds, there is a diffusion of fluid exudates into the open wound and away from the wound margins. This process results in a soft, flattened wound facilitating closure without tension [84]. This process eliminates wound edema in minutes instead of days.

The use of hyaluronidase has been evaluated in the treatment of bite wounds in the orofacial area. In the cases reviewed, 2 to 3 mL of hyaluronidase were injected into the wound margins, with pressure being held for at least 10 minutes. All wounds healed uneventfully between 17 days and 1 month after injury. Hyaluronidase is not available currently for wounds treated in the ED.

Summary

To treat wounds properly, the emergency physician needs knowledge of basic wound physiology along with host and wound factors affecting healing. Although many options are available for wound closure, the choice of closure needs to be appropriate for the wound. Wound and host factors affect the type of closure that is best for different types of wounds. The ultimate goal is to obtain the ideal functional and cosmetic result without complications.

References

[1] National Hospital Ambulatory Medical Care Survey. Emergency department summary. Advance data from vital and health statistics; no. 293. National centre for health statistics. 1996 Available at: http://www.cdc.gov/nchs/data/ad/ad293.pdf, page 12, table 10. Accessed March 2007.

[2] Trott A. Surface injury and wound healing. In: Wounds and lacerations emergency care and closure. St. Louis (MO): Mosby; 1991. p. 12–23.

[3] Cruse PJE, Foord R. A five-year prospective study of 23,649 surgical wounds. Arch Surg 1973;107:206–9.

[4] Stamou SC, Maltezou HC, Psaltopoulou T, et al. Wound infections after minor limb lacerations: risk factors and the role of antimicrobial agents. J Trauma 1999;46(6):1078–81.

[5] Pulaski EJ, Meleney FL, Spacth WL. Bacterial flora of acute traumatic wounds. Surg Gynecol Obstet 1941;72:982–8.

[6] Robson MC, Duke WF, Krizek TJ, et al. Rapid bacterial screening in the treatment of civilian wounds. J Surg Res 1973;14:426–30.

[7] Berk WA, Osbourne DD, Taylor DD. Evaluation of the 'golden period' for wound repair: 204 cases from a third world emergency department. Ann Emerg Med 1988;17(5):496–500.

[8] Berk WA, Welch RD, Bock BF. Controversial issues in clinical management of the simple wound. Ann Emerg Med 1992;21(1):72–80.

[9] Pascual FB, McGinley EL, Zanardi LR, et al. Tetanus surveillance–United States, 1998-2000. MMWR Morb Mortal Wkly Rep 2003;52(SS03):1–8.

[10] Centers for Disease Control. Morbidity and mortality weekly report. Available at: www.cdc.gov/mmwr/preview/mmwrhtml. Accessed March 2007.

[11] Hollander JE, Singer AJ, Valentine SM, et al. Risk factors for infection in patients with traumatic lacerations. Acad Emerg Med 2001;8:716–20.

[12] Chisholm CD. Wound evaluation and cleansing. Emerg Med Clin North Am 1992;10(4): 665–72.

[13] Lammers RL, Magill T. Detection and management of foreign bodies in soft tissue. Emerg Med Clin North Am 1992;10(40):767–80.

[14] Anderson MA, Newmeyer WL, Kilgore ES. Diagnosis and treatment of retained foreign bodies in the hand. Am J Surg 1982;144:63–7.

[15] Singer AJ, Stark MJ. Pretreatment of lacerations with lidocaine, epinephrine, and tetracaine at triage: a randomized double-blind trial. Acad Emerg Med 2000;7(7):751–6.

[16] Kelly AM, Cohen M, Richards D. Minimizing the pain of local infiltration anesthesia for wounds by injection into the wound edges. J Emerg Med 1994;12:593–5.

[17] Bartfield JM, Sokaris SJ, Raccio-Robak N. Local anesthesia for lacerations: pain of infiltration inside vs. outside the wound. Acad Emerg Med 1998;5:100–4.

[18] Edlich RF, Rodeheaver GT, Morgan RF, et al. Principles of emergency wound management. Ann Emerg Med 1988;17:1284–302.

[19] Bartfield JM, Gennis P, Barbera J, et al. Buffered versus plain lidocaine as a local anesthetic for simple laceration repair. Ann Emerg Med 1990;19(12):1387–9.

[20] Brogan GX Jr, Giarrusso E, Hollander JE, et al. Comparison of plain, warmed, and buffered lidocaine for anesthesia of traumatic wounds. Ann Emerg Med 1995;26(2):121–5.

[21] Bartfield JM, Lee FS, Raccio-Robak N, et al. Topical tetracaine attenuates the pain of infiltration of buffered lidocaine. Acad Emerg Med 1996;3:1001–5.

[22] Sacchetti A, Senula G, Strickland J, et al. Procedural sedation in the community emergency department: initial results of the ProSCED registry. Acad Emerg Med 2007;14: 41–6.

[23] Sinha M, Christopher NC, Fenn R, et al. Evaluation of nonpharmacologic methods of pain and anxiety management for laceration repair in the pediatric emergency department. Pediatrics 2006;117(4):1162–8.

[24] Hamer ML, Martin CR, Krizek TJ, et al. Quantitative bacterial analysis of comparative wound irrigations. Ann Surg 1975;181(6):819–22.

[25] Dire DJ, Welsh AP. A comparison of wound irrigation solutions used in the emergency department. Ann Emerg Med 1990;19:704–8.

[26] Hollander JE, Singer AJ. Laceration management. Ann Emerg Med 1999;34(3):356–67.

[27] Stevenson TR, Thacker JG, Rodeheaver GT, et al. Cleansing the traumatic wound by high pressure syringe irrigation. JACEP 1976;5(1):17–21.

[28] Singer AJ, Hollander JE, Quinn JV. Evaluation and management of traumatic lacerations. N Engl J Med 1997;337(16):1142–8.

[29] Dulecki M, Pieper B. Irrigating simple acute traumatic wounds: a review of the current literature. J Emerg Nurs 2005;31(2):156–60.

[30] Peterson LW. Prophylaxis of wound infection. Arch Surg 1945;50(4):177–83.

[31] Knapp JF. Updates in wound management for the pediatrician. Pediatr Clin North Am 1999;46(6):1201–13.

[32] Hollander JE, Richman PB, Werblud M, et al. Irrigation in facial and scalp lacerations: does it alter outcome? Ann Emerg Med 1998;31(1):73–7.

[33] Ernst AA, Gershoff L, Miller P, et al. Warmed versus room temperature saline for laceration irrigation: a randomized clinical trial. South Med J 2003;96(5):436–9.

[34] Moscati RM, Reardon RF, Lerner EB, et al. Wound irrigation with tap water. Acad Emerg Med 1998;5:1076–80.

[35] Moscati R, Mayrose J, Fincher L, et al. Comparison of normal saline with tap water for wound irrigation. Am J Emerg Med 1998;16:379–81.

[36] Bansal BC, Wiebe RA, Perkins SD, et al. Tap water for irrigation of lacerations. Am J Emerg Med 2002;20:469–72.

[37] Haury B, Rodeheaver G, Vensko J, et al. Debridement: an essential component of traumatic wound care. Am J Surg 1978;135(2):238–42.

[38] Schultz GS, Sibbald RG, Falanga V, et al. Wound bed preparation: a systematic approach to wound management. Wound Repair Regen 2003;11:1–28.

[39] Seropian R, Reynolds BM. Wound infections after preoperative depilation versus razor preparation. Am J Surg 1971;121:251–4.

[40] Perelman VS, Francis GJ, Rutledge T, et al. Sterile versus nonsterile gloves for repair of uncomplicated lacerations in the emergency department: a randomized controlled trial. Ann Emerg Med 2004;43:362–70.

[41] Markovchick V. Suture materials and mechanical after care. Emerg Med Clin North Am 1992;10(4):673–89.

[42] Singer AJ, Quinn JV, Thode HC Jr, et al. Determinants of poor outcome after laceration and surgical incision repair. Plast Reconstr Surg 2002;110(2):429–35.

[43] Trott A. Basic laceration repair principles and techniques. In: Falk KH, editor. Wounds and lacerations emergency care and closure. St. Louis (MO): Mosby; 1997. p. 132–53.

[44] Khan A, Dayan PS, Miller S, et al. Cosmetic outcome of scalp wound closure with staples in the pediatric emergency department: a prospective, randomized trial. Pediatr Emerg Care 2002;18(3):171–3.

[45] George TK, Simpson DC. Skin wound closure with staples in the accident and emergency department. J R Coll Surg Edinb 1985;30(1):54–6.

[46] Kanegaye JT, Vance CW, Chan L, et al. Comparison of skin stapling devices and standard sutures for pediatric scalp lacerations: a randomized study of cost and time benefits. J Pediatr 1997;130:808–13.

[47] Lo S, Aslam N. A review of tissue glue use in facial lacerations: potential problems with wound selection in accident and emergency. Eur J Emerg Med 2004;11(5):277–9.

[48] Singer AJ, Quinn JV, Clark RE, et al. Closure of lacerations and incisions with octylcyanoacrylate: a multicenter randomized controlled trial. Surgery 2002;131:270–6.

[49] Quinn J, Wells G, Sutcliffe T, et al. A randomized trial comparing octylcyanoacrylate tissue adhesive and sutures in the management of lacerations. JAMA 1997;277(19): 1527–30.

[50] Simon HK, McLario DJ, Bruns TB, et al. Long-term appearance of lacerations repaired using a tissue adhesive. Pediatrics 1997;99:193–5.

[51] Perron AD, Garcia JA, Hays EP, et al. The efficacy of cyanoacrylate-derived surgical adhesive for use in the repair of lacerations during competitive athletics. Am J Emerg Med 2000; 18(3):261–3.

[52] Simon HK, Zempsky WT, Bruns TB, et al. Lacerations against Langer's lines: to glue or suture? J Emerg Med 1998;16(2):185–9.

[53] Zempsky WT, Parrotti D, Grem C, et al. Randomized controlled comparison of cosmetic outcomes of simple facial lacerations closed with Steri strip skin closures or Dermabond tissue adhesive. Pediatr Emerg Care 2004;20(8):519–24.

[54] Katz KH, Desciak EB, Maloney ME. The optimal application of surgical adhesive tape strips. Dermatol Surg 1999;25(9):686–8.

[55] Lin M, Milan M. Managing scalp lacerations. ACEP News 2007;30.

[56] Trott A. Special anatomic sites. In: Falk KH, editor. Wounds and lacerations emergency care and closure. St. Louis (MO): Mosby; 1997. p. 178–207.

[57] Armstrong BD. Lacerations of the mouth. Emerg Med Clin North Am 2000;18(3): 471–80.

[58] Zukin DD, Simon RR. Regional care. In: Emergency wound care principles and practice. Rockville (MD): Aspen Publishers, Inc; 1987. p. 77–109.

[59] de Alwis W. Fingertip injuries. Emerg Med Australas 2006;18:229–37.

[60] Quinn J, Cummings S, Callaham M, et al. Suturing versus conservative management of lacerations of the hand: randomized controlled trial. BMJ 2002;325:299–300.

[61] Via RM. Suturing unnecessary for hand lacerations under 2 cm. J Fam Pract 2003;52(1): 23–4.

[62] Hattori Y, Doi K, Ikeda K, et al. A retrospective study of functional outcomes after successful replantation versus amputation closure for single fingertip amputations. J Hand Surg [Am] 2006;31:811–8.

[63] Richards A, Crick A, Cole R. A novel method of securing the nail following nail bed repair. Plast Reconstr Surg 1999;103(7):1983–5.

[64] Hassan MS, Kannan RY, Rehman N, et al. Difficult adherent nail bed dressings: an escape route. Emerg Med J 2005;22:312.

[65] Pasapula C, Strick M. The use of chloramphenicol ointment as an adhesive for replacement of the nail plate after simple nail bed repairs. J Hand Surg [Br] 2004;29(6):634–5.

[66] Roser SE, Gellman H. Comparison of nail bed repair versus nail trephination for subungual hematomas in children. J Hand Surg [Am] 1999;24:1166–70.

[67] Dire DJ. Cat bite wounds: risk factors for infection. Ann Emerg Med 1991;20:973–9.

[68] Chen E, Hornig S, Shepherd SM, et al. Primary closure of mammalian bites. Acad Emerg Med 2000;7:157–61.

[69] Burke JF. The effective period of preventive antibiotic action in experimental incisions and dermal lesions. Surgery 1961;50:161–8.

[70] Edlich RF, Kenney JG, Morgan RF, et al. Antimicrobial treatment of minor soft tissue lacerations: a critical review. Emerg Med Clin North Am 1986;4(3):561–80.

[71] Sacks T. Prophylactic antibiotics in traumatic wounds. J Hosp Infect 1988;11(Suppl A): 251–8.

[72] Roberts AHN, Teddy PJ. A prospective trial of prophylactic antibiotics in hand lacerations. Br J Surg 1977;64:394–6.

[73] Cummings P, Del Beccaro MA. Antibiotics to prevent infection of simple wounds: a meta-analysis of randomized studies. Am J Emerg Med 1995;13:396–400.

[74] Whittaker JP, Nancarrow JD, Sterne GD. The role of antibiotic prophylaxis in clean incised hand injuries: a prospective randomized placebo controlled double blind trial. J Hand Surg [Br] 2005;30(2):162–7.

[75] Zubowicz VN, Gravier M. Management of early human bites of the hand: a prospective randomized study. Plast Reconstr Surg 1991;88(1):111–4.

[76] Stevenson J, McNaughton G, Riley J. The use of prophylactic flucloxacillin in treatment of open fractures of the distal phalanx within an accident and emergency department: a double-blind randomized placebo-controlled trial. J Hand Surg [Br] 2003;28(5):388–94.

[77] Callaham M. Prophylactic antibiotics in common dog bite wounds: a controlled study. Ann Emerg Med 1980;9:410–4.

[78] Wu T. Simple techniques for closing skin defects and improving cosmetic results. Aust Fam Physician 2006;35(7):492–6.

[79] Lowe T, Paoloni R. Sutured wounds: factors associated with patient-rated cosmetic scores. Emerg Med Australas 2006;18(3):259–67.

[80] Bar-Meir E, Zaslansky R, Regev E, et al. Nitrous oxide administered by the plastic surgeon for repair of facial lacerations in children in the emergency room. Plast Reconstr Surg 2006; 117:1571–5.

[81] Gassner HG, Brissett AE, Otley CC, et al. Botulinum toxin to improve facial wound healing: a prospective, blinded, placebo-controlled study. Mayo Clin Proc 2006;81(8):1023–8.

[82] Kragh JF, Basamania CJ. Surgical repair of acute traumatic closed transection of the biceps brachii. Journal of Bone & Joint Surgery 2002;84-A(6):992–8.

[83] Crow BD, Haltom JD, Carson WL, et al. Evaluation of a novel biomaterial for intrasubstance muscle laceration repair. J Orthop Res 2007;25:396–403.

[84] Baurmash HD, Monto M. Delayed healing human bite wounds of the orofacial area managed with immediate primary closure: treatment rationale. J Oral Maxillofac Surg 2005; 63:1391–7.

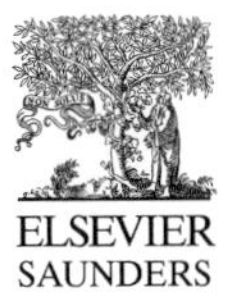

ELSEVIER
SAUNDERS

Emerg Med Clin N Am 25 (2007) 901–914

EMERGENCY
MEDICINE
CLINICS OF
NORTH AMERICA

Injury Prevention and Control

Marian Betz, MD[a,*], Guohua Li, MD, DrPH[b]

[a]*Harvard Affiliated Emergency Medicine Residency, Department of Emergency Medicine, Beth Israel Deaconess Medical Center, One Deaconess Road, West Clinical Center 2, Boston, MA 02215, USA*

[b]*Department of Emergency Medicine, John Hopkins University School of Medicine, 1830 East Monument Street, Suite 6-100, Baltimore, MD 21205, USA*

Injuries remain the leading cause of death for Americans from ages 1 to 44 years and the fifth leading cause of death for all ages combined [1,2]. Young people are affected disproportionately, with injuries accounting for almost one third of all years of potential life lost before age 65—a proportion greater than cancer and heart disease combined [3]. The economic burden of injury also is significant. In 2000, injuries accounted for 10% of total United States medical expenditures. If rehabilitation, lost wages, and productivity are included, total costs exceed over $224 billion per year [2,4].

Emergency physicians deal with a broad spectrum of injuries daily, from simple lacerations to multisystem trauma. For every injury death, there are more than 200 emergency department (ED) visits [5–7], amounting to 41.3 million visits in 2004 or 14.4 visits per 100 persons [8]. Injury-related visits accounted for 37.3% of all ED visits, and 40% of these injury visits were for unintentional falls, motor vehicle crashes, or being struck by an object or person [8]. Although emergency physicians are skilled in the medical care of injuries, most receive little training in injury epidemiology and prevention.

The field of injury prevention is young; it was only in the middle of the last century that its theories and approaches were introduced. Injuries traditionally have been viewed as "accidents" (ie, unpredictable, unavoidable, random events) [9]. The pioneers of the injury prevention field argued that injuries were the product of interaction between a host, environment, and vector—much like infectious diseases—and, therefore, might be prevented by interventions targeted toward any of the contributing factors. Efforts often begin with changes in education, engineering, and legislation, and as awareness of a specific injury risk grows, public perception changes.

* Corresponding author.

E-mail address: mbetz@bidmc.harvard.edu (M. Betz).

0733-8627/07/$ - see front matter
doi:10.1016/j.emc.2007.06.009 ***emed.theclinics.com***

Injury epidemiology

An appreciation of injury risk and causation must be grounded in epidemiology. There are a variety of classification methods for injuries, and within each there are certain demographic patterns. Injury data come from many sources. The most effective injury-prevention approaches use epidemiologic findings in the design of interventions targeting multiple contributory factors.

Injury classification

An understanding of the epidemiology of injury and prevention approaches requires awareness of the basic classification schemes. Perhaps the most intuitive to emergency physicians is describing injuries in terms of body location. For injury-related visits to EDs, the upper extremity (wrist, hand, or finger) is the most commonly mentioned site of injury (11.3%), followed by the lower extremity (4.3%) and face (4.1%) [8].

Injuries also may be classified by severity. Falls are the most common nonfatal injury treated in EDs for all ages—except among patients 15 to 24 years of age—and yet are the leading cause of injury death only for those 65 years and older [1,10]. Conversely, motor vehicle crashes rank only fourth among all causes of nonfatal injuries treated in EDs, but are the most common fatal injury for persons ages 1 to 64 years and for all ages combined [1,10]. Approximately 50% of fatal injuries cause immediate death, 30% cause death within 48 hours of the injury, and the remaining 20% cause death from complications over the subsequent weeks [11]. Injury severity also can be measured in terms of case fatality rates, with high rates for firearm violence, or in terms of resultant morbidity, with high morbidity for brain and spinal cord injuries [9]. There are a variety of scales used for assessing injury severity, including the Abbreviated Injury Scale, the Injury Severity Score, New Injury Severity Score, the Anatomic Profile, the Revised Trauma Score, the Functional Independence Measure, and *International Classification of Diseases, Ninth Revision*–based systems [6]. Each scale has different advantages and disadvantages for evaluating the impact of an injury, illustrating the difficulty in finding a single comprehensive system.

Often, injuries are classified by mechanism, such as motor vehicle crashes, drowning, and gunshot wounds. A related classification scheme is by intentionality, which is less intuitive to most clinicians, because it has less clinical importance than body region, severity, or mechanism. Unintentional injuries include traffic-related injuries, falls, poisonings, overexertion, burns, and other events that traditionally would have been called "accidents." Intentional injuries consist of self-inflicted and assaultive injuries, such as deaths from suicide and homicide. Of injuries treated in United States EDs in 2004, 67.9% were classified as unintentional and 5.6% were intentional, with the remaining injuries of undetermined intent or due to adverse effects of medical treatment [8]. Of the approximately 145,000 injury deaths in the United States each year, about 63% are categorized as unintentional, 34%

as intentional, and 3% as undetermined. The rates of injury morbidity and mortality vary by age group, with children more at risk for suffocation and drowning and young adults more at risk for suicide and firearm violence [1,12].

Demographic patterns

The incidence and severity of injuries vary among different demographic groups, with particular risks among children and adolescents. Fifty-one percent of injury deaths and 44% of injury-related hospitalizations occur among those younger than 45 years of age [3], and those aged 15 to 24 years have the highest risk for minor injuries of any age group [11]. The death rate from homicide for children is higher in the United States than in any other industrialized nation [13]. Homicide remains the most common cause of death for African Americans aged 10 to 24 years and the second most common cause of death for Hispanics in the same age group [14]. Sexual violence also is prevalent during childhood, with one third of lifetime rapes occurring by age 12 years and one half by age 18 years [15]. From ages 1 to 14 years, more deaths each year are due to unintentional and intentional injuries than to the combined total of the remaining top ten causes of death [3]. Adolescents aged 16 to 19 years face the highest risk for motor vehicle crashes, especially during the first year of driving, and boys in this age group have a crash death rate twice that of girls [16].

At the opposite end of the age spectrum, the elderly also face unique injury risks. Those 65 years and older accounted for 25% of injury deaths and 33% of injury-related hospitalizations in 2000, although they represented only 13% of the total United States population [3,17]. The elderly also have the highest rates of any age group for death or hospitalization from an injury and for ED visits for injuries [11,18]. Falls are the leading cause of injury-related deaths among the elderly older than age 75 years, whereas motor vehicle crashes are the most common cause for patients between the ages of 1 and 74 years [3]. Although some of these falls result in immediate death, others may cause long-term morbidity and a slow decline in independence. Twenty-five percent of independent elderly patients with hip fractures require institutional care for at least 1 year after their injury, and only half return to their prior level of independence [9,19].

In all age groups, annual male fatal injury rates are higher than female fatal injury rates (79 per 100,000 compared to 34 per 100,000, respectively) [3]. Boys and men accounted for 86% of homicides among 10- to 24-year-olds in 2003 and for 80% of suicides in 1998, although there were more suicide attempts among women [2,14]. Nonfatal injury rates are also higher among men than women, with 10,500 per 100,000 men compared to 8,996 per 100,000 women for all ages combined [3].

Certain occupations also are associated with a higher risk for injury. In 1999, ED providers treated 3.9 million occupational injuries and illnesses

[20], and half of the reported occupational injuries in 2003 resulted in loss of productivity [21]. The highest rates of fatal and nonfatal injuries occur in mining, agricultural, fishing, forestry, and construction industries [20,22]. Health care providers face special risks themselves; hospitals and nursing and residential facilities were among the 14 industries that accounted for almost half of reported occupational injuries in 2004, and health care and social services accounted for 15.9% of all nonfatal occupational injuries [21].

Data sources

The lack of comprehensive national data on injuries has been a major obstacle in injury research; however, the recognition of injury as a public health problem has improved injury surveillance significantly. Vital statistics, compiled from death certificates, are often thought of as the chief source of mortality data, but they may have limited details about injuries because of variations in completion and reporting [11,23]. There are more than 30 other national systems maintained by the US Government for recording injury data, each with different details about the severity, mechanism, treatment, and outcome of injuries [24]. Examples include the Fatality Analysis Reporting System, a public-access database of fatal traffic crashes managed by the National Highway Traffic Safety Administration, and the Youth Risk Behavior Surveillance System, a compilation of data on youth behavior from surveys administered by the Centers for Disease Control and Prevention [25]. Other national surveys also provide abundant information on injuries treated in the United States, including the mechanism, body site, and severity of the injury as well as demographic characteristics of the injury victim [26,27]. Specific information on injuries treated in EDs is available from individual hospital databases and from national surveys, such as the National Hospital Ambulatory Medical Care Survey and the National Electronic Injury Surveillance System-All Injury Program, both of which include data on fatal and nonfatal injuries [26,28].

Prevention approaches

Injury data are useful for understanding basic epidemiology and form the scientific basis for injury-prevention programs. The central tenet of the injury field is that rather than being unpreventable "accidents," injuries, like diseases, occur because of the complex interactions among the human host, agent (ie, a vector of energy), and the environment. Each of these three elements is potentially modifiable through interventions. In the 1960s, Dr. William Haddon formulated a conceptual framework for injury prevention and control. The conceptual framework, now widely known as the Haddon Matrix, relates the three elements in the epidemiologic model (host, agent, and environment) to the three phases of the injury sequence (pre-event, event, and postevent). Because all injuries are caused by acute and uncontrolled transfer of energy, the Haddon Matrix guides the development of strategies to influence the risk and consequences of energy transfer from the vector to the human host. Preventive measures at the three phases of the injury sequence correspond to primary, secondary, and tertiary preventions, respectively. As an example, an injury from a motor vehicle collision results from interactions among a host (driver), agent (moving car), and environment (highway). Primary prevention is prevention of the crash itself and results from modifying factors leading to the crash ("pre-event"), such as driver education, car handling, or highway design. Secondary prevention—or prevention of injury given a crash—includes changing "event" factors, such as driver seatbelt use, airbag deployment, or crash-absorbing barrels on highway shoulders. Finally, tertiary prevention is prevention of poor outcomes once the injury has occurred and is the form of injury prevention most familiar to emergency physicians. Interventions in the realm of tertiary prevention include advances in medical care, car designs that allow rapid extraction, and improved emergency medical services response times. Although each of these individual tactics may seem small in scope, the overall effect on injury morbidity and mortality is substantial. Organized trauma systems, smoke detectors, collapsible automobile steering columns, window guards, childproof medication packaging, protective sporting equipment, safety phlebotomy needles, and graduated driver licensing are examples of interventions that have been shown to decrease injury mortality and morbidity [29,30].

National goals for injury reduction

Various goals for injury prevention and reduction have been set at local, state, national, and global levels. Perhaps the most comprehensive are the objectives specified in Healthy People 2010, the United States national health agenda for the first decade of the twenty-first century. Several measurable targets for improving health and preventing illness related to injury are included in Healthy People 2010 [31], which acknowledges that reduction of injury morbidity and mortality requires collaboration between many different sectors, from health care to transportation and law to social services [13]. Although many of the prevention strategies are based on government, community outreach, or industry activities, others are applicable to ED settings. Specifically, emergency physicians have important roles to play in patient education, surveillance system improvement, and ongoing research in treatment and outcomes.

Patient education

The period directly after an injury—including care provided in EDs—is a time when many patients may be most susceptible to interventions for prevention of repeat injuries. Once a patient has been stabilized for admission or discharge, ED physicians, nurses, and social workers have an ideal opportunity to educate patients on the importance of prevention strategies applicable to the situation. ED staff also can screen certain populations for particular injury risks easily and quickly and offer education or social services referral as appropriate.

Motor vehicle crashes are the fourth leading cause of nonfatal injuries treated in EDs [10] and the leading cause of injury deaths in the United States [1]. Healthy People 2010 includes goals for reducing fatal and nonfatal injuries sustained by vehicle occupants and pedestrians. The national goal for seatbelt use is 92% by 2010, and approaches for reaching this goal include state seatbelt laws and increased traffic checkpoints [13,32]. ED staff and other medical professionals who care for injuries can help to achieve this target by reinforcing the importance of seatbelt and child restraint use.

Usage rates are lower for helmets than for seatbelts, although helmets are effective in reducing injury mortality and morbidity for motorcyclists, bicyclists, and athletes. A motorcyclist wearing a helmet has a 29% decreased risk for death and a 67% decreased risk for traumatic brain injury during a crash compared with one not wearing a helmet [13], and helmets reduce the risk for head injury in bicyclists by 85%. Overall, states without helmet laws have fatality rates from head injuries that are at least twice the rates of states with helmet laws [13]. Mandatory helmet use laws have been contentious for motorcycles, but Healthy People 2010 includes the goal that all states pass laws for mandatory bicycle helmet use for those under age 15 years. Whether or not such laws are enacted, care providers treating motorcycle- and bicycle-related injuries should stress the importance of future helmet use, especially among children and teens.

Children have high rates of particular injuries, and parents should be educated about risks and prevention. For example, immediate use of a poison center hotline after a potentially toxic ingestion—90% of which occur at home—can reduce the risk for a significant poisoning and avoid an ED visit. Health care professionals should provide parents with hotline numbers and should use these resources themselves when treating patients with ingestions, because many poison centers depend on call volume for funding [13]. The proper use of child car restraints, home smoke alarms, and protective sports equipment also are effective injury-prevention tools that require education of caregivers.

Surveillance system enhancement

Quality data are fundamental to understanding injury epidemiology and designing appropriate interventions for decreasing mortality, morbidity, and incidence. In 1998, only 12 states had statewide surveillance systems in EDs for recording the causes of injuries, and only 23 states used hospital discharge data to collect data on these causes [13]. Healthy People 2010 goals include increasing both of these to all states because understanding how injuries occur is the key to prevention [13]. Emergency physicians can work with hospital and government administrators to improve these surveillance systems as well as ensure that their patient charts include mention of the injury mechanism to facilitate correct coding.

Research

Ongoing research in injury epidemiology, treatment, and outcome is fundamental to effective and efficient injury prevention. Clinical studies of injuries treated in EDs provide useful information about patient demographics and prehospital care. Current understanding of the best surgical and medical treatment options of particular injuries has come from the experience and research of physicians in emergency medicine, critical care, and trauma surgery. Close collaboration between these groups will remain important to optimization of care of the injured patient.

Injury prevention in the emergency department

Emergency physicians and other care providers can work to prevent injuries in many ways, from injury surveillance to risk factor identification to policy development. Some examples of ED-based injury-prevention programs include interventions on violence, falls, traffic injuries, and alcohol abuse.

Violence

Physical and emotional violence toward children, intimate partners, and the elderly remain common in the United States. Homicide is the second leading cause of death for persons aged 15 to 24 years [33]; youth involved in violence are at high risk for injury in the future and have up to 44% readmission rates for later assaults [34]. Youth violence also occurs at home; in 1996 there were close to 1 million child victims of maltreatment and more than 1000 fatalities [13]. Physicians need to be able to recognize injuries suspicious for child abuse, and EDs should have systems in place for assisting victims with evidence collection and social services.

Domestic violence against adults also remains a significant problem; each year approximately 1.5 million women and 834,7000 men are physically assaulted or raped by an intimate partner [13]. Estimates of lifetime prevalence of intimate partner violence against women range from 25% to 30%, and more than one third of women presenting to EDs have experienced some form of abuse [35]. Many victims of abuse visit EDs for injuries or other complaints; one study found that almost two thirds of women identified by police records as victims of intimate partner violence had visited at least one ED within the year [36].

The various manifestations of interpersonal violence—child, intimate partner, and elder abuse and violence between youth or adults—have similar origins and are connected in a "cycle of violence" [37], suggesting that general ED interventions may be valuable. Screening for safety at home and in relationships is common in many EDs [38], often completed as part of the standard triage documentation. Although injury-related visits are more likely to have domestic violence screening documented, most ED visits by victims of violence are for noninjury complaints [36]. Screening patients is a simple and quick way to offer victims help and is a natural extension of health care providers' questions about other risk factors, like smoking and exercise [34].

Physicians are legally responsible for reporting suspected cases of child or elder abuse to appropriate authorities. For domestic abuse, posters in restrooms and hallways and pamphlets in rooms can provide help to domestic abuse victims not wanting to identify themselves. EDs can serve as safe refuges for victims seeking shelter overnight and can provide them with referrals, including social worker evaluations, local resource listings, and assistance contacting the police [35]. Such referrals also can be useful for youth involved in violence [39], especially when parents are present and can be involved.

Violence from firearms is a particularly difficult problem because of the political issues surrounding regulations for purchase and use. In 1998, 19% of the United States population had loaded, but unlocked, guns in their homes [13]. Health care professionals can work to decrease firearm violence through direct counseling of patients about proper home storage and firearm safety, as well as through support of changes in gun design, sale, and legal use.

Fall prevention

EDs already treat large numbers of patients with injuries sustained during falls, and these injuries will continue to increase in prevalence as the United States population ages; by 2050, an estimated 23% of the population will be older than age 65 years [40]. Gait disorders, dementia, and osteoporosis place the elderly at high risk for falls and significant injuries, including spine, hip, and extremity fractures. Each year, one third of United States elderly adults sustain a fall, and 20% to 30% of these will have an injury that places them at risk for premature death [40]. Women have a significantly higher rate of hospitalization for hip fractures; a Healthy People 2010 goal is to decrease this rate from 1356 to less than 880 per 100,000 [13,40].

Most emergency physicians are used to screening for home safety as part of criteria for discharge or hospital admission; an elderly individual who lives alone in a third floor apartment and requires a walker is at much higher risk for a repeat fall than one who lives with family in a single-level home and can walk unassisted. Recognition of risk factors for falls, such as age, falls in the past, environmental hazards, balance problems, dementia, functional limitations, and psychoactive medication use [40], is the first step in the prevention of fall-related injuries. Research has demonstrated that effective interventions to prevent falls target environmental and behavioral factors [41]. Such strategies use removal or reduction of hazards in homes, avoidance of medications likely to cause sedation or lightheadedness, exercise for balance and strength, and health education about risk factors [40]. Emergency physicians can help to prevent falls by providing patients and families with hazard checklists, by communicating with primary care doctors about medication regimens, and by collaborating with case managers or social workers to provide necessary home services for patients.

Traffic safety

Assessment of seatbelt and airbag use is a standard part of the assessment of a patient after a motor vehicle collision, because these protective devices are indicators of the severity and type of injuries expected. Similarly, emergency personnel ask injured bicyclists or motorcyclists about helmet use in assessing the likelihood of head injury. A natural extension of such questioning is the education of patients once stabilized—either the positive reinforcement for having used protective equipment or the encouragement to use equipment in the future to prevent repeated injuries. Patients who have just experienced a significant or frightening injury may be particularly receptive to such education, and even brief counseling may have great impact.

The elderly are a high-risk population for traffic injuries because the fatality rate for motor vehicle crashes is nine times higher in those older than 70 years of age [13]. Although questioning driving ability is a difficult issue related to the maintenance of independence and acceptance of the aging process, ED staff have the opportunity to identify and potentially intervene with patients and their families.

Alcohol-related injuries

Alcohol is the foremost risk factor for injury, and an estimated 27% of injured adults visiting EDs are intoxicated or abuse alcohol [42]. Overall, 100,000 preventable deaths in the United States each year are due to alcohol or illicit drug misuse [42]. Approximately 40% of fatal traffic crashes are alcohol related [32], and patients who survive a crash may—once sober—be especially susceptible to counseling or interventions to reduce drinking and risky behavior. Numerous studies have shown that brief screening and interventions in the ED or inpatient setting may reduce recidivism and the number of drinks consumed per week [42–44]. Such programs also may reduce health care costs [42]. Prevention programs can be difficult to implement in emergency care settings because of resource limitations and staff attitudes about the likelihood of an individual's ability to change [43]. However, there is strong evidence that such programs do have significant effects on individuals and communities; screening, interventions, and treatment referrals should be a routine part of trauma care for intoxicated patients [44]. Although not using a seatbelt or helmet places the individual at risk, driving a motor vehicle while intoxicated places others in the community at risk, and health care professionals should work to protect the public's health.

Current status, future directions

Although injuries remain the leading cause of death in the United States for persons aged 1 to 44 years, there have been significant reductions in mortality and morbidity. With the acceptance of injuries as a public health problem—rather than the result of unpreventable "accidents"—has come a growing body of research concerning the epidemiology of injuries and the design, implementation, and effectiveness of targeted interventions. Injury prevention requires a multidisciplinary approach, including community mobilization, engineering design, policy development, and law enforcement. As public awareness of a particular injury problem grows, behavior patterns can change; examples include consumer demand for safer cars and use of helmets by professional athletes [29].

Physicians have an integral role to play in injury prevention. First, physicians can counsel patients directly about injury risks and prevention. In their daily interactions with patients in the ED, physicians interface with a broad segment of the population. Brief screening for risk factors, such as alcohol abuse, can offer opportunities for behavior reinforcement and health education. This is especially important in the pediatric population, through education and anticipatory guidance for parents; examples include correct car seat use and the particular injury risks that arise at each developmental stage.

Second, physicians can refer high-risk patients to appropriate resources. Brief screening for injury risk factors allows ED personnel to identify patients who would benefit from assistance. Social workers and case managers can help to connect patients with these resources, including domestic violence programs, legal assistance, detoxification centers, home assistance for the elderly, and youth counseling.

A third opportunity for involvement is the design and implementation of ED-based interventions. In 2000, the Public Health Task Force of the Society for Academic Emergency Medicine systematically reviewed 17 preventive interventions previously reviewed by the US Preventive Services Task Force [45]. Of the 17 interventions, 8 related to injuries: alcohol screening and intervention, geriatric fall prevention, smoke detector counseling, child physical abuse screening, domestic violence screening, firearm safe storage counseling, helmet and motorcycle use counseling, and youth violence counseling. All received B or C ratings, with insufficient evidence for or against ED-based interventions because of the lack of studies evaluating such interventions in an ED setting [45]. Clearly, more research is needed, including trials evaluating program implementation and outcomes and examination of cost-effectiveness and resource use.

Research aimed at identifying risk factors and developing effective interventions is the fourth area of potential involvement in injury prevention for emergency physicians. Physicians should continue to study the treatment and outcomes of particular injuries through clinical research, but physicians also can be involved in research oriented at interventions on injury risk and program evaluation. The approach to any public health issue should be through multiple steps—each requiring its own type of focused research—and injury prevention is no exception. The scope of the injury problem must be defined adequately with surveillance and epidemiologic studies, which also will identify risk factors. Prevention efforts begin with a broad examination of possible intervention options, and programs are selected based on their effectiveness, feasibility, and public acceptance. Community involvement and feedback are important at this stage and throughout the implementation of any injury intervention. Well-designed studies are necessary to evaluate the effectiveness of an intervention, because these results are used frequently to argue for or against policy changes.

A fifth area for physician involvement in injury prevention is policy development. This can occur at multiple levels, from advocating for state and federal regulations that reduce the public's exposure to risk factors and foster safe environment and behavior to working with local government and employers to address occupational, recreational, traffic, and home injury risks. The gap between science and policy often has been a barrier to the translation of research findings into evidence-based laws, and physicians can help to bridge this chasm through education of the public and lawmakers about injury issues. Past successes include legislation for vehicle restraints, helmets, and graduated driver licensing, all of which have had an impact on injury morbidity and mortality.

Although the past half-century has seen dramatic reductions in injury morbidity and mortality in the United States, there is much work to be done. Firearms and youth violence may be the two greatest challenges facing the injury field. The political nature of the firearm debate makes intervention more difficult, and the multifactorial etiology of youth violence requires multidisciplinary collaboration. As the population ages, injury issues facing the elderly, including fall risks and elderly driver licensing, will become increasingly important. Ultimately, all of these problems require community-supported solutions; emergency physicians' role in the treatment of injuries and the identification of at-risk individuals makes them important stakeholders throughout the spectrum of the public health approach to injury prevention and control, from injury surveillance to program evaluation.

References

[1] 10 Leading causes of injury death by age group highlighting unintentional injury deaths, United States – 2003. Office of Statistics and Programming, National Center for Injury Prevention and Control, Centers for Disease Control and Prevention. Available at: http://www.cdc.gov/ncipc/osp/charts.htm. Accessed December 15, 2006.
[2] Injury fact book 2001–2002. Atlanta (GA): National Center for Injury Prevention and Control, Centers for Disease Control and Prevention; 2001. p. 6.
[3] WISQARS, National Center for Injury Prevention and Control, Centers for Disease Control and Prevention. Available at: http://www.cdc.gov/ncipc/wisqars/. Accessed December 15, 2006.
[4] Finkelstein EA, Fiebelkorn IC, Corso PS, et al. Medical expenditures attributable to injuries–United States, 2000. Morb Mortal Wkly Rep 2004;53:1–4.
[5] Office of Statistics and Programming, National Center for Injury Prevention and Control, Centers for Disease Control and Prevention. National estimates of nonfatal injuries treated in hospital emergency departments–United States, 2000. MMWR Morb Mortal Wkly Rep 2001;50:340–6.
[6] Bonnie RJ, Fulco CE, Liverman CT. Reducing the burden of injury: advancing prevention and treatment 1999. Washington, DC: National Academy Press; 1999.
[7] Vyrostek SB, Annest JL, Ryan GW. Surveillance for fatal and nonfatal injuries–United States, 2001. MMWR Surveill Summ 2004;53:1–57.
[8] McCaig LF, Nawar EW. National hospital ambulatory medical care survey: 2004 emergency department summary. Adv Data 2006;372:1–29.
[9] Fowler C. Injury prevention. In: McQuillan KA, Von Rueden K, Hartsock R, et al, editors. Trauma nursing: from resuscitation through rehabilitation. 3rd edition. Philadelphia: W.B. Saunders Company; 2002. p. 73–93.
[10] National estimates of the 10 leading causes of nonfatal injury treated in hospital emergency departments, United States, 2004. Office of Statistics and Programming, National Center for Injury Prevention and Control, Centers for Disease Control and Prevention. Available at: http://www.cdc.gov/ncipc/osp/charts.htm. Accessed December 1, 2006.
[11] Mackenzie EJ, Fowler C. Epidemiology of trauma. In: Mattox KJ, Feliciano DV, Moore EE, editors. Trauma. 5th edition. Stamford (CT): Appleton & Lange; 2004. p. 21.
[12] 10 Leading causes of injury death by age group highlighting violence-related injury deaths, United States – 2003. Office of Statistics and Programming, National Center for Injury Prevention and Control, Centers for Disease Control and Prevention. Available at: http://www.cdc.gov/ncipc/osp/charts.htm. Accessed January 19, 2007.
[13] United States Department of Health and Human Services. Healthy people 2010. 2nd edition. With understanding and improving health and objectives for improving health, vol. 2. Washington, DC: U.S. Government Printing Office; 2000.
[14] Youth violence: fact sheet. National Center for Injury Prevention and Control, Centers for Disease Control and Prevention. Available at: http://www.cdc.gov/ncipc/factsheets/yvfacts.htm. Accessed September 7, 2006.
[15] Hambidge SJ, Davidson AJ, Gonzales R, et al. Epidemiology of pediatric injury-related primary care office visits in the United States. Pediatrics 2002;109:559–65.
[16] Teen drivers: fact sheet. National Center for Injury Prevention and Control, Centers for Disease Control and prevention. Available at: http://www.cdc.gov/ncipc/factsheets/teenmvh.htm. Accessed September 7, 2006.
[17] U.S. interim projections by age, sex, race, and Hispanic origin. United States Census Bureau. Available at: http://www.census.gov/ipc/www/usinterimproj/. Accessed December 12, 2006.
[18] National Center for Health Statistics. Health, United States, 1996–7 and injury chartbook. Hyattsville (MD): National Center for Health Statistics; 1997.

[19] Falls and hip fractures among older adults, National Center for Injury Prevention and Control, Centers for Disease Control and Prevention. Available at: http://www.cdc.gov/ncipc/factsheets/falls.htm. Accessed October 10, 2006.

[20] Worker health chartbook 2004, National Institute for Occupational Safety and Health, Centers for Disease Control and Prevention. NIOSH Publication No. 2004–146. Available at: http://www.cdc.gov/niosh/docs/chartbook. Accessed October 10, 2006.

[21] Workplace injuries and illnesses in 2004. Bureau of Labor Statistics, United States Department of Labor. Available at: http://www.bls.gov/iif/home.htm. Accessed January 19, 2007.

[22] Census of fatal occupational injuries summary, 2005. Bureau of Labor Statistics, United States Department of Labor 2006. Available at: http://www.bls.gov/news.release/cfoi.toc.htm. Accessed September 21, 2006.

[23] Fingerhut LA, McLoughlin E. Classifying and counting injury. In: Rivara FP, Cummings P, Koepsell TD, et al, editors. Injury control: a guide to research and program evaluation. New York: Cambridge University Press; 2001. p. 15–31.

[24] Segui-Gomez M, Mackenzie EJ. Measuring the public health impact of injuries. Epidemiol Rev 2003;25:3–19.

[25] Youth risk behavior surveillance system. National Center for Chronic Disease Prevention and Health Promotion, Centers for Disease Control and Prevention. Available at: http://www.cdc.gov/HealthyYouth/yrbs/index.htm. Accessed September 21, 2006.

[26] Ambulatory health care data. National Center for Health Statistics, Centers for Disease Control and Prevention. Available at: http://www.cdc.gov/nchs/about/major/ahcd/ahcd1.htm. Accessed January 19, 2007.

[27] National hospital discharge and ambulatory surgery data. National Center for Health Statistics, Centers for Disease Control and Prevention. Available at: http://www.cdc.gov/nchs/about/major/hdasd/nhds.htm. Accessed September 21, 2006.

[28] The national electronic injury surveillance system (NEISS). National Center for Injury Prevention and Control, Centers for Disease Control and Prevention. Available at: http://www.cdc.gov/ncipc/wisqars/nonfatal/datasources.htm#5.2. Accessed September 21, 2006.

[29] Hemenway D. Success stories in injury prevention. Harvard Injury Control Research Center, Harvard School of Public Health 2006. Available at: http://www.hsph.harvard.edu/hicrc/success.html. Accessed September 21, 2006.

[30] Nathens AB, Jurkovich GJ, Cummings P, et al. The effect of organized systems of trauma care on motor vehicle crash mortality. JAMA 2000;283:1990–4.

[31] Healthy people 2010. National Center for Health Statistics, Centers for Disease Control and Prevention. Available at: http://www.cdc.gov/nchs/hphome.htm#Healthy%20People%202010. Accessed January 21, 2007.

[32] Beato CV. Injury and violence prevention. U.S. Department of Health and Human Services, Public Health Service 2003.

[33] 10 Leading causes of death by age group, United States – 2003. Office of Statistics and Available at: http://www.cdc.gov/nchs/about/otheract/hpdata2010/focusareas/fa15-injury.htm. Accessed October 10, 2006. Programming, National Center for Injury Prevention and Control, Centers for Disease Control and Prevention. Available at: http://www.cdc.gov/ncipc/osp/charts.htm. Accessed December 15, 2006.

[34] Denninghoff KR, Knox L, Cunningham R, et al. Emergency medicine: competencies for youth violence prevention and control. Acad Emerg Med 2002;9:947–56.

[35] Wathen CN, MacMillan HL. Interventions for violence against women: scientific review. JAMA 2003;289:589–600.

[36] Kothari CL, Rhodes KV. Missed opportunities: emergency department visits by police-identified victims of intimate partner violence. Ann Emerg Med 2006;47:190–9.

[37] Hill JE. Healthcare professionals and the prevention of youth violence: where do we go from here? Am J Prev Med 2005;29:182–4.

[38] Degutis LC, Greve M. Injury prevention. Emerg Med Clin North Am 2006;24:871–88.

[39] Zun LS, Downey LV, Rosen J. Violence prevention in the ED: linkage of the ED to a social service agency. Am J Emerg Med 2003;21:454–7.

[40] Stevens JA, Olson S. Reducing falls and resulting hip fractures among older women. MMWR Recomm Rep 2000;49:3–12.

[41] Weigand JV, Gerson LW. Preventive care in the emergency department: should emergency departments institute a falls prevention program for elder patients? A systematic review. Acad Emerg Med 2001;8:823–6.

[42] Maier RV. Controlling alcohol problems among hospitalized trauma patients. J Trauma 2005;59:S1–2.

[43] Diclemente CC. The challenge of change. J Trauma 2005;59:S3–4.

[44] Hungerford DW. Recommendations for trauma centers to improve screening, brief intervention, and referral to treatment for substance use disorders. J Trauma 2005;59: S37–42.

[45] Babcock Irvin C, Wyer PC, Gerson LW. Preventive care in the emergency department, part II: clinical preventive services–an emergency medicine evidence-based review. Society for Academic Emergency Medicine Public Health and Education Task Force Preventive Services Work Group. Acad Emerg Med 2000;7:1042–54.

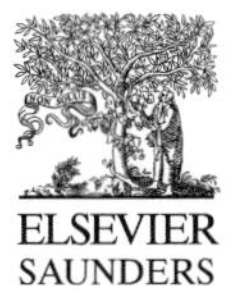

ELSEVIER
SAUNDERS

EMERGENCY MEDICINE CLINICS OF NORTH AMERICA

Emerg Med Clin N Am 25 (2007) 915–920

Index

Note: Page numbers of article titles are in **boldface** type.

A

B

doi:10.1016/S0733-8627(07)00094-6

O

P

R

S